AVIAN IMMUNOLOGY

ADVANCES IN EXPERIMENTAL MEDICINE AND BIOLOGY

Recent Volumes in this Series

AVIAN IMMUNOLOGY

Edited by
Albert A. Benedict
University of Hawaii at Manoa

PLENUM PRESS • NEW YORK AND LONDON

Library of Congress Cataloging in Publication Data

International Conference on Avian Immunology, University of Hawaii, 1977.
    Avian immunology.

    (Advances in experimental medicine and biology; v. 88)
    Includes index.
    1. Chickens—Diseases. 2. Veterinary immunology. I. Benedict, Albert Alfred,
1921-   II. Title. III. Series.
SF995.I57 1977   636.5'08'96079   77-2732
ISBN 0-306-32688-4

Proceedings of the International Conference on Avian Immunology held
at the University of Hawaii, Honolulu, Hawaii, March 12–13, 1977

© 1977 Plenum Press, New York
A Division of Plenum Publishing Corporation
227 West 17th Street, New York, N.Y. 10011

Printed in the United States of America

Preface

Many participants at this conference often have been asked the question, "Why do you work with chickens?". We agree with the argument that people are just curious, and like Mt. Everest chickens are here. In a more practical sense, the answer to that question makes reference to the clear-cut delineation of the T and B cells in birds. Indeed, the birth of chicken immunology probably occurred with the discovery of the immunological importance of the bursa of Fabricius. A justification for working with chickens no longer elicits a paranoid response, for the value of a phylogenetic approach for an understanding of the immune system is now obvious. The papers in this volume illustrate why the chicken is a valuable model for so many major concepts that are of general importance in immunology; such as, the ontogeny of T and B cells, the GVH reaction, the genetic basis of disease resistance, tumor immunity and regulation of the immune response.

Heard at this conference were views of avian immunology derived from diverse perspectives. The occasion afforded an opportunity for people with a common bond but from backgrounds as varied as medical schools, molecular biology and genetic institutes, animal disease research institutes, poultry research laboratories, animal science and biological science departments to review data, ask questions, and plan future experiments. We heard exchanges between those who were associated with the development of chicken breeds resistant to Marek's disease for commercial purposes with those involved in dissecting the major histocompatibility complex. The theorists also were given opportunity to propose theories.

The summation talks given by Jeanette Thorbecke, Max Cooper and Al Benedict will serve as the basis for these introductory remarks. We have made no attempt at being comprehensive, but we hope the flavor of the meeting is imparted. A. A. Benedict takes full responsibility for any inaccuracies in transcription from tape of the summations.

The ontogeny of lymphoid cells seems the most appropriate
place to start. The early events in T and B cell ontogeny are
still confusing. There seems to be no agreement on the data and
on the semantics of the question of progenitor vs. stem cells.
Nevertheless, we are beginning to understand more about progenitor
cells which are committed to particular cell lines, and about stem
cells in the sense of having almost unlimited capability of giving
rise to undifferentiated progeny. An important future development
will be to determine the nature of the substances that attract
stem cells and which are produced by specialized thymus epithelium,
and perhaps by the bursa. The way stem cells recognize these signals
is an important question to answer.

Not predictable from mammalian models has been the observation
that there is a lack of cells called into the bursa even before the
signal for entry of stem cells has been shut off. A likely model
suggested that after a certain point in development there were no
longer any cells capable of migrating into the bursa and becoming
B cells. A fascinating possibility is the suggestion that a cell
comes into the bursa, is not committed, then can still wander into
the thymus. This cell does not appear to have B cell characteristics; that is, immunoglobulin is not expressed on its surface.

Detection of some of the earlier stages in the B cell generation is now possible, and this is one of the main uses of the
chicken model. Chickens have proved to be a source of pure B cells
at a very early and defined stage in their life history, thus
making available biological clues to analyze molecular events.
It is going to be interesting to determine the physiological
significance of the secretory phase early in the development of
at least some B cells.

The combined data of papers on suppression answered at least
tentatively some questions on the regulation of immunoglobulin
synthesis. B cells are found in chickens adoptively transferred
with suppressor cells (spleen cells) from bursectomized birds, but
immunoglobulin secretion is depressed. Suppressor cells probably
mediate their effects by acting directly on B cells; however, it
was interesting that plasma cells and germinal centers disappear
in recipients rapidly after transfer of suppressor cells. Neither
the nature of the suppressor cells nor the B cell factor which
recognizes the suppressor is known. In this connection, cells
which suppress GVH reactivity and blastogenic responses to PHA
are present in a subset of chicken thymus cells. Whether the
suppressor cells are B cells which have taken up residence in the
thymus is a prospect which needs looking into.

Disturbed immunoglobulin regulation is suggested in birds which
have an inherited dysgammaglobulinemia, but suppressor factors have
not been reported in these birds. This disease is characterized by
a 7S immunoglobulin deficiency which occurs after several weeks of
normal 7S immunoglobulin synthesis; thus this condition in birds
may be a model for inherited, common variable ("late onset") immunodeficiency in humans.

Immune unresponsiveness also may be induced by antigen-antibody
complexes, with the structure of the complexes being important in
maintenance of tolerance. Both adherent cells and at least one
other cell type seem to be susceptible to this kind of unresponsiveness.

The pervading influence of the major histocompatibility complex
(MHC) in mammalian immunology is no less involved in avian immunology.
It is not surprising that the B antigen is structurally similar to
the mammalian counterparts, HLA and H-2. With the discovery of
increasing numbers of serological, histogenetic, and GVH recombinants,
and the finding of additional functions and cellular antigens
associated with the MHC, a primitive map of the B complex is now
possible. The region of the chromosome involved is divided into two
parts, B-F and B-G. Compared to the H-2 of mice, the frequency of
recombination in the B complex is lower, and there seems to be
asymmetry in the arrangement of the chicken MHC. In some ways, the
B complex arrangement corresponds more to the human than to the mouse
MHC. The phylogenetic implications of these studies are exciting.

The poultry industry has known for many years that hatchability,
viability, and egg production have a genetic basis, and this was
proved later to be somehow associated with B alleles. In the 1960's
Marek's disease became a serious problem to the poultry industry.
Through the efforts of a number of poultry research laboratories,
resistance to Marek's disease was found to be influenced by certain
B alleles. This was one of the earliest observations on the relationship between disease resistance and histocompatibility. As in
other animal species, we heard that synthetic antigens are being
used to characterize the MHC associated immune responses and,
unlike results obtained in mammals, the immune response to the
copolymer (T,G)-A--L in chickens exquisitely delineated the antigenic determinants of this immunogen based on responses controlled
both by genes associated and unassociated with the B complex. The
high degree of development of the chicken immune system to dissect
the (T,G)-A--L determinants, and to respond to poly-glutamic acid
which is essentially non-immunogenic in rabbits and mice (unpublished
data) is curious in view of the finding that 7S antibodies synthesized to certain haptens do not have the high binding capacity of
horse and rabbit antibodies. The later finding on the antibody
binding site is more in line with phylogenetic expectations.

It was pointed out that it is an oversimplification to expect immune responses to be controlled by a single gene associated with the MHC. As mentioned earlier in regard to the anti-(T,G)-A--L response, many immune responses to a variety of immunogens probably will be shown to be controlled by two or more genes, some of which are not MHC associated. This is borne out in the pathogenesis of spontaneous autoimmune thyroiditis in the Obese strain of chicken in which many genetic traits seem to play a role. Perplexing are the East Lansing inbred line 6 chickens which are highly resistant to Marek's disease, whereas the East Lansing inbred line 7 chickens with the identical B allele are highly susceptible. These lines also differ quantitatively in their ability to respond to certain immunogens, and some of these quantitative differences in antibody production are associated with two autosomal loci, Bu-1 and Th-1, which determine alloantigens of B and T cells, respectively. Finally, for an immune response, the cooperation between T and B cells requires some histocompatibility identity. This later point needs clarification in view of reports of cooperation across the histocompatibility barrier.

The chicken model has been unique in tumor immunity as Marek's disease is the only naturally occurring malignancy that can be prevented by vaccination. Chickens vaccinated with the herpes virus of turkey develop a cell mediated cytotoxic response to tumor-associated surface antigen. Cell mediated immunity seems to be the chief factor in protecting against clinical manifestations of Marek's disease. In an attempt to develop a procedure to be used under field conditions to control lymphoid leukosis tumors, an androgen analog was fed to chickens. This treatment causes a progressive involution of the bursa, and therefore prevents development of lymphoid leukosis tumors.

In the chicken, cooperation between specific immune T cells and normal monocytes results in inhibition of growth of a carcinogen-induced transplantable fibrosarcoma. Particularly significant is the finding that tumor-specific immunity occurs locally even when induced with a delayed-type hypersensitivity reaction to antigens which do not cross-react with the tumor antigens.

"What chicken line are you working with?" was often asked at the conference. As expected, disparate findings may result from genetic differences. It seems that our current work with chicken lines is approaching the degree of sophistication evidenced in mouse genetics. Viable homozygous chicken lines are available for experimental purposes from a number of sources. We believe that it is crucial for the development of chicken immunogenetics that further efforts be made to characterize lines genetically, and to produce congenic lines. In view of the long generation time of the chicken compared to the mouse, clever methods must be developed to enhance the rate of production of congenic lines.

It was good to hear that a committee is working on an internationally acceptable nomenclature for the B locus as this is urgently needed to classify inbred lines.

The structural and genetic identification of immunoglobulin allotypes has made available additional stable and easily detected genetic markers to characterize inbred lines. A system of nomenclature for both the 7S and 17S immunoglobulin allotypes was proposed. Perhaps not surprising was the observation that the genetic polymorphism of the 7S immunoglobulin allotype gene (CS-1) was about that observed for the Ig-1 gene of inbred mice. It appears that intracistronic recombination may account for the generation of the genetic polymorphism of the CS-1 gene alleles. It is pertinent to note that the chicken may be quite useful for studies on the genetic mechanism responsible for allotype expression because in several inbred lines low levels of inappropriate or "unexpected" allotypes were found. The presence of pseudoalleles has been proposed, which is in accord with a regulatory gene hypothesis for allotype expression.

Several uses of the chicken model were not discussed, some of which are experiments dealing with constraints on genetic models of immunoglobulin synthesis, kinetics and cellular events of in vivo immune responses, and idiotype explorations. Particularly important will be idiotype studies because of the value of looking at the generation of clonal diversity in the chicken model. We hope to have a Second International Conference on Avian Immunology when these and other subjects will be discussed.

This conference was made possible through the generous financial help of the University of Hawaii Foundation; the Graduate Division, College of Arts and Sciences, and Department of Microbiology of the University of Hawaii; the Hawaii Egg Producers Association and the Hawaii Fryer Council; also by the devoted care of Ms. Dolores Springer throughout the stages of planning, meeting, and book preparation. Our deepest gratitude to all of you.

Mahalo and Aloha

Honolulu, Hawaii
May, 1977

Contents

LYMPHOID DEVELOPMENT

Ontogeny

B Cell Maturation

Disease

Inbred Lines

TUMOR IMMUNITY

IMMUNOGLOBULINS

Allotypes

Binding Site

Lymphoid Development

ONTOGENY OF MYELOPOIETIC PRECURSOR CELLS IN THE CHICKEN EMBRYO

A. Szenberg

The Walter and Eliza Hall Institute of Medical Research
Post Office, Royal Melbourne Hospital, Victoria 3050,
Australia

SUMMARY

The agar culture technique which enables enumeration of myeloid precursor cells was used to establish the time of appearance and further development of these cells in chick embryos. Yolk mesenchyme is the largest producer of precursor cells from day 6 to day 17 of incubation.

In circulating blood precursor cells probably from the yolk appear at day 9 and stay at fairly high levels till day 17.

Spleen and bone marrow have high percentage of precursor cells from day 10 till hatching, but afterwards rapid fall takes place to normal young adult levels.

Thymus contains very few precursor cells during whole period of incubation.

Bursa of Fabricius shows a very sharp peak of precursor activity on day 14 and 15 of incubation.

INTRODUCTION

In 1966 a technique was developed for growing myelopoietic cells in soft agar culture (1, 2).   In this technique the specific progenitors of granulocytes and macrophages form colonies of maturing granulocytes and/or macrophages.

The growth of the colonies depends on the presence of adequate concentration of a factor called colony stimulating factor (CSF). The system can also be used for human haemopoietic cells.

The progenitors forming colonies in agar are the immediate progeny of multipotential haemopoietic stem cells able to form spleen colonies in mice (Till and McCulloch assay).

A detailed description of CSF from different sources has been given in a review by Metcalf (3).   There have been reports (4, 5) that chicken yolk, bone marrow and spleen will produce colonies in soft agar culture.

In this paper I have used a modified agar culture technique to study the development of the granulocyte-macrophage precursor cells in chick embryos.

MATERIALS AND METHODS

Fertile eggs (White Leghorn-Australorp cross) were obtained commercially.   Chickens used in this study were hatched from these eggs and reared in our animal facilities.   Cell suspensions were prepared sterile from spleen, bursa, thymus, bone marrow and yolk of embryos, newly hatched or young adult chickens. Known numbers of cells were put into agar culture.   Depending on the expected frequency of granulocyte-macrophage colony forming cells (CFC) between 2×10^3 and 10^5 cells were put into one culture dish;   circulating blood was cultured by adding 0.05 ml per dish.

Culture Conditions

Double strength Weymouth's Medium (MB 752/1) was prepared from dry powder (Wellcome Reagents) dissolved in DDW[*] containing 10% of chicken serum and 10% of FCS.   Penicillin (400,000 units) and Streptomycin (200, 000 μg) were added per 1 l. of medium. Medium was sterilized by filtration through a Milipore filter. An appropriate volume of medium was warmed to 37°C, mixed with an equal volume of 0.6% agar in DDW (40°C) and then the cells were added and the mixture distributed in 1 ml volumes to each 35 mm Falcon petri dish.

Before addition of the cells in agar-medium, the petri dishes were charged with an appropriate amount of CSF in 0.1 ml volume. After the agar solidified, the dishes were incubated for 7 days in a CO_2 incubator (10% CO_2 in air) at $39-40^{\circ}$C.

Colonies were counted with a binocular dissection microscope, total magnification 40x, scoring aggregates of 4-20 cells as clusters and > 20 cells as colonies. Five replicate culture dishes were counted for each cell suspension. Experiments in which control bone marrow cells from 18 day embryos produced colony counts significantly different from average, were discarded.

Sources of CSF

Mouse CSF does not stimulate chicken colonies and vice versa. Preliminary experiments were done using an underlayer of buffy coat cells. Then I tried lung conditioned medium (LCM) prepared by incubation of chicken lungs for 3-4 days, exactly like mouse LCM (3). Finally I discovered a very rich source of CSF in eggwhite of non fertile eggs. CSF is also present in yolk, but is much more difficult to extract.

Egg white was diluted 3x with DDW, spun at 2000 g for 30 minutes and then precipitated with ammonium sulfate. The fraction precipitating between 40% and 90% saturation was used as the source of CSF. If we consider the amount of CSF which has to be added to 1 culture dish to produce maximal number of colonies as 1 unit, 1 ml of egg white contains appr. 80 units. I have been using supramaximal concentration, appr. 2 units per culture.

* DDW- distilled deionized water

RESULTS

Tables 1 - 5 show the time of appearance and frequency of granulocyte-macrophage progenitor cells detected as colony-forming cells in agar.   Table 5 indicates the total number of these cells in several organs at indicated time points.

What can be seen immediately is that the first appearance of precursor cells takes place in the mesenchyme of the yolk (blood islands) (Table 1) at day 6, and that yolk is the largest producer of precursor cells till day 17 of incubation.   After that day all haemopoietic activity in the yolk is reduced considerably, and disappears completely between day 18 and 19.

The first precursor cells in spleen and blood (Tables 2 and 3) appear in very small numbers at day 9 of incubation.   The highest frequency in the spleen is observed on days 13 - 16, maximal level being appr. 2%.   In circulating blood high numbers of precursor cells appear on day 11, and stay at this level till day 17.

As soon as the central cavity appears in the bone marrow, a few precursor cells can be found.   Their number stays at a level of 0.8 - 2% during the whole embryonic development but decreases rapidly after hatching to adult level of 0.1%.   Of the primary lymphoid organs, thymus shows (Table 6) uniformly extremely low frequency of precursor cells, most probably migrants from the circulation.

Bursa (Table 7) presents quite a different picture.   Starting with a very low percentage and total number of precursor cells at day 12 and 13, over eight fold increase in % and eighty-five fold increase in total number takes place between days 13 and 14. Further, nearly two-fold increase in total number takes place between days 14 and 15.   Afterwards a very rapid decrease in proportion of precursor cells (appr. 10 fold from day 15 to 16) takes place.

Table 1

YOLK CFC IN %

Day	4	5	6	7	8	9
	0	0	0.001	0.018	0.025	0.023

Day	10	11	12	13	14	18
	0.041	0.022	0.028	0.037	0.012	0

Cells were collected from 5 - 30 embryos for each experiment.
Each experiment was performed 20 - 40 times. For each time
point and each organ, 5 culture dishes were counted in each
experiment. The total number of precursor cells per organ was
calculated from average number of colonies and average total
number of white cells per organ. Bone marrow was always
obtained from the left tibia.   To calculate the total number of
bone marrow cells in the embryo, the number of cells in the
tibia was multiplied by 8.

Table 2

SPLEEN CFC IN %

Day	9	11	12	13	14	15	16
	0.4	1.2	1.3	2	1.3	2	1.5

Day	17	18	19	20	+3	Adult	
	1	0.8	1.2	0.5	0.1	0	

Same as for Table 1.

Table 3

CFC per 0.1 ml OF EMBRYONIC BLOOD

Day	9	11	12	13
	0.6	60.8 ± 4	86 ± 4	57 ± 6
Day	14	15	16	17
	60 ± 10.5	49.5 ± 11	60 ± 7	52 ± 2.75

Same as for Table 1.

Table 4

BONE MARROW CFC IN %

Day	10	11	12	13	14	15	16
	Few	0.7	1.7	2	1.3	0.9	0.8
Day	17	19	20	+3	Adult		
	0.75	0.8	0.8	0.25	0.1		

Same as for Table 1.

Table 5

TOTAL NO. OF CFC IN EMBRYONIC ORGANS

	YOLK	SPLEEN	BONE MARROW
11 d.	72×10^3	5.8×10^3	9.5×10^3
13 d.	96×10^3	20×10^3	11×10^3
14 d.	120×10^3	20×10^3	25×10^3

Same as for Table 1.

Table 6

CFC IN EMBRYONIC THYMUS

Day	10	12	13	14	15
%	0.01	0.002	0.009	0.001	0.02
Day	17	19	20	Adult	
%	0.001	0.002	0.001	0	

Same as for Table 1.

Table 7

CFC IN EMBRYONIC BURSA

Day	12	13	14	15	16
%	0.05 ± 0.03	0.07 ± 0.03	0.59 ± 0.21	0.33 ± 0.24	0.04 ± 0.016
Total No.	6	14	1180	1980	440
Day	17	18	19	+3	Adult
%	0.02	0.02	0.005	0.002	0
Total No.	600	1100	290	140	

Same as for Table 1.

DISCUSSION

The data presented pose several interesting questions. With the exception of yolk, and circulating blood, it is difficult to establish whether the precursor cells are produced locally from the stem cells or whether they are progeny of the precursor cells arriving from circulation.

It seems to be reasonable to accept that after day 16, stem cells are present in the spleen and bone marrow. In the thymus rudiment the first stem cells are present at day 8 of incubation, but at no time can any significant number of precursor cells be found in this organ.

Bursa presents a very special case. Here the very rapid increase in numbers of precursor cells corresponds exactly to the largest influx of stem cells. Between day 13 and 14 of incubation, the total number of cells in this organ shows a ten-fold increase and majority of these cells (80%) do not have detectable immunoglobulins on their surface (6). It is therefore possible to assume that some of the stem cells arriving in the bursal rudiment are diverted to a myelopoietic line of development before they can reach bursal epithelium.

Another interesting point is that even though stem cells are present in the yolk probably from the first day of incubation (because erythropoiesis is already in progress), and the CSF is present in the egg, myelopoiesis cannot be detected before day 6. It seems then that another non identified factor is necessary to transform stem cells into myelopoietic precursor cells.

ACKNOWLEDGMENTS

Technical assistance of Miss Wendy Carter and Miss Ann Dunstan was greatly appreciated. I am very grateful to Dr. D. Metcalf for introducing me to the technique of growing colonies in agar and for helpful discussions and advice during the progress of this work.

This project was supported by a grant from N.H.M.R.C. (Canberra), and by a grant from Volkswagenschtiftung to Prof. G. Nossal.

REFERENCES

1. Bradley, T.R. and Metcalf, D., Aust. J. Exp. Biol. Med. Sci., 44 : 287 (1966).

2. Ichikawa, Y., Pluznik, D.H., Sachs, L., Proc. Nat. Acad. Sci. (USA) 56 : 488 (1966).

3. Metcalf, D., Exp. Hemat. 1: 185 (1973).

4. Dodge, W.H. and Moscovici, C., J. Cell.Physiol. 81 : 371 (1973).

5. Dodge, W.H., Silva, R.F. and Moscovici, C. J. Cell. Physiol. 85 : 25 (1975).

6. Szenberg, A., in Comparative Immunology (J.J.Marchalonis, ed.) (Blackwell Scientific Publications, Oxford, 1976).

ONTOGENY OF HEMOPOIETIC COLONY-FORMING UNITS IN THE CHICK

EMBRYO SPLEEN

Gordon Keller, Calliopi Havele, Michael Longenecker and
Erwin Diener

Medical Research Council Transplantation Group and the
Department of Immunology, University of Alberta, 845E
Medical Sciences Bldg., Edmonton, Alberta, Canada T6G 2H7

SUMMARY

Inoculation of spleen cells of chicken embryos onto the chorio-
allantoic membrane (CAM) of other chicken embryos led to the formation of white (granulocytic) and pink (mixed erythrocytic and
granulocytic) hemopoietic colonies. The number of CAM colonies
formed was a linear function of the number of cells inoculated indicating that each colony originated from a single colony-forming
unit (CAM-CFU). CAM-CFU's consist of an aggregate of primitive
undifferentiated cells which penetrate the ectodermal layer of the
CAM, then proliferate and differentiate into mature granulocytes
or erythrocytes. Deaggregated CAM-CFU's failed to form colonies
indicating that cell interaction may be required for colony formation. The genetic constitution of the host embryo has no effect
on colony formation but mixtures of donor cells from inbred embryo
spleen were found to be more efficient colony formers than mixtures
of donor cells from non-inbred embryo spleens. Ontogeny studies
demonstrated that the chick embryo spleen contains peak hemopoietic activity between fifteen and seventeen days of incubation
declining thereafter to undetectable levels two days post hatching.
At this time the inoculation of spleen cell suspensions leads to
the formation of lymphoid colonies which increase in number with
age of the donor.

INTRODUCTION

Our knowledge of the mammalian hemopoietic stem cell has been
greatly advanced by two assay systems. The CFU-S assay (1,2)
identifies the progeny of pluripotent stem cells in the form of

discrete, macroscopically visible colonies in the spleen of an irradiated recipient. The CFU-C assay (3,4,5) is based on the formation of colonies *in vitro* and is thought to provide an estimate of
the relative number of progenitor cells committed to granulocytic-,
macrophage- or lymphoid-cell differentiation.

These two assays have provided evidence concerning the importance of the microenvironment for the development of hemopoietic colonies. Thus, the type of microenvironment that a stem
cell encounters has been shown to determine the type of colony produced. In the irradiated spleen, the microanatomical environment
which propagates the growth of a hemopoietic colony has been called
hemopoietic inductive environment (HIM) (6,7). The type of colony
produced is regarded as a direct reflection of the surrounding HIM.
Similarly, the development of colonies, *in vitro*, from precursor
cells, has been shown to depend on the presence of colony-stimulating factors (CSF) in the culture medium (3,8,9).

Unlike the mammalian system, very little is known about the
ontogenic development of the hemopoietic stem cell in birds. This
deficiency is largely due to the lack of a suitable assay for the
quantitative analysis of avian hemopoietic precursor cells. A
recent study by Jankovic *et al.* (10) suggests that the chorioallantoic membrane (CAM) of the chicken embryo might support the growth
of hemopoietic colonies and could therefore provide a basis for the
development of an experimental model comparable to the CFU-S assay
in mammals. With this in mind, we have characterized the conditions
for such an assay in the chicken embryo. In this communication, we
report on the kinetics of hemopoietic colony formation on the chorio-
allantoic membrane, using embryonic spleen as a source of colony-
forming units. Our experimental evidence suggests that the individual hemopoietic colony on the CAM is derived from a cell aggregate.
Furthermore, we found that hemopoietic colony-forming units are
restricted to the embryonic spleen. Shortly after birth, the
colony-forming units disappear from the spleen and are succeeded
by precursors of lymphoid colonies.

MATERIALS AND METHODS

Inbred SC and FP eggs were purchased from Hyline International,
Johnston, Iowa. SC embryos carry the major histocompatibility
alleles B^2/B^2 and FP embryos carry the alleles B^{15}/B^{21}. Random
bred eggs were obtained from the University of Alberta Poultry
Research Farm, Edmonton. Japanese quail eggs were supplied by
the University of Alberta Animal Farm, Ellerslie, Alberta. Unless

otherwise stated, spleen cells from fourteen-day-old embryos were used as the source of colony-forming units. Cell suspensions were prepared by gently pressing the tissue through a wire sieve. Large macroscopically visible clumps were allowed to settle for 7.5 minutes and the supernatant containing single cells and small aggregates was used as the inoculum. Viable cell counts were determined by dye exclusion. Erythrocytes were excluded from the count. After preparation, the donor cells were inoculated onto the CAM in a 0.1 ml volume. Twelve day embryos were prepared for CAM inoculation in essentially the same manner as described by Longenecker *et al.* (11). After inoculation of donor cells, the hole in the shell of the host was covered with tape, sealed with paraffin, and the egg was reincubated in a horizontal position. At the appropriate time after inoculation, the host embryos were sacrificed, the CAM removed and the colonies counted. All membranes were coded prior to counting. Hanks balanced salt solution (GIBCO) and RPMI 1640 (GIBCO) media both supplemented with 10% FC were used for the preparation of cell suspensions. Colonies, along with the adjacent portion of the CAM, were fixed in 10% formalin, processed and cut at a thickness of 5μ. Hematoxylin and Eosin stain was used for morphological identification of the cells in the colony. Feulgen stain (12) was used to distinguish quail cells from chicken cells (13,14). Cells and embryos were irradiated in a Cs^{137} gamma cell 40 (Atomic Energy of Canada) at a dose rate of 100 rads/min. Colony size was determined using an optical grid in the eyepiece of a Wild microscope at a magnification of 15X. Colonies from each membrane in a group were included in the size analysis. Statistical analysis was carried out on an AMDAHL 470 V6 computer using the public library program for analysis of variance, Student's t-test and Duncan's New Multiple Range test.

RESULTS

Inoculation of embryonic spleen cells (ESC) onto the CAM of twelve-day-old syngeneic or allogeneic recipients results in the formation of discrete white and pink colonies. The number of colonies obtained seven days post inoculation was found to be directly proportional to the number of cells in the inoculum (Figure 1). Regression analysis revealed that the points between 10^5 and 10^7 inoculated cells form a straight line on a $\log_{10}$ - $\log_{10}$ plot with a slope that does not differ significantly from the ideal slope of 1.00. This suggests that each colony is initiated by a single, limiting, colony-forming unit. If donor cell proliferation is required for colony formation, then irradiation of donor cells prior to inoculation onto the recipients CAM is expected to result in a characteristic radiation-survival curve with a D_{37} between 70 - 150. Similar curves have been

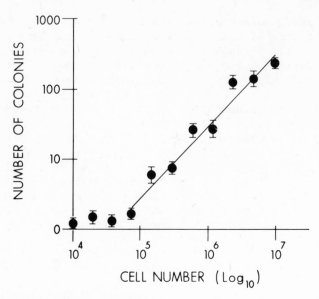

Figure 1 Relationship between the number of embryonic spleen cells
          inoculated and the number of hemopoietic colonies formed
          on the CAM.   Each point represents the mean number of
          colonies obtained from 12 recipients.   Vertical bars
          represent standard error of the mean.

obtained with the CFU-S assay in the mouse where the cells com-
prising each colony appear to represent the progeny of a single
hemopoietic stem cell (1).   Two aspects of our radiation-survival
curve (Figure 2) differ from that obtained following irradiation
of CFU-S in the mouse.   First, we have observed a D_{37} of approximately 170 rad which is slightly above the upper limit expected
for a system which depends on cell proliferation alone.   Second,
approximately 10% of CAM-colonies were found to resist doses of
irradiation as high as 1000 rad.   For these reasons, the kinetics
of colony formation were observed following irradiation of donor
ESC at a dose of 1000 rad.   Embryos were sacrificed 0.5, 1, 2, 3,
4, 5 and 7 days after cell inoculation of irradiated or non-
irradiated ESC and the number as well as the sizes of the colonies
were determined.

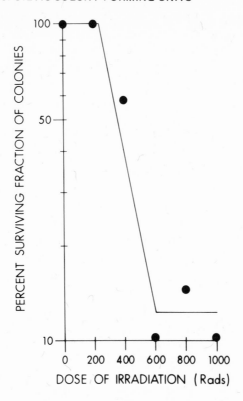

Figure 2   Effect of irradiating the embryonic spleen cells on
their capacity to generate hemopoietic colonies on the
CAM. Ordinate represents the $\log_{10}$ percentage of
colonies obtained relative to control values. Each
point represents the value obtained from 10 recipients.

To our surprise, colonies could be detected as early as 12 hours
post inoculation and the number (Figure 3) as well as the size
(Figure 4) of these colonies were similar regardless of whether
the donor cells had been irradiated prior to inoculation. The
number of colonies initiated by unirradiated ESC reached near
maximum by 12 hours post inoculation and remained relatively constant throughout the observation period of seven days. On the other
hand, the number of colonies formed by irradiated ESC decreased
progressively after 12 hours to a minimum at seven days, repre-
senting about 15% of the number initially present. The sizing
data show that by 48 hours, when the mean size of the colonies in
both groups had reached a maximum, unirradiated colonies were

significantly larger than irradiated ones, differing from the
latter on the average by 35 ± 1 μ. Since the early increase in
size of CAM-colonies within the first 24 hours after inoculation
is irradiation resistant, we suggest such early colony growth is
due to aggregation of cells rather than the cellular proliferation.

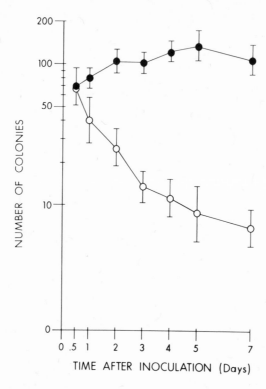

Figure 3   Effect with time of irradiating the embryonic spleen
           cells on their capacity to sustain growth of hemopoietic
           colonies on the CAM. Closed circles represent mean
           values obtained from 12 recipients inoculated with un-
           irradiated donor cells. Open circles represent mean
           values obtained from 12 recipients inoculated with ir-
           radiated donor cells. Differences between the groups
           significant (p<0.01) for all time points after 2 days
           post inoculation, according to the Duncan New Multiple
           Range test. Vertical bars represent standard error of
           the mean. Irradiation dose: 1000 rad.

     Next, we designed a series of experiments to characterize the
colony-forming unit. Results from these preliminary studies show
that a spleen cell suspension loses its colony-forming ability if

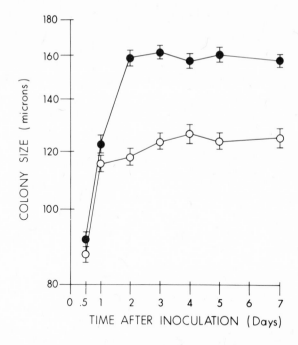

Figure 4   Effect of irradiating the embryonic spleen cells on the
size of colonies on the CAM at various time points post
inoculation.   Closed circles represent mean values obtained from at least 200 colonies derived from unirradiated donor cells.   Open circles represent mean values
obtained from at least 200 colonies derived from irradiated donor cells.   Differences between the groups
significant (p<0.01) for all time points after two days
post inoculation, according to the student's t-test.
Vertical bars represent standard error of the mean.
Irradiation dose: 1000 rad.

the aggregates are allowed to settle out prior to inoculation.
Also, deaggregation of the aggregates by trypsinization abrogates
colony-forming activity and reaggregation *in vitro* restores colony-
forming capacity.   These results suggest that, in all likelihood,
colonies on the CAM derive from cell aggregates rather than a
single cell.   Hereafter, these aggregates will be referred to as
CAM-colony-forming units (CAM-CFU).

Histological analysis of colonies revealed (Figure 5a) that,
at 12 hours post inoculation, CAM-CFU's consist of aggregates of

undifferentiated cells which appear on the epithelial surface of
the CAM.   This undifferentiated cell type predominates between 12
and 72 hours post inoculation.   During this time the colonies
penetrate the ectodermal epithelium and grow into the mesodermal
layer of the CAM (Figure 5b).   Three days after inoculation, immature and mature granulocytes and erythrocytes are seen to emerge
and increase in number until day 5 at which time approximately 90%
of the cells in a typical colony appear differentiated, the remaining 10% of the cells failing to differentiate (Figure 5c).   Two
types of colonies were distinguishable at this time: white colonies composed of granulocytes and undifferentiated cells, and pink
colonies composed of erythrocytes, granulocytes and undifferentiated cells (Figure 6,7).

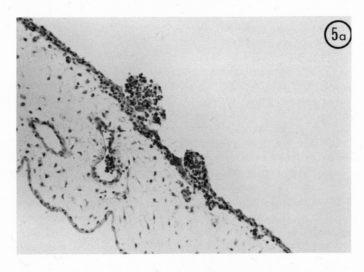

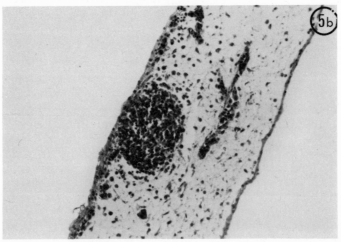

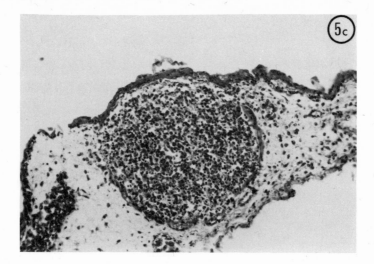

Figure 5 Developmental sequence of hemopoietic colonies on the CAM.
a) Two CFU's appear as cell aggregates on the outer epithelium of the CAM, 12 hours post inoculation (x 190).
   Hematoxylin - Eosin stain.
b) Hemopoietic colony has penetrated the mesenchyme of
   the CAM, 2 days post inoculation (x 190). Hematoxylin - Eosin stain.
c) Fully developed hemopoietic colony in the mesenchyme
   of the CAM, 5 days post inoculation (x 190). Hematoxylin - Eosin stain.

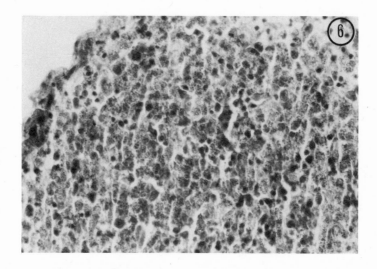

Figure 6 Section of a "white" hemopoietic colony on the CAM
showing granulopoietic activity, 7 days post inoculation
(x 480). Hematoxylin - Eosin stain.

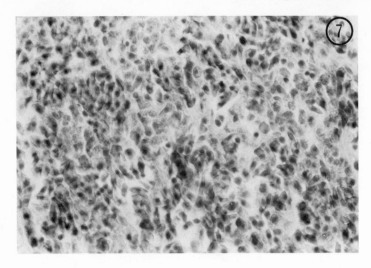

Figure 7   Section of a "pink" hemopoietic colony on the CAM
           showing predominantly erythropoietic and some granulo-
           poietic activity, 7 days post inoculation (x 480).
           Hematoxylin - Eosin stain.

In order to verify the donor origin of the colonies observed,
quail embryo spleens were used as a source of CAM-CFU's. Interphase quail cells can easily be distinguished from chicken cells
on the basis of a chromatin marker (13,14). The majority of cells
in one-day-old colonies resulting from the inoculation of 12-day-
old quail spleen cells were found to contain the quail chromatin
marker (Figure 8). Furthermore, irradiation of the host embryo
(Table I), prior to inoculation, did not alter the size or the
number of colonies induced by unirradiated donor ESC. These data
strongly suggest that CAM colonies are derived from donor cells
with no significant contribution by the host.

A series of experiments was designed to determine whether the
CAM-CFU assay detects a genetic influence on colony formation,
either from point of view of colony support by the CAM or with regard to the number of CAM-CFU's detected per spleen. Inbred B^2/B^2
and random bred embryos were compared as hosts and donors for
colony formation in each possible combination. Table II shows that
random bred and inbred B^2/B^2 host embryos support colony formation
equally well. Interestingly, however, B^2/B^2 donors yielded con-

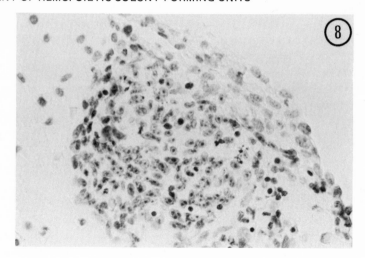

Figure 8   Section of a hemopoietic colony, derived from 12-day-old
           embryonic quail spleen, on the CAM of the chicken, 1 day
           post inoculation (x 480). Feulgen Stain.

Table 1:   Effect of irradiating the host embryo on colony number
           and size.

days after inoculation [a]	irradiated host (500 rad)	mean number ± S.E. of colonies (log 10)	mean size ± S.E. of colonies (log 10)
1	–	1.94 ± 0.70 (87) [b]	2.14 ± 0.01 (138)
1	+	1.77 ± 0.09 (59)	2.12 ± 0.01 (123)
7	–	2.06 ± 0.06 (115)	2.25 ± 0.01 (178)
7	+	2.09 ± 0.06 (123)	2.24 ± 0.01 (174)

(a) 1.5×10^6 donor spleen cells were inoculated onto each CAM.

(b)   Values in parentheses represent the arithmetic mean.

      Note: None of the values between the irradiated and non-
      irradiated hosts were found to be significantly different
      from each other (student's t-test).

siderably more colonies than did randomly bred donors. Since the
latter are segregating for several *B* alleles, and since spleen
cells from many embryos were mixed prior to inoculation in these
experiments, the data suggest that embryonic spleen cells of

divergent histocompatibility types might not interact as well as do syngeneic cells to form aggregates of efficiently interacting elements.

Table 2: Effect of host and donor genotype on colony number.

donor genotype [a]	host genotype	Mean number $\pm$ S.E. of colonies (log 10) [b]
B^2/B^2	B^2/B^2	1.86 $\pm$ 0.08 (72) [c]
B^2/B^2	random bred	1.82 $\pm$ 0.09 (66)
random bred	B^2/B^2	1.34 $\pm$ 0.13 (22)
random bred	random bred	1.27 $\pm$ 0.12 (19)

(a) 3×10^6 donor spleen cells were inoculated onto each CAM.

(b) Values between syngeneic and allogeneic donor cell mixtures significantly different from each other (p<0.01; analysis of variance).

(c) Values in parentheses represent arithmetic mean.

     Having established an assay for the study of CAM-CFU's, we proceeded to carry out time course studies on the ontogenic development of hemopoiesis in the chicken spleen, an organ which in birds is thought to represent the main hemopoietic organ equivalent to the mammalian fetal liver. Spleens from chickens ranging from 11 days of embryonic life to six days post hatching were used as a source of donor cells for inoculation (Figure 9). Approximately 42 CAM-CFU's per organ were detected in the spleen of the eleven-day-old embryo and this rose to a maximum of 136 CAM-CFU's per embryonic spleen between 15 and 17 days of age. The number of CAM-CFU's then decreased until shortly after hatching at which time little or no CAM-CFU activity was found. However, upon inoculation of spleen cells from two-day-old chickens, the formation of small (100μ), white colonies was observed. These did not result from a graft-versus-host reaction in response to histoincompatibility since they were present when the donor spleen cells were syngeneic with the host embryo. Histological studies revealed that the majority of cells within these colonies are lymphocytes (Figure 10). The number of these colonies on syngeneic hosts increased rapidly with increasing age of the donor.

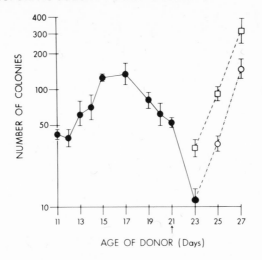

Figure 9   Content of CFU's and of lymphoid precursor cells in the
            spleen of the chicken during ontogenic development.
            Colonies counted four days post inoculation.   Closed
            circles represent the mean numbers of CFU's per spleen.
            Open circles represent the mean numbers of lymphoid
            colonies per spleen.   Donors and recipients were both
            B^2/B^2.   Arrow along the abscissa indicates the day of
            hatching.   Vertical bars represent standard error of
            the mean.

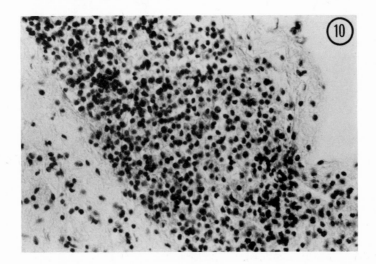

Figure 10   Section of lymphoid colony, derived from a 2-day-old
            chicken spleen, on the CAM of a chicken embryo.   The
            majority of cells in this colony have the characteris-
            tics of lymphocytes (x 480).   Hematoxylin - Eosin stain.

DISCUSSION

The development of an avian hemopoietic colony assay has en-
abled us to study the ontogeny of hemopoietic colony-forming units
within the spleen of the chicken embryo. The assay identifies
hemopoietic colonies on the CAM of the chicken embryo upon inoculation of embryonic spleen cells. Using quail cells as the inoculum, we have been able to show that such colonies were of donor
origin. Throughout mammalian embryonic development, the majority
of hemopoietic stem cells is found in the fetal liver. Shortly
after birth, these cells migrate to the spleen and bone marrow,
where they are found throughout adult life (15). In the chicken,
the spleen, rather than the liver, appears to represent the major
transitory hemopoietic organ during embryogenesis, the peak hemopoietic activity of which we have found to occur between days 15-
17 of incubation. Thereafter, it decreases gradually until shortly
after hatching, at which time little or no hemopoietic activity is
detectable. Around the time of hatching, the spleen ceases to be
hemopoietic and becomes lymphoid instead. The beginning of this
transition is marked by the appearance of lymphoid colony-forming
units which we have found to develop into colonies on the CAM.
These colonies are not to be confused with the pocks characteristic
of graft-versus-host reactivity; the former develop when donor cells
and the recipient CAM are histocompatible whereas the latter derive from allogeneic immunocompetent lymphocytes. Furthermore,
syngeneic lymphoid colonies consist of healthy looking lymphocytes
throughout, whereas allogeneic pocks contain a characteristic
centre of necrosis.

In vivo and *in vitro* assays for the identification and quantitative analysis of mammalian CFU's have greatly increased our knowledge of the developmental sequence of blood-forming tissue from
a presumably multipotential stem cell to the mature end cell of
specialized function (1,3,4). Such assays have furthermore yielded
evidence for the existence of an inductive milieu provided by the
stromal tissue of the irradiated spleen in the mouse (7) or *in
vitro* by the colony-stimulating factor (3). One of the most striking
examples has been the demonstration in some strains of mice, of an
incapacity of the spleen to support and propagate the growth of
CFU's (16). Work on human peripheral blood has led to the identification of an adherent cell which may be associated with such
growth promoting function when tested *in vitro* (17). The significance of an *in situ* inductive milieu for hemopoiesis is indicated
by our data which suggest that the CAM-CFU in the chicken spleen
consists of a cell aggregate rather than of a single stem cell.
The results from the irradiation experiments suggest that during
the first 24 hours post inoculation, colony formation on the CAM
by embryonic spleen cells is primarily due to cell aggregation
rather than cell division, although the latter contributes to the

increase of colony size, once aggregation has occurred. More
directly, CAM-CFU's were found among cell aggregates rather than
among the singly dispersed cells of a spleen cell suspension.
Furthermore, our data suggest that some reaggregation of disrupted
CFU's may even have taken place on the CAM subsequent to inoculation of splenic tissue. In conclusion, the data we have reported
in this communication emphasize the unique opportunity to dissect
the embryonic CAM-CFU into its functional elements which, in part,
control hemopoiesis.

REFERENCES

1. Till, J.E. and McCulloch, E.A., Rad. Res., 14:213 (1961).

2. Becker, A.J., McCulloch, E.A. and Till, J.E., Nature, 197:
   452 (1963).

3. Bradley, T.R. and Metcalf, D., Aust. J. Exp. Biol. Med. Sci.,
   44:287 (1966).

4. Pluznik, D.H. and Sachs, L., J. Cell and Comp. Physiol.,
   66:319 (1965).

5. Metcalf, D., Warner, N.L., Nossal, G.J.V., Miller, J.F.A.P.
   and Shortman, K., Nature, 255:630 (1975).

6. Curry, J.L. and Trentin, J.J., Develop. Biol., 15:395 (1967).

7. Wolf, N.S. and Trentin, J.J., J. Exp. Med., 127:205 (1968).

8. Metcalf, D. and Foster, R. Jr., Proc. Soc. Exp. Biol. Med.,
   126:758 (1967).

9. Metcalf, D., Bradley, T.R. and Robinson, W., J. Cell Physiol.,
   69:93 (1967).

10. Jankovic, B.C., Isakovic, K., Lukec, M.L., Uujanovic, N.L.,
    Spomenka, P. and Markovic, B.M., Immunology, 29:497 (1975).

11. Longenecker, B.M., Sheridan, S., Law, G.R.J. and Ruth, R.F.,
    Transpl., 9:544 (1970).

12. Feulgen, R. and Rossenbeck, H. in Histochemie Normale et
    Pathologique, Vol. 1, pp. 356 (Gauthier-Villars, Paris,
    Ed. 1924).

13. LeDouarin, N., Bull. Biol. Fr. Belg., 103:435 (1969).

14. LeDouarin, N., Develop. Biol. 30:217 (1973).

15.   Metcalf, D. and Moore, M.A.S., Haemopoietic Cells, 172 pp.
      (North-Holland Publishing Company, Amsterdam · London, 1971).

16.   McCulloch, E.A., Siminovitch, L., Till, J.E., Russell, E.S.
      and Bernstein, S.E., Blood 26:399 (1965).

17.   Messner, H.A., Till, J.E. and McCulloch, E.A., Blood 42:701
      (1973).

ACKNOWLEDGEMENTS

      This work was supported by Medical Research Council of Canada
(No. 55-42201 and No. 55-42302) and by the National Cancer Institute of Canada (No. 55-45018).

      Dr. Longenecker is a research associate of the National Can-
cer Institute of Canada.

DIFFERENTIATION OF THE PRIMARY LYMPHOID ORGANS IN AVIAN EMBRYOS : ORIGIN AND HOMING OF THE LYMPHOID STEM CELLS

N.M. LE DOUARIN[x], E. HOUSSAINT[‡] and F. JOTEREAU[‡]

[x]Inst. d'Embryologie du CNRS et du Collège de France
Nogent s/Marne 94130 - FRANCE
[‡]Lab. d'Embryologie de la Faculté des Sciences de
Nantes - FRANCE

The avian embryo provides a convenient model to investigate the ontogeny of the primary lymphoid organs since birds are the only vertebrates in which the sites of differentiation of both T and B lymphocytes are known. On the other hand, the accessibility of the avian embryo during the whole developmental period makes it an elective experimental material for studying problems related to morphogenesis and organogenesis. For instance, the role of cell migrations on certain histogenetic processes could be particularly demonstrated in birds owing to the availability of cell markers systems such as sex chromosomes (1, 2, 3) and interspecific combinations of tissues from quail (Coturnix coturnix japonica) and chick (Gallus gallus). The latter system is based on a peculiarity in the structure of the interphase nucleus of the quail which makes it possible to distinguish unequivocally quail from chick cells in chimaeric tissues of these species.

By parabiosis experiments on chick embryos involving vascular anastomosis of chorioallantoic or yolk-sac blood vessels, Moore and Owen (1, 3) demonstrated the immigration of cells into the thymus, and the bursa of Fabricius, suggesting that the lymphoid population which develops in these organs is at least partly derived from blood-borne stem cells. This view was confirmed and extended by a series of experiments carried out by our group using the quail-chick marker system (6, 7, 8, 9, 10, 11, 12). We were able to demonstrate 1) the inability of either

the epithelial or the mesenchymal components of the thymic and
bursic rudiments to give rise to lymphocytes ; 2) the extrinsic
origin of the whole lymphoid population which develops in the
thymus and the bursa ; 3) the stage of development at which the
thymic and bursal primordia become populated by stem cells.

Thymuses and bursas were taken from quail and chick embryos at various developmental stages :
- from 30-somite stage to 10 days of incubation for the thymus
- from 5 to 15 days of incubation in the case of the bursa.

These rudiments were grafted heterospecifically in the somatopleure of 3-day hosts (quail hosts for chick organs and chick
hosts for quail organs). The grafts were observed when they had
reached the total age of 14 days for the thymus and 19 to 20 days
for the bursa. The cell type of the lymphocytes was observed
after Feulgen staining.

For the quail thymus, the lymphocytes were entirely of host
origin in the explants taken from the donor before the end of the
5th day of incubation. In explants taken from quails during the
6th day, the lymphocytes were a mixture of host and donor cells
while they were all of host type when the thymuses were grafted
after the end of the 6th day. It could thus be concluded that the
colonization of the thymus in the quail embryo occurs during the
6th day of incubation and lasts about 24 hours.

Similar investigations showed that in the chick the invasion
of the thymus takes place from 6 1/2 to 8 days of incubation and
lasts about 36 hours while the bursal primordium is colonized by
precursor cells later in development, between 7 to 11 days of
incubation in the quail and between 8 to 14 days in the chick
(Table 1).

The inflow of stem cells which invades the thymus at the early
stages of its ontogeny is followed by a short period during which
no or very few cells home in the organ. However, by grafting in
chick embryos already colonized quail thymuses (i. e. taken from
quail embryos at 7 and 8 days of incubation onward), one can see
chick haemocytoblasts appearing in the external cortex 4 to 5 days
after the implantation. From 9 days onward, chick lymphocytes
progressively replace the initial quail lymphoid population. The
replacement proceeds from the external to the internal cortex
and reaches the medulla after 12 to 15 days in graft (8).

TABLE 1 - Time of colonization of the thymus and the bursa of Fabricius by lymphoid stem cells in chick and quail embryos.

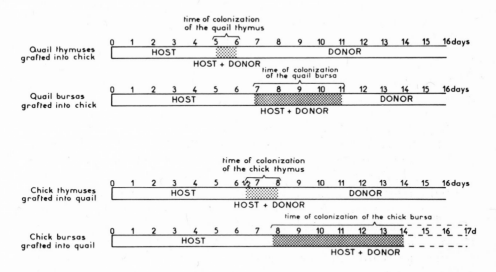

1. INVESTIGATIONS ON THE MECHANISMS CONTROLLING THE ONSET AND THE ARREST OF STEM CELL HOMING IN THE EARLY THYMIC RUDIMENT.

The first problem investigated was the question as to whether the onset of the stem cell inflow in the thymus depends on the availability of haemocytoblasts in the blood or on the intrinsic capacity of the thymic rudiment to retain them.

By transplanting a 4-day quail thymic primordium into a 3-day chick host for 2 days and then into a quail host we were able to show that stem cells ready to colonize the thymus are present in the chick circulation as early as 3-4 days of incubation (8). Therefore, stem cells are available in the embryo about 2 1/2 days before they enter the thymic epithelium. It is thus clear that the onset of stem cell immigration is regulated by

an intrinsic thymic property and does not depend on the availability of haemocytoblasts.

This being established, it seemed interesting to investigate
the mechanism by which the inflow of stem cells is limited in
time and almost completely stops for a while after 24 hours in
the quail and 36 hours in the chick : we asked the question as to
whether the thymic rudiment loses its capacity to retain the stem
cells at the same stage as in normal conditions (6 days of incubation in quail and 8 days in chick), when the homing process is experimentally prevented.

Thymic rudiments taken before the time where their colonization starts (at 4 days in the quail and 6 days in the chick) were
cultured for 4 to 6 days in a diffusion chamber on the CAM of 8-
day chick embryos for 4 to 6 days. No stem cells could penetrate
the primordium and the colonization period was over at the end
of the culture time. The explant was then transplanted heterospecifically into the somatopleure of 3-day hosts and observed after
10 days in grafts. In all cases, normal thymic histogenesis occurred and the lymphoid population which developed in the explants
was of host type.

This experiment indicates that the ability to retain the haemocytoblasts which develops in the thymus at a precise stage (5 days
for the quail and 6 1/2 days for the chick) is maintained in the
epitheliomesenchymal rudiment isolated in culture. Moreover the
mechanism which reduces the homing capacity of the rudiment
in normal development appears regulated by the number or cells
which enter it.

2. PRODUCTION OF A CHEMOTACTIC FACTOR BY THYMIC
AND BURSIC RUDIMENTS : A POSSIBLE MECHANISM TO EX-
PLAIN THE STEM CELL INVASION.

Several types of experiment have been devised to see whether
the thymic and bursic anlagen attract the circulating haemocytoblasts through the production of a chemotactic substance. The
general experimental design consisted in the interspecific association of thymic and bursic rudiments ready to be colonized with
various sources of stem cells which were either thymuses or
bursas already populated but in which lymphoid differentiation
had not yet started or was only just beginning. Such a situation
occurs in the thymus at 6 to 8 days in the quail and 8 to 10 days

in the chick and in the bursa, around 11 days in the quail and 12-
14 days in the chick. In the latter case, lymphoid differentiation
is in fact already in progress as attested by the presence of surface immunoglobulin in a small number (~ 0.1 %) of differentiating lymphocytes from the 12th day of incubation (13). However
most of the lymphoid cells present in the bursa at this stage have
not begun to express Ig genes. On the other hand at these developmental stages, both thymus and bursa have been shown incapable
of being colonized by a significant amount of new stem cells.

   In a first series of experiments, the organs were cultured
side by side either in the soma topleure of a 3-day chick host or
on the CAM of a chick embryo for 6 days and observed after
Feulgen staining. The chimaerism found in the organ at the end
of the graft attested that a traffic of lymphoid cells has occurred
between them. It is important to notice that in these experimental
conditions both organs remain individualized and that no fusion
occurs even if they are in close contact at the time of transplantation.

   The results, reported in table 2, show that, when taken after
they have been populated, neither the thymus nor the bursa was
able to receive extrinsic lymphoid cells throughout the duration
of the graft. This confirm the previous findings summarized in
table 2.

   On the other hand, when a "non-colonized" rudiment is associated with an "already-colonized" one, be it a thymus or a bursa,
cells of the latter invade the former in a certain number of cases.
This suggests that the "non-colonized" rudiment is actually attractive for lymphoid cells and that this attraction is exerted not only
on the circulating host stem cells but also on the haemocytoblasts
which have already homed in either a thymus or a bursa.

   In a second experimental series, the thymic and bursic primordia were associated in in vitro culture : 6-day chick thymuses and 11-day quail bursas were placed on each side of a nucleo-
pore filter with a pore diameter of 5 μm and cultured for 2 to 4
days. Then the thymus was either fixed and observed histologically or grafted into the somatopleure of a 3-day chick host to allow
subsequent lymphoid differentiation to occur. After 2 to 4 days in
culture, a number of quail cells were found in the chick thymus
(Fig. 1). If retransplanted into a chick host for 6 days the chick
thymus contained a mixture of lymphocytes from both species

TABLE 2 - Association of rudiments of the primary lymphoid organs.

Lymphoid rudiment at the attractive period	Lymphoid rudiment colonized by lymphoid stem cells	Number of cultures	Chimerism	
			Chick	Quail
6-day chick thymus	11-day quail bursa	13	10	0
6-day chick thymus	8-day quail thymus	6	4	0
7-day chick bursa	11-day quail bursa	8	1	0
Both lymphoid rudiments colonized by lymphoid stem cells				
10-day chick thymus	8-day quail thymus	10	0	0
10-day chick thymus	11-day quail bursa	28	0	0

The organ specificity of the thymic attraction was tested as follows : explants of thymus, liver or mesonephros taken from 6-day old chick embryos, were associated in transfilter cultures with 11-day quail bursas.

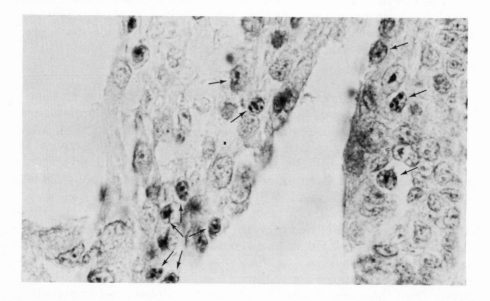

Figure 1 : Transfilter culture of a 6-day chick thymus and an 11-day quail bursa of Fabricius. The thymus epithelium is colonized by quail cells originating from the bursa. The quail cells (arrows) are widespread in the whole thymic rudiment. Duration of the culture : 2 days. Feulgen-Rossenbeck's staining.   x 1250.

showing that lymphoid stem cells which had homed in the quail
bursa and had crossed the filter have completed their lymphoid
differentiation in the thymic environment (Fig. 2).

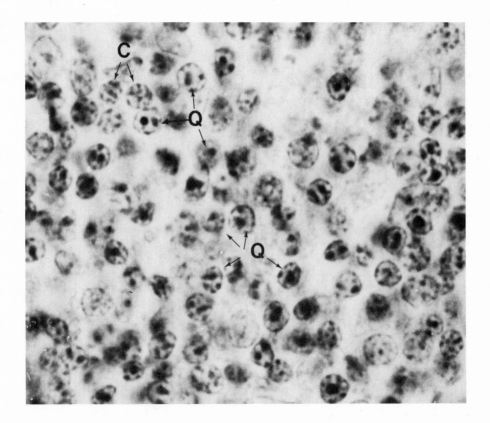

Figure 2 : Same experiment as in figure 1, but the thymic rudiment has been grafted into a 3-day chick host for 6 days. CL :
chick lymphocytes deriving from host stem cells ; QL : quail lymphocytes originating from bursic stem cells which have migrated
into the thymic epithelium during the in vitro culture. Feulgen-
Rossenbeck's staining.   x 2000.

TABLE 3 - Migration of quail cells in transfilter cultures of 11-day quail bursa and 6-day chick organ rudiments (The number of quail cells was counted in 10 sections of each culture. Six cultures were observed for each organ).

6-day chick-organs	Number of quail cells after 48 hours of culture. mean/culture
Thymus	291
Liver	85
Mesonephros	3

The number of quail cells which had crossed the filter was counted after 48 hours in culture. The results reported in table 3 show that practically no cells migrated into the kidney tissue, a certain number of cells migrated into the liver while a great many cells were found in the thymic rudiment. In addition, in thymus transfilter cultures, the quail cells colonized the whole explant (Fig. 1) while in liver cultures, they were found predominantly in contact with the filter.

DISCUSSION AND CONCLUSIONS

The last experiment reported strongly suggests that the seeding of stem cells in the thymic rudiment is regulated through a chemotactic mechanism. Our hypothesis is that from 6 1/2 days of incubation in the chick the epithelium of the thymic rudiment produces a chemotactic substance which diffuses around the organ, arrests the stem cells and causes them to cross the wall of the blood vessel and migrate actively into the epithelium through the basement membrane. When settled in the organ, the stem cells make close membrane contacts with the epithelial cells. When a certain number of stem cells have seeded the thymic epithelium the latter becomes unattractive probably because the production of the substance responsible for the attraction has stopped. Then the stem cells can, for a while, leave the organ if they are experimentally subjected to the attraction of another lymphoid rudiment.

In addition, it appears that the embryonic lymphoid stem cells are undistinctly attracted by both the bursic and the thymic rudiments. This suggests that the attractive mechanism and very likely the diffusible substances responsible for the chemotactic attraction of the hemocytoblasts is the same for the bursa and for the thymus. Once seeded in the lymphoid organs the stem cells proliferate and undergo the process of differentiation into B or T cells according to the microenvironment to which they are subjected. The experiments in which bursic stem cells can be transferred to the thymus and inversely can provide a model for studying the stage from which the stem cells become committed to the B-cell or T-cell differentiating pathways. For example, one can ask the question as to whether the cells which are transferred from the bursa to the thymus in our experimental conditions, were already committed to become B cells by their initial stay in the bursa.

This work was supported by a grant from D.G.R.S.T. n°76-7-0972.

REFERENCES

1. Moore, M.A.S. and Owen, J.J.T., Nature (Lond.), 208:956 (1965).

2. Moore, M.A.S. and Owen, J.J.T., Developm. Biol., 14:40 (1966).

3. Moore, M.A.S. and Owen, J.J.T., J. exp. Med., 126:715 (1967).

4. Le Douarin, N., Bull. biol. Fr. Belg., 103:435 (1969).

5. Le Douarin, N., Developm. Biol. 30:217 (1973).

6. Le Douarin, N. and Jotereau, F., Nature New Biol., 246:25 (1973).

7. Le Douarin, N. and Houssaint, E., C. R. Acad. Sci. (Paris) (Sér. D), 278:2975 (1974).

8. Le Douarin, N. and Jotereau, F., J. exp. Med., 142:17 (1975).

9. Le Douarin, N., Houssaint, E., Jotereau, F. and Belo, M., Proc. nat. Acad. Sci. (Wash.), 72:2701 (1975).

10. Houssaint, E., Belo, M. and Le Douarin, N.M., Developm. Biol., 53:250 (1976).

11. Le Douarin, N.M., Jotereau, F.V. and Houssaint, E., in Phylogeny of Thymus and Bone Marrow - Bursa Cells (R.K. Wright and E.L. Cooper, Eds) (Elsevier/North-Holland Biomedical Press, Amsterdam, 1976).

12. Le Douarin, N.M., Jotereau, F.V., Houssaint,E. and Belo, M., Ann. Immunol., 127C:849 (1976).

13. Grossi, C.E., Lydyard, P.M. and Bockmann, D.E., Feder, Proc., 35:400 (1976).

CELL TRANSPLANTATION INTO IMMUNODEFICIENT CHICKEN EMBRYOS

Reconstituting Capacity of Different Embryonic Cells[1]

Jussi Eskola and Paavo Toivanen

Department of Medical Microbiology, Turku University

SF-20520 Turku 52, Finland

The findings to be described in this paper form a step in our studies on the B cell development in the chicken. In these studies we have largely used the cyclophosphamide model of immune deficiency first described by Lerman and Weidanz (1). Based on a series of experiments we have characterized the postbursal and bursal stages of B cell development (2-6). As a postbursal cell we have defined a cell which is capable of further function and maturation without any influence by the bursa of Fabricius, i.e., this cell can be transferred into cyclophosphamide-treated surgically bursectomized newly-hatched recipients and a full functional restoration of immune functions occurs in the recipients. Postbursal cells appear in significant numbers in the bursa around the third and fourth week after hatching, and shortly thereafter in the spleen, bone marrow and also in the thymus. In contrast, a cell type defined in functional terms as a bursal stem cell needs the bursal microenvironment for further maturation. This cell is capable of inducing a full functional as well as morphological reconstitution only when the bursal rudiment is available. No effect occurs if this cell is transferred into cyclophosphamide-treated surgically bursectomized recipients. The bursal stem cell is present in the bursa during the late embryonic development and shortly after the hatching.

In the search for the source and occurrence of prebursal stem cells, we have utilized the same cyclophosphamide model. In the first of these experiments we transplanted different embryonic cells from different stages of development into 4-day-old cyclo-

---

[1] Supported by grants from the Sigrid Jusélius Foundation and the Lääke Oy Research Foundation, and by NIH Contract NO1-CB-43971.

phosphamide-treated recipients (7). It appeared that the only
cells capable of a functional and morphological reconstitution
were bursa cells. There was no effect with cells from spleen,
bone marrow, thymus, liver or even from yolk sac. However, we realized that perhaps the 4-day-old bursal rudiment of cyclophosphamide-treated recipients is too old to harbor and educate the primitive embryonic stem cells. There must be a mutual interaction between the microenvironment of the bursa and the cells to be edu-
cated (2, 7). In order to avoid a mismatch between the microenvironment and the cells, an embryonic model of immune deficiency
was developed (8).

In this model, chicken embryos are treated with three consecutive injections of cyclophosphamide, given on days 15, 16 and 17
of incubation. On the next day, the embryos are injected intravenously with cells from different embryonic sources. The effects
of the transplantation are studied by morphological and functional
criteria at 4-6 weeks posthatching.

When 18-day embryonic cells were injected into 18-day cyclophosphamide-treated recipients, the only cells among bursa, spleen,
bone marrow, thymus and liver cells used were bursa cells which
were capable of reconstituting the body and organ weights of the
recipients (Table 1) or the antibody formation against sheep red
blood cells and *Brucella* (Table 2). Previously, the relative
weight of the bursa has been found to be a reliable indicator of
the number of well-developed follicles in the bursa (2).

Table 1

Transplantation of 18-day embryonic cells into cyclophosphamide(CY)-
treated embryos; effect on body and organ weights measured at the
age of 36 days. Mean values are given.

CY	Cells	Body weight[+]	Bursa weight[§]	Spleen weight[§]	Thymus weight[§]
+	-	229[*]	80[*]	187[*]	175[*]
+	Bursa	274	341	235	272
+	Spleen	241	81	189	195
+	Marrow	237	96[‡]	259[‡]	201
+	Thymus	222	83	193	159
+	Liver	251[‡][*]	90[*]	185[*]	181[*]
-	-	313	408	234	286

[+] In grams
[§] Mg/100 g of body weight
[‡] P < 0.05   } when compared to CY-treated controls
[*] P < 0.001

Table 2

Transplantation of 18-day embryonic cells into cyclophosphamide(CY)-treated embryos; effect on agglutinin response to SRBC and *Brucella* (mean $\log_2$ titers).

CY	Cells	SRBC		*Brucella*	
		1^0	2^0	1^0	2^0
+	–	0.6	0.8	0.5	0.9
+	Bursa	1.9	4.1	2.2	6.8
+	Spleen	0.2	0.9	0	0.4
+	Marrow	0.4	1.0	0	0
+	Thymus	0.6	1.1	0	0
+	Liver	0.7	0.8	0.1	0.4
–	–	2.2	4.3	4.0	8.7

Bleedings for the primary and secondary responses were carried out at the age of 31 and 36 days, respectively.

It is worthwhile to point out that transplantation of embryonic bursa cells resulted also in an increased thymus weight and in a restored thymus morphology. However, we rather would like to interprete this finding due to the restored general condition of the birds than to the existence of bursa-derived thymus cells.

When 15-day embryonic cells were injected into 18-day-old embryos the results were very much the same. (In this situation we did not have age-matched cells and cell-recipients since cyclophosphamide treatment given before the day 15 resulted in such a mortality that this kind of experiments were impossible.) Here, the bursa cells resulted again in a morphological (Table 3) and functional restoration of the humoral immunity. However, the effects were not as clear as those obtained with 18-day embryonic cells. Secondly, bone marrow cells as well as spleen cells induced a slight but significant restoration of the bursal weight indicating restoration of the bursal morphology. However, there was no evidence for a functional restoration by bone marrow or spleen cells. For instance, the average of secondary antibody titers against *Brucella* was after transplantation of bone marrow cells 0.8, which is the same as in untransplanted cyclophosphamide-treated birds; in those transplanted with bursa cells the value was 3.8. Transplantation of embryonic cells from the liver did not result in any effect by any of the criteria used.

We also used yolk sac cells from 9, 11, 13, 15 and 18 days of incubation. With these cells no effect either on the morphology (Table 4) or on immune functions of the cell recipients was obtained.

Table 3

Transplantation of 15-day embryonic cells into cyclophosphamide(CY)-treated embryos; effect on body and organ weights measured at the age of 36 days. Mean values are given.

CY	Cells	Body weight[+]	Bursa weight[§]	Spleen weight[§]	Thymus weight[§]
+	-	214	82*	209	145
+	Bursa	268	199*	212	209[‡]
+	Marrow	233	110*	209	180
+	Spleen	225	119*	239	166
+	Thymus	223	91	195	145
+	Liver	228*	91	190	136*
-	-	309*	402	230	274*

[+] In grams
[§] Mg/100 g of body weight
[‡] P < 0.05 ⎫
[*] P < 0.001 ⎭ when compared to CY-treated controls

Table 4

Transplantation of yolk sac cells into cyclophosphamide(CY)-treated embryos; effect on body and organ weights measured at the age of 36 days. Mean values are given.

CY	Age of donors[+]	Body weight[§]	Bursa weight[‡]	Spleen weight[‡]	Thymus weight[‡]
+	-	220	83	187	162
+	9	233	89	204	150
+	11	211*	92	179**	169
+	13	185*	74	157**	135
+	15	222	82	211	158
+	18	233**	96**	180**	179**
-	-	316**	425**	230**	278**

[+] Days of incubation
[§] In grams
[‡] Mg/100 g of body weight
[*] P < 0.05 ⎫
[**] P < 0.01 ⎭ when compared to CY-treated controls

Table 5

Transplantation of embryonic bursa cells into cyclophosphamide(CY)- or testosterone(TE)-treated chicken embryos; effect on body and organ weights measured at the age of 36 days. Mean values are given.

Treatment	Bursa cells[+]	Bursa weight[§]	Spleen weight[§]	Thymus weight[§]
-	-	419	241	308
CY[‡]	-	74	159	133
CY[*]	+	362	234	272
TE[*]	-	10	182	131
TE	+	13	174	129

[+] On the day 18 of incubation, 2×10^6 cells were injected intra-venously
[§] Mg/100 g of body weight
[‡] 1.0 mg/embryo/day on the days 13, 14 and 15 of incubation
[*] 2.5 mg/embryo on the 10th day of incubation

Table 6

Transplantation of embryonic bursa cells into cyclophosphamide(CY)- or testosterone(TE)-treated chicken embryos; effect on the production of anti-*Brucella* antibodies at the age of 36 days. Mean values are given.

Treatment	Bursa cells	Anti-*Brucella* antibodies		
		IgM[+]	IgG[+]	Agglutinins[§]
-	-	102	89	10.9
CY	-	6	6	0.8
CY	+	57	51	9.8
TE	-	26	42	0
TE	+	25	55	0

[+] The concentrations are indicated as percentage of a standard plasma, measured by radioimmunoassay
[§] $\log_2$ titer

Table 7

Transplantation of embryonic bursa cells into cyclophosphamide(CY)-
or testosterone(TE)-treated chicken embryos; effect on the plasma
immunoglobulins at the age of 36 days. Mean values are given.

Treatment	Bursa cells	Total immunoglobulins (mg/ml)	
		IgM	IgG
-	-	3.2 ± 1.7	13.2 ± 6.8
CY	-	0.5 ± 0.6	0.9 ± 0.4
CY	+	3.9 ± 0.9	8.6 ± 4.7
TE	-	2.0 ± 2.1	5.6 ± 6.2
TE	+	2.5 ± 1.9	5.1 ± 4.3

The negative results obtained with the yolk sac cells prompted
us to entertain the possibility that perhaps cyclophosphamide de-
stroys something crucial in the bursal microenvironment rendering
it unsuitable to harbor and educate the primitive stem cell. Therefore, another model of embryonic immune deficiency was also used.
For a comparison, birds treated with testosterone were transplanted
with bursa cells on day 18 of incubation (9). It appeared that
testosterone-treated birds showed no signs of reconstitution by the
morphological and functional criteria used (Tables 5-7). The only
group which was reconstituted were birds treated with cyclophosphamide and transplanted with bursa cells. These findings indicate
that the testosterone model of immune deficiency is not suitable
for reconstitution studies. It seems that testosterone affects the
stromal cells of the bursa (9, 10), and that cyclophosphamide de-
stroys only the lymphoid population undergoing differentiation and
leaves the bursal stroma intact (9).
    On the basis of the experiments described, three conclusions
are available. First, at 18 days of incubation, the bursa cells
are the only cells capable of the long-term restoration of humoral
immunity when transferred into 18-day-old cyclophosphamide-treated
recipients. Secondly, when 15-day embryonic donors were used, also
spleen and marrow cells showed, in addition to bursa cells, a slight
restorative effect on the bursal morphology, however, without any
signs of functional restoration. It remains to be established
whether this slight morphological reconstitution really represents
presence of prebursal stem cells in the embryonic bone marrow at
an early stage of development. Thirdly, yolk sac cells did not
have any reconstituting effect when transplanted into 18-day old
embryonic recipients. This finding is in disagreement with the
suggestion about the yolk sac origin of lymphoid stem cells (11).

However, the question whether the mutual interaction between the microenvironment and the cells depends on a developmental match is effective also here.

REFERENCES

1.   Lerman, S. P. and Weidanz, W. P., J. Immunol., 105: 614 (1970).

2.   Toivanen, P. and Toivanen, A., Eur. J. Immunol., 3: 585 (1973).

3.   Toivanen, P., Toivanen, A. and Tamminen, P., Eur. J. Immunol., 4: 405 (1974).

4.   Toivanen, P., Toivanen, A. and Tamminen, P., Eur. J. Immunol., 4: 220 (1974).

5.   Sorvari, T., Toivanen, A. and Toivanen, P., Transplantation, 17: 584 (1974).

6.   Sorvari, T. E. and Toivanen, A., Scand. J. Immunol., 5: 317 (1976).

7.   Toivanen, P., Toivanen, A. and Good, R. A., J. Immunol., 109: 1058 (1972).

8.   Eskola, J. and Toivanen, P., Cell. Immunol., 13: 459 (1974).

9.   Eskola, J., Ruuskanen, O., Fräki, J. E., Viljanen, M. K. and Toivanen, A., Scand. J. Immunol., 6: 185 (1977).

10. Glick, B., Perkins, W. D. and Holbrook, K., J. reticuloendoth. Soc., 20: 2a (1976).

11. Metcalf, D. and Moore, M. A. S., Haemopoietic Cells, (North-Holland, Amsterdam, 1971).

MIGRATION PATTERNS OF AVIAN EMBRYONIC BONE MARROW CELLS AND THEIR DIFFERENTIATION TO FUNCTIONAL T AND B CELLS

W. T. Weber and R. Mausner

University of Pennsylvania

Philadelphia, Pennsylvania   19104

Previous studies by Moore and Owen (1,2) as well as more recent experiments with interspecific chimeras (3,4) support the concept that blood-borne lymphoid cell precursors immigrate into the bursa as well as into the thymus. These precursors presumably are multipotential stem cells that according to some investigators origi- nate in the yolk sac (5), whereas others propose certain intraembryo- nic hematopoietic islands as the first recognizable source of stem cells (4,6). By 14-18 days of embryonation, stem cells capable of migrating to the thymus and bursa have been detected in additional hematopoietic sites such as spleen and bone marrow (2). None of the above experiments, however, have formally demonstrated that this migration of cells to the thymus and bursa is in all instances fol- lowed by functional differentiation to T and B cells respectively. This is simply assumed and extensively quoted as if it were estab- lished fact. It is not without challenge, however, and a recent study concluded that embryonic bone marrow does not harbor bursal precursor cells and suggested that the previously demonstrated mi- gration of 14-18 day embryonic spleen and bone marrow to the bursa may have been of no physiological significance and probably repre- sented nonspecific trapping (7). It is apparent that considerable confusion and controversy exists in relation to early events in T and B cell ontogeny.

We decided to reexamine the question of the presence or absence of precursor cells for thymic and bursal lymphocytes in certain hematopoietic sites at specific stages of embryonic development, to formally establish the capacity of precursor cells to differenti- ate to T and B cells in their respective microenvironments and to examine whether the thymus and bursa displayed significant differ- ences in regulating the influx of precursor cells and their differ-

entiation at different stages of development. The latter question
was prompted by several observations which suggested a definite
functional difference between bursa and thymus in this regard. The
most important of these was the demonstrated failure of the bursa,
in striking contrast to the thymus, to regenerate its lymphoid cell
population following either localized irradiation (8) or following
repeated administration of cyclophosphamide in the newly hatched (9)
as well as in the late embryonic period (10). This could be interpreted as a differential sensitivity of the bursal and thymic microenvironment to these agents, resulting in a selective failure to
support cell differentiation in the bursa. The observed difference
could, however, also result from 1) a selective failure of precursor
cells to gain entrance to the bursal microenvironment beginning in
the late embryonic period, 2) the existence of separate populations
of precursor T (PT) and precursor B (PB) cells with a selective nume-
rical decrease or disappearance of the latter in the late embryonic
or newly hatched period or 3) a combination of these two.

These considerations led to the construction of several models
with hypothetical functional differences between thymus and bursa
and allowing for multipotential stem cells versus separate lineages
of precursor T and precursor B cells respectively. The models could
be subjected to experimentation and results obtained analyzed for
compatibility with any one model. One model which gained special
significance in light of subsequent experimental results is shown
in figure 1. This model predicts a migration pattern and differentiation to functional T and B cells following the transfer of precursor cells of a designated developmental stage to recipients of a
given age as illustrated. For example, precursor cells of 14 day
old embryos transferred to embryos 18 days or older would be expected
to differentiate into functional T cells following the migration of
PT cells through the thymus. Few or no B cells would develop, however, as the transferred PB cells could no longer gain entrance into
the bursa at that stage.

Materials and methods. White Leghorn chick embryos of the SC
line (Hy-Line International, Dallas Center, Iowa) homozygous for the
major histocompatibility locus, genotype B_2B_2 were used in all experiments. 30×10^6 viable, sex chromosomally marked bone marrow or
spleen cells obtained from embryos or chicks at specific stages of
development were injected intravenously into recipients at specific
stages of development. Recipient embryos had been exposed 24 hrs
previously to 750 R γ-irradiation from a Cs 137 source. At varying
intervals after hatching the appropriate chimeras were killed and
cell suspensions from the thymus, bursa, bone marrow and spleen prepared for direct chromosome preparations. In addition, aliquots
of these cell suspensions were cultured for 48 hours in serum-free
medium with a) specific T cell stimulants Concanavalin A (Con A) and
Phytohemagglutinin (PHA), b) specific B cell stimulants anti-immunoglobulin (R-antiCIg) and dextran sulfate (DxS) and c) appropriate

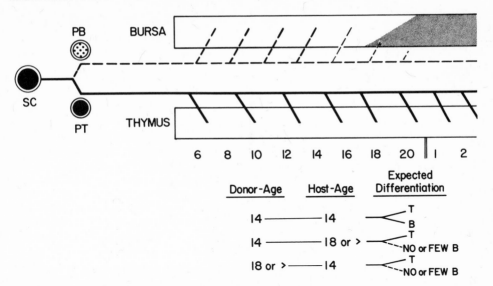

Figure 1. Proposed model of migration patterns of embryonic precursor T (PT) and precursor B (PB) cells into the thymus and bursa. Specifically the model proposes: 1) separate lineages of PT and PB cells, 2) only a temporary presence of PB cells during embryonic development (up to day 18-19), but continuous presence of PT cells during the embryonic and post embryonic period, 3) decreasing influx of PB cells into the bursa beginning approximately on the 16th-17th day of embryonation, with complete exclusion by day 20 (indicated by stippled area). PT cells have the potential to immigrate into the thymus at any time during the embryonic and the post embryonic period.

unstimulated control cultures. Details for preparation of cell suspensions, chromosome analysis, culture conditions and specificity of respective stimulants have been published previously (11,12). Following culture, the net number of functional donor (host) T cells per 10^4 cells in appropriately stimulated cultures was determined. It represents the number of donor (host) T cells/10^4 cells in stimulated cultures minus the value obtained in controls. Individual values for each culture were determined by multiplying the percentage of donor (host) cells x mitotic index x 10. The net number of donor (host) B cells in cultures stimulated by specific B cell stimulants was determined in the same way. These experiments therefore traced not only the migration pattern of transferred cells, but they simultaneously and in quantitative terms revealed whether injected cells differentiated to 1) T cells, 2) B cells, 3) T and B cells or 4) failed to differentiate. Migration patterns of bone marrow and spleen cell populations and their potential to differentiate to functional T and B cells were determined for the following separate cell transfer combinations: 1) transfer of cells of 14,17,19 day

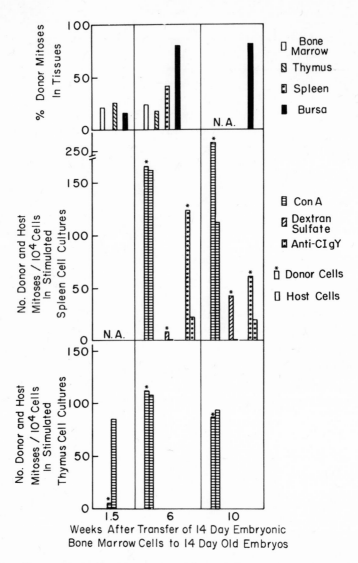

Figure 2. Top: Distribution of cells of donor karyotype in bone marrow, thymus, spleen and bursa of recipients at different intervals after cell transfer. Mid-Bottom: Net number of dividing Con A responsive T cells of donor (host) origin, as well as the number of dividing Anti-CIg and Dextran Sulfate responsive B cells of donor (host) origin per 10^4 cells in spleen and thymus cell cultures of recipients. Net number represents respective values in stimulated minus values in control cultures.

embryos and 2 day old hatched chicks to 14 day old embryos, 2) transfer of cells of 14 day embryos to 2 day old hatched chicks.

Results. The data obtained after transfer of 14 day embryonic bone marrow cells (EBMC) to 14 day embryos are shown in Fig. 2. At 1.5, 6 and 10 weeks after transfer, spontaneously dividing donor cells were found in significant numbers in the bone marrow, thymus, bursa and spleen of recipients. Differentiation of donor cells to T cells was first detectable in Con A-stimulated thymus cell cultures at 1.5 weeks. It was not possible to determine if T cells of donor origin had already migrated from the thymus to the spleen, as the spleen at that time was too small and did not yield a sufficient number of cells for culture. At 6 and 10 weeks after cell transfer, large numbers of Con A responsive donor T cells were found in spleen cell cultures and donor T cells exceeded those of host origin. Similar observations were made for the thymus. The number of anti-Ig responsive B cells of donor origin in spleen cell cultures at 6 and 10 weeks was approximately 2-4 times higher as compared to the number of B cells of host origin. This was corroborated by similar findings in DxS-stimulated cultures. Thus, 14 day EBMC transferred to 14 day old embryos were shown to migrate to the thymus and bursa and direct evidence was obtained for their differentiation to T and B cells respectively. The same conclusion was reached in experiments (not shown) involving the transfer of 14 day embryonic spleen cells to 14 day old embryos. It should be pointed out here that 14-19 day embryonic bone marrow and spleen as well as marrow of 2 day old hatched chicks did not contain detectable numbers of Con A responsive or anti-Ig responsive cells, indicating that in the above experiments and in those described later, the transferred cell populations did not contain significant numbers of differentiated T or B cells.

Following the transfer of 17 day EBMC or spleen cells to 14 day old embryos, donor cells were again found in large numbers in bone marrow, thymus and bursa at 8-9 weeks after cell transfer. The extent of donor T cell differentiation in spleen and thymus was at levels comparable to those observed after transfer of 14 day EBMC to 14 day old embryos. Anti-CIg responsive B cells of donor origin were readily detected in spleen cell cultures, but the number of donor B cells was approximately half the number of host B cells, suggesting a decreasing potential of B cell differentiation upon transfer of 17 day EBMC.

Figure 3 shows the results obtained after the transfer of 19 day EBMC to 14 day old embryos. It is evident that cells of donor origin had almost completely replaced the host cell population in the bone marrow and the thymus. In contrast, the number of donor mitoses in the bursa was extremely variable with values of 53% at 4 weeks and less than 2% at 9 weeks. Significantly, B cells of donor origin were not detected in the spleen. The highest value obtained was

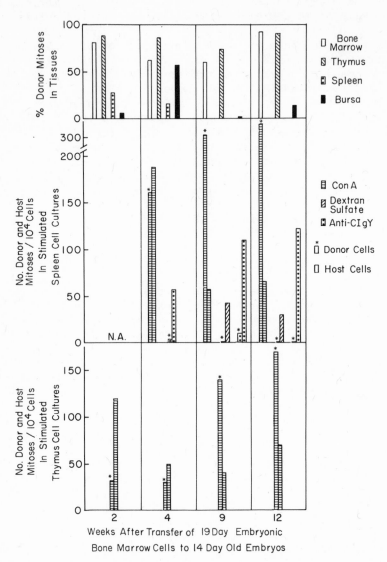

Figure 3. Top: Distribution of cells of donor karyotype in bone
marrow, thymus, spleen and bursa of recipients at different intervals after cell transfer. Mid-Bottom: Net number of dividing Con A
responsive T cells of donor (host) origin, as well as the number of
dividing Anti-CIg and Dextran Sulfate responsive B cells of donor
(host) origin per 10^4 cells in spleen and thymus cell cultures of
recipients. Net number represents respective values in stimulated
minus values in control cultures.

8 donor B cells per 10^4 cells at 9 weeks after transfer. This value
is barely above background and it correlated with an absence of donor
mitoses in the bursa at this time interval. Equally important are
the findings at the 4 week interval, at which time more than 50%
donor mitoses were detected in the bursa without a significant number of anti-Ig responsive donor B cells being found in the spleen.
These data indicate clearly, that the mere presence of dividing
donor cells in a given lymphoid organ, in this case the bursa, cannot
be taken as evidence for the differentiative capacities of these
cells. In contrast, there was no impairment of differentiation to
T cells, with the number of Con A responsive T cells of donor origin
in spleen cell cultures being nearly equal to or exceeding the number
of host T cells by a factor of 5-6. Observations in the thymus
closely paralleled those in the spleen. Therefore, 19 day EBMC
transferred to 14 day old embryos migrated to the thymus, and this
was followed by unimpaired differentiation and extensive production
of functional T cells. The ability of EBMC to immigrate and proliferate in the bursa became quite variable, however, and even when
it did occur it was not followed by significant differentiation to
B cells.

The decreased potential of donor BM cells of 19 day embryos
to enter the bursa and their failure to differentiate to B cells
after transfer to 14 day old embryos was further supported by results obtained after injection of bone marrow of 2 day old hatched
chicks into 14 day old embryos. Cells of donor origin were found
in large numbers in bone marrow and thymus of recipients and there
was no detectable impairment of differentiation to T cells. In
contrast, donor cells were not detected in the bursa and there was
complete failure of donor cells to differentiate to functional anti-
CIg responsive B cells.

In order to determine whether the bursa and thymus exerted a
differential effect on the influx of precursor cells during the
immediate postembryonic period, 14 day EBMC were transferred to 2 day
old hatched chicks. As shown in figure 4, cells of donor origin were
readily detected in bone marrow and thymus. Differentiation of donor
cells to Con A responsive T cells was detectable in the thymus as
early as 1.5 weeks after cell transfer and there were large numbers
of Con A responsive T cells of donor origin in the spleen at 6, 7 and
13 weeks after cell transfer. Strikingly, dividing donor cells were
not found in the bursa at any of these time periods investigated
and there was a complete failure of differentiation to B cells.
These results indicate that by 1-2 days after hatching the bursa had
acquired a unique role in that it, in contrast to the thymus, selectively excluded further immigration and prevented differentiation
of potential precursor cells. A summary of the major findings are
shown in table 1.

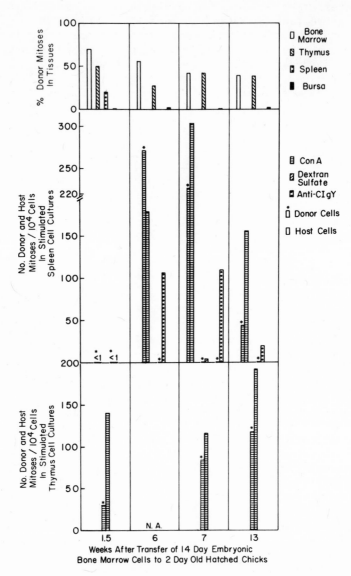

Figure 4. Top: Distribution of cells of donor karyotype in bone marrow, thymus, spleen and bursa of recipients at different intervals after cell transfer. Mid-Bottom: Net number of dividing Con A responsive T cells of donor (host) origin, as well as the number of dividing Anti-CIg and Dextran Sulfate responsive B cells of donor (host) origin per 10^4 cells in spleen and thymus cell cultures of recipients. Net number represents respective values in stimulated minus values in control cultures.

Table 1.   Donor Cell Migration and Differentiation to T and B cells in Cell Transfer Recipients.

Age and Source of Donor Cells	Age of Recipients at Time of Cell Transfer	Donor Cell Migration to		Donor Cell Differentiation	
		Thymus	Bursa	T	B
14 day EBMC*	14 day embryo	+++	+++	+++	+++
17 day EBMC	14 day embryo	+++	++	+++	++
19 day EBMC	14 day embryo	+++	+/-	+++	-
2 day BMC post hatching	14 day embryo	+++	-	+++	-
14 day EBMC	2 day post hatching	+++	-	+++	-

*EBMC = embryonic bone marrow cells

Discussion. These experimental results are compatible with the model presented at the outset. Specifically, the data support the concept of separate lineages of PT and PB cells with the additional qualification that PB cells decrease numerically, beginning on the 16th - 17th day of embryonation, and can no longer be found in bone marrow or spleen by the second day after hatching. In contrast, PT cells are present at undiminished levels in the marrow and spleen during the embryonic period and are still readily detected in the marrow during the postembryonic period. Furthermore, a striking difference between thymus and bursa with regard to the regulation of precursor cell influx was found. Here, the bursa revealed a distinct pattern in that at 14 days of embryonation it readily accepted influx of PB cells present in 14 day embryonic marrow, whereas at 1-2 days after hatching the bursa no longer permitted influx and differentiation of these same PB cells. A definitive explanation for the exclusion of PB cell immigration into the bursa is presently not available. It may reflect an exquisitively sensitive recognition between membrane receptors on PB cells and developing cellular elements of the bursal microenvironment. This recognition and exclusion could be regulated at the endothelial cell level of the bursal microvasculature or in the extravascular bursal tissue where it may be influenced by levels of a bursal humoral factor.

The apparent disappearance of PB cells from late embryonic BM and spleen seems to coincide temporally with the developing exclusion

of PB cell influx into the bursa. However, these apparently are
independent events as suggested by a similar rate of PB cell disappearance from late embryonic marrow of in ovo testosterone treated
chicks which lack a bursal structure (unpublished data). It is also
conceivable that PB cells may in fact not disappear entirely but may
be sequestered at some as yet unidentified site, other than marrow
or spleen, although this is considered unlikely.

In contrast to the bursa, the thymus clearly accepted influx
of PT cells in the embryonic as well as in the postembryonic period
and supported their differentiation to functional T cells. Previous
investigations utilizing interspecific chimeras had suggested that
the chick thymus is colonized by inflow of stemcells at about the
7th day of embryonation, followed by another inflow around the time
of hatching which completely renews the first lymphoid population (4).
It is not clear whether this latter inflow pattern is a peculiarity
related to the use of interspecific chimeras or is indeed a true
reflection of the developing chick thymus under normal physiological
conditions. On the basis of our results we favor the interpretation
that the thymus is certainly capable of accepting an influx of PT
cells during the embryonic as well as the postembryonic periods.
Under normal physiological conditions this influx may well be intermittent and it certainly need not be continuous. However, if influx
of PT cells can occur subsequent to specific events such as after
radiation induced or drug induced (cyclophosphamide, cortisone)
partial depletion of the existing thymus cell population, this would
have obvious implications in those clinical situations which result
in temporary thymus atrophy.

The concept of separate populations of PT and PB cells especially with a selective disappearance of PB cells at a given stage
of embryonation is difficult to accept. Although it would still
permit the existence of a pool of multipotential stem cells, it would
imply that the eventual expansion of the total B cell repertoire is
dependent on the proliferation of those cells that had seeded into
the bursa by the time of hatching. No additional influx would occur.
This would suggest furthermore that after bursal involution there
may be no new source of uncommited virgin B cells and continued
B cell function would be dependent on long-lived B cells. This must
be contrasted with the suggestion that after bursal involution the
bone marrow may be a location for continued production of B cells
from progenitor cells which have migrated through the bursa earlier,
became committed to B cell differentiation and retained their proliferative and differentiative capacity in an extrabursal location
(13). If this were correct, one should still be able to detect,
after bursal involution, a sequential development of the B cell
lineage with gradual acquisition of Ig and other B cell membrane
markers down to the functional B cell level in a proportion of bone
marrow cells. This has not been demonstrated to date but is worthy

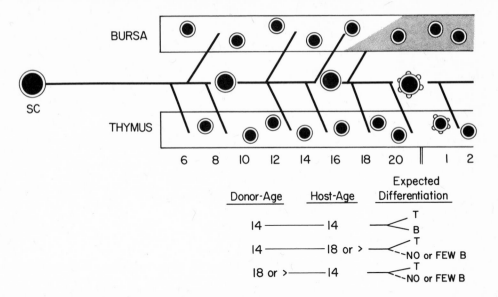

Figure 5. Proposed model of migration patterns of multipotential
stem cells (SC) into the thymus and bursa. Specifically this model
proposes: 1) SC with changing membrane characteristics during embryonic development = early embryonic SC significantly different from
late embryonic or post-embryonic SC. 2) Bursa highly discriminating,
accepting only SC of early type, followed by total exclusion of SC
immigration into the bursa after 18-19 days of embryonation.
3) Thymus non-discriminating during the embryonic or postembryonic
period. SC have the potential to enter the thymus at any time
during the embryonic and postembryonic period.

of further investigation. The reported induction of Bu-1[+] antigen
in 20-30% of bone marrow cells of newly hatched chicks after incubation with bursal extract would suggest that PB cells are still
present in bone marrow (14), which is contrary to the interpretation
of our data within the discussed model. However, the induction of
one type of bursa cell related antigen on cells is insufficient proof
for differentiation of such cells to fully functional B cells. At
this point, the concept of separate lineages of PT and PB cells
during the embryonic period can serve as one working hypothesis.
It may be possible to selectively eliminate or drastically reduce
one of the two precursor cell pools during embryonic development.
This should reflect itself detectably in suitable transfer experiments, as have been employed in this series of experiments.

    Although the experimental results are compatible with the model
discussed, we also attempted to reconcile the data with a model which
considered multipotential stem cells, rather than separate lineages

of PT and PB cells as progenitor cells. The characteristics of this
model, reflecting the experimental results, is shown in figure 5.
To fit the results within this model it was necessary to postulate
that there may be one (or several?) changes in the membrane characteristics of multipotential cells during embryonic development,
resulting in a distinct difference between the stem cell pool in
early (10-16 days) as compared to late (18 and >) stages of embryonation. In addition, the bursa would not only be highly selective,
allowing inflow only of early but not of late stem cell type, but
in addition, the bursa would exclude any stem cell influx beginning
in the late embryonic period. The thymus on the other hand would
not be discriminating and, as in the other model, would be capable
of accepting stem cell influx under certain conditions at any embryonic and post-embryonic period. In this model, the observed pattern
and regulation of stem cell influx into the bursa would be determined
by an interaction of changing membrane characteristics of stem cells
and an independently developing functional change in the bursa.
Thus, the failure of stem cells present in bone marrow of 2 day old
hatched chicks to enter and differentiate in the normal bursa of a
14 day embryo could be explained by a postulated membrane change in
the late stem cell pool and the selectivity of the bursa for stem
cells of only early type. Conversely, the failure of stem cells
present in 14 day embryonic marrow to enter the bursa of 2 day old
hatched chicks could be based on the development of a bursa-regulated
shut-off of stem cell influx by that time. It should be pointed out
here, that the variable ability of stem cells of 19 day embryonic
marrow to enter the bursa of 14 day embryos but their failure to
differentiate, could be interpreted within this model as a possible
defect of late stem cells to complete differentiation in a normal
bursal microenvironment. Another possibility of course is that the
donor cells found proliferating in the bursa in that specific transfer combination were myeloid cells or T cells and not bursal lymphocytes.

At this point, the available data does not allow a definitive
selection of one model. However, both models presented suggest a
series of experiments which should lead to further elucidation of
T and B cell ontogeny in the avian system and hopefully to a selection and further characterization of one of these models.

Acknowledgement. This research was supported by USPHS grant
AM 11693 from the Institute of Arthritis, Metabolism and Digestive
Diseases. The excellent technical assistance of Ms. Jane Alexander
is gratefully acknowledged.

REFERENCES

1. Moore, M. A. S. and Owen, J. J. T., Develop. Biol. 14:40 (1966).

2. Moore, M. A. S. and Owen, J. J. T., Nature (London) 215:1081 (1967).

3. Le Douarin, N. M., Houssaint, E., Jotereau, F. V. and Belo, M., Proc. Nat. Acad. Sci. 72:2701 (1975).

4. Le Douarin, N. M., and Jotereau, F. V., J. Exp. Med. 142:17 (1975).

5. Hemmingsson, E. J. and Alm, G. V. Acta Pathol. Microbiol. Scand. A, 81:79 (1973).

6. Dieterlen-Lievre, F., Annee Biol. 12:481 (1973).

7. Eskola, J. and Toivanen, A., Cell. Immunol. 26:68 (1976).

8. Weber, W. T. and Weidanz, W. P., J. Immunol. 103:537 (1969).

9. Glick, B., Transplantation 11:433 (1971).

10. Eskola, J. and Toivanen, P., Cell. Immunol. 13:459 (1974).

11. Weber, W. T., Clin. Exptl. Immunol. 6:919 (1970).

12. Weber, W. T., Transplantation Rev. 24:113 (1975).

13. Toivanen, P. and Toivanen A., Europ. J. Immunol. 3:585 (1973).

14. Brand, A., Gilmour, D. G. and Goldstein, G., Science 193:319 (1976).

UNIQUE ASPECTS OF IMMUNOGLOBULIN EXPRESSION DURING EARLY B CELL

DIFFERENTIATION IN THE CHICKEN

C. E. Grossi, P. M. Lydyard, and M. D. Cooper

Departments of Microbiology and Pediatrics
and the Comprehensive Cancer Center
University of Alabama in Birmingham
Birmingham, Alabama   35294

Perhaps the most significant events during the life history of B cells are changes in the expression of immunoglobulin genes. In this regard, results of studies in birds and mammals suggest that B cell development can be conveniently divided into 3 principle stages. The first is primarily concerned with the generation of clonal diversity; during this stage, non-Ig producing stem cells differentiate and divide to form large numbers of B lymphocytes, each expressing IgM antibodies of a single specificity. Next, the generation of isotype diversity occurs within B cell clones; limited numbers of cells within each clone switch from IgM synthesis only to the surface expression of other immunoglobulin classes without a change in antibody specificity (or V-region gene expression). Lastly, clones are selected for stimulation by antigen, or clones may be stimulated by polyclonal mitogens to divide and differentiate into plasma cells. Helper and suppressor T cells participate primarily in regulating the latter events.

We will be mainly concerned in this paper with the first of these arbitrarily defined stages, during which two interesting differences are notable between representative birds and mammals: (i) B cell clones in birds are normally generated within the bursa of Fabricius (1-3), whereas generation of clones of B cells in mammals begins in fetal liver and continues thereafter within the bone marrow (4-12). (ii) While B cells in the avian bursa express IgM detectable by immunofluorescence both in the cytoplasm(cIgM) and on the surface(sIgM) (2), the youngest cells of B cell lineage in mammalian fetal liver and bone marrow contain cIgM but lack stable sIgM receptors (9,12-14). These mammalian cells are generally referred to as pre-B cells. Large pre-B cells

61

divide frequently and ultimately give rise to small sIgM$^+$ B
lymphocytes lacking detectable cIgM (4,6,15,16). Newly formed or
baby B lymphocytes in mammals have been shown to be highly susceptible to modulation of sIgM by exposure to bivalent anti-μ antibodies (8,17,18) and, correspondingly, to tolerance induction by
exposure to multivalent antigens in the absence of T cell help
(10,19,20). By contrast, adult B lymphocytes are less easily
inhibited by cross-linkage of their surface antibodies.

In this paper we describe results of recent experiments aimed
at defining some of the characteristics of IgM expression in the
cytoplasm and on the surface of young B cells in chickens. Our
data suggests that: (i) the bursa is the exclusive site of B-cell
generation during normal development; (ii) during ontogeny, IgM
in bursal cells is expressed in a characteristic sequence of distinct cytoplasmic distribution patterns; (iii) these patterns of
cIgM distribution are related to an age-dependent difference in
susceptibility of sIgM to modulation by anti-IgM antibodies and
(iv) in ovo treatment with anti-IgM antibodies arrests the normal
development of bursal cells via a mechanism involving modulation
of sIgM.

PATTERNS OF cIgM EXPRESSION IN BURSAL CELLS

For analysis of cIgM expression, suspensions of bursal cells
were obtained from donors of different ages (from day 12 of incubation up to 15 weeks after hatching), washed, cytocentrifuged
onto glass slides, fixed, and stained with fluorochrome-labeled
purified antibodies to μ-chain determinants. In some birds older
than 4 weeks, cortical and medullary bursal lymphocytes were
mechanically separated before staining for cIgM.

As was previously shown (21), in donors of all ages examined,
bursal cells expressing cIgM expressed sIgM as well. Therefore,
to avoid interference of sIgM in determining the pattern distribution of cIgM, viable cells were stripped of sIgM by pronase
treatment prior to cytoplasmic staining. The three general patterns of cIgM localization detected in bursal cells are illustrated in Fig. 1.

In bursal cells designated as type 1, diffuse cytoplasmic
localization of IgM, often accentuated in the perinuclear region
and the nuclear notch, was noted. Type 2 bursal cells were
stained either in the perinuclear cisterns or in the Golgi region,
or in both. Type 3 cells contained IgM in small vesicles that
were randomly dispersed in the cytoplasm.

Figure 1

(See text for description of cIgM distribution represented in these drawings of characteristic bursal cell types.)

PATTERNS OF cIgM EXPRESSION DURING BURSAL CELL DEVELOPMENT *

cIgM PATTERN	STAGE OF FOLLICULAR DEVELOPMENT: 12-16 DAY OLD EMBRYO +	HATCHING ‡	MATURE FOLLICLE X: CORTEX	MEDULLA
TYPE I	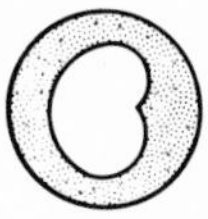	NP++	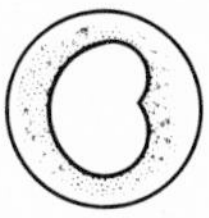	NP
TYPE 2	NP	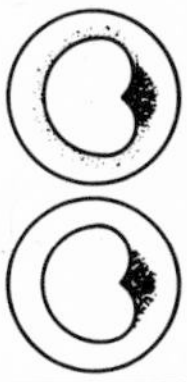	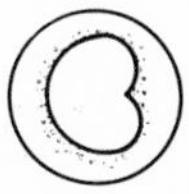	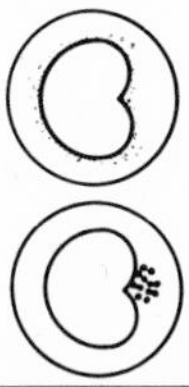
TYPE 3	NP	NP	NP	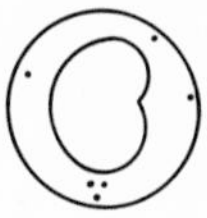

* The normal sequence of development is from type I to type 3.
\+ At this stage only the medullary compartment is present.
‡ Cortex begins to develop soon after hatching.
x The two separate compartments, cortex and medulla, are fully developed.
++NP = not present in percentages >1 %.

During normal B cell ontogeny, sequential development of bursal cells with the differing patterns of cIgM distribution was observed. Type 1 cells appeared at 12 days of incubation and were the only B cell type present until the 16th day of incubation. Type 2 cells appeared after the 16th day of incubation and became the predominant cell type until the 2nd week of hatching. Type 3 cells appeared soon after hatching and increased in number with the maturation of bursal follicles. In the cortical and medullary populations separated from mature bursal follicles, type 1 cells were predominant in the cortical fraction while type 3 cells prevailed in the medullary population. That type 3 bursal cells represent a secretory phase during B cell development was suggested by the demonstration of extracellular IgM in the medulla of bursal follicles and supported by demonstration of the loss of IgM from the vesicles in type 3 cells when they were incubated for an hour at 37°C. This *in vitro* release of cIgM was greatly reduced when cytochalasin B was included in the incubation medium (21).

In mammals, early cells of B cell lineage are not as easily examined since they are a minority population in the hemopoietic tissues in which they are formed. However, we have noted that patterns of cIgM resembling those described in the chicken are present in human fetal liver and bone marrow pre-B cells (unpublished). This suggests that an early secretory phase is common to both avian and mammalian B cells, and is involved in the transition to cIgM⁻/sIgM⁺ B cells.

IN VITRO MODULATION CHARACTERISTICS OF sIgM
ON YOUNG AND OLD B CELLS.

IgM on the surface of B lymphocytes can be removed by treatment with anti-IgM antibodies of viable cells in suspension. In mouse and human, this stripping of sIgM, usually termed modulation, requires increasing concentrations of anti-μ antibodies as a function of B cell maturation (8,17, Gathings, unpublished observations).

In the present study, lymphocytes from several sources were treated with purified goat antibodies specific for chicken μ-chain determinants. A concentration range of antibodies from 0.05 μg to 10 μg/ml was used. Following incubation with anti-μ antibodies at 37°C for 30 min., the percentage of cells stainable for sIgM by fluorochrome-labeled antibodies was determined and the percent inhibition was expressed as the percentage decrease of control values of sIgM-positive cells preincubated in media alone.

As shown in Fig. 2, the doses of antibody required to modulate sIgM on B lymphocytes vary considerably with the organ source and the age of the donor. Antibody concentrations required for efficient modulation of sIgM on peripheral blood and bone marrow lymphocytes were 10 to 100 times greater than for modulation of sIgM on bursal cells from 15 day old embryos. Lymphocytes from bursae of older donors required progressively higher concentrations of anti-IgM antibodies for sIgM modulation, up until 3 weeks of age. However, modulation of sIgM on a proportion of bursal lymphocytes obtained from 12-15 week old birds, appeared to be more susceptible to the lower antibody concentrations. Analysis of the requirements for modulation of sIgM on separated cortical and medullary bursal cells revealed that the cortical but not the medullary fraction contained cells that were more susceptible to anti-IgM antibodies.

Figure 2

Modulation characteristics of sIgM on B cells as a function of age
and organ source. The % inhibition was determined by the reduction
in numbers of lymphocytes stainable with fluorochrome-labeled antibodies to μ-chain determinants after treatment for 30 min. at 37°C
to various concentrations of anti-μ antibodies as compared to the
number of sIgM+ cells in untreated control samples.

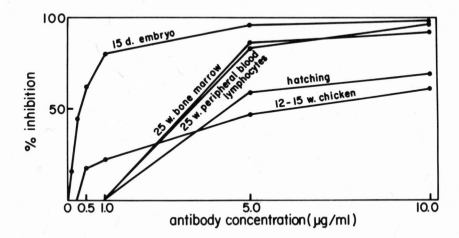

The modulation characteristics of IgM on bursal cells at
different ages thus appear to be related to the pattern of cIgM
expression. Type 1 cells, found in early embryonic development
and in the cortex of the mature follicle are more susceptible to
antibody modulation of their sIgM. Type 2 and type 3 cells are
more resistant to sIgM stripping by antibody. Since type 3 cells
appear to be capable of secreting their IgM, the possibility
existed that secreted IgM might partially neutralize the effect
of anti-IgM antibodies on sIgM, thus reducing the effective dose.
To approach this problem, we studied the modulation characteristics of medullary cells previously incubated at 37°C for 1 hour.
Under these conditions, medullary cells released most of their
cIgM contained in vesicles. However, no significant differences
were observed for sIgM modulation requirements for these cells as
compared to those for cells held at 4°C before analysis. This
suggests that the IgM secretion is insufficient to have a significant effect on the doses of anti-IgM antibodies required for
modulation of sIgM on bursal medullary cells.

Thus avian and mammalian B cells are alike in that with
increasing maturation their sIgM becomes progressively more resistant to modulation by cross-linking ligands. Unlike the situation
in mammals, B cells in the chicken bone marrow have the sIgM modu-

lation characteristics of mature B cells, thus supporting other evidence which indicates that the bursa and not bone marrow is the normal production site for B cells in birds. Another significant difference in B cell differentiation in birds and mammals is that avian B cells express stable sIgM antibodies as soon as they begin to express cIgM, whereas mammalian B cells do not. This suggested that avian B cells would be susceptible to inhibition by sIgM modulation at the earliest recognizable point in differentiation, and this idea was confirmed by results of experiments described below.

ARREST OF B LYMPHOCYTE DEVELOPMENT BY ANTI-IgM ANTIBODY GIVEN DURING EMBRYONIC LIFE

Treatment of 13 day old embryos with purified goat antibodies to chicken IgM, followed by bursectomy at hatching, impairs B cell development and results in permanent agammaglobulinemia (22-24). In the present experiments, we studied the effects of anti-IgM antibodies on B cell generation by analysis of sIgM and cIgM detectable in bursal cells 4 and 8 days after anti-μ injection. Whereas body and spleen weights were unaffected by antibodies to chicken IgM, both bursal weights and cell recoveries were reduced in treated embryos (Table I); bursal lymphocyte depletion was confirmed by histologic examination of stained bursal sections. No sIgM positive cells were present in bursae obtained from 3 anti-IgM treated embryos 4 days after antibody injection; very low percentages of sIgM positive cells were detectable 8 days after anti-μ treatment. However, cIgM positive cells in low but significant numbers were found both at 4 and 8 days (13.5% and 9.5 to 43.6% respectively) following anti-μ treatment (Table II).

TABLE I

EFFECT OF ANTI-μ TREATMENT OF 13 DAY EMBRYOS ON BURSAL AND SPLEEN GROWTH*

Treatment	17th Embryonic Day				At Hatching			
	Body	Spleen	Bursa		Body	Spleen	Bursa	
	Wt. (gm)	Wt. (mg)	Wt. (mg)	Cell No. (x 10^{-6})	Wt. (gm)	Wt. (mg)	Wt. (mg)	Cell No. (x 10^{-6})
None	22.8** (1.1)	15.5 (1.1)	26.2 (1.6)	2.2 (0.7)	47.4 (2.3)	14.3 (1.6)	63.4 (3.5)	30.0 (3.2)
Anti-μ	22.2 (1.0)	13.0 (1.7)	25.8 (2.3)	0.48*** (0.4)	42.4 (2.2)	14.6 (1.9)	27.6*** (3.2)	2.8*** (1.6)

*Embryos were injected intravenously with 2.6 mg of purified goat anti-chicken-μ antibodies and sacrificed 4 days later or at hatching.

**Mean values for groups of 3-5 embryos (± SE).

***p=<0.1.

TABLE II

EXPRESSION OF SURFACE AND CYTOPLASMIC IgM IN BURSAL CELLS

FROM NORMAL AND ANTI-μ TREATED CHICK EMBRYOS*

Days after injection	Treatment	% of cells expressing IgM (surface/cytoplasmic)
4 (day 17)	None	56.5/56.5
	anti-μ	0/13.5
8 (at hatching)	None	80.5/80.5
	anti-μ	3.3/43.6
		3.7/20.1
		1.5/ 9.5

*13-day-old chick embryos were injected intravenously with 2.6 mg of purified goat antibodies to chicken μ-chains and sacrificed 4 days later or at hatching.

Analysis of cIgM in bursal cells from anti-IgM treated embryos revealed a delay in the normal sequence of appearance of bursal cells having different patterns of cIgM distribution. At 17 days of incubation, bursae from anti-μ treated embryos contained only cells with the type 1 pattern, whereas the type 2 perinuclear pattern predominated in bursal cells from age-matched controls. At hatching, only cells with type 1 and, occasionally, type 2 perinuclear patterns were observed in anti-μ treated birds, whereas localization in the Golgi region was the most frequent pattern observed in bursal cells from controls (Fig. 3).

Bursal cells treated in vitro and in vivo with goat antibodies to chicken IgM and stained subsequently for intracellular localization of goat IgG, contained goat IgG within cytoplasmic vesicles. This suggests that the sIgM stripping occurred primarily through endocytosis and that the arrest of the normal ontogeny of cIgM expression in bursal cells was mediated by the intracytoplasmic IgM immune complexes via a mechanism yet to be precisely defined.

Figure 3

PATTERNS OF cIgM EXPRESSION IN BURSAL CELLS FROM NORMAL AND ANTI μ- TREATED CHICK EMBRYOS +

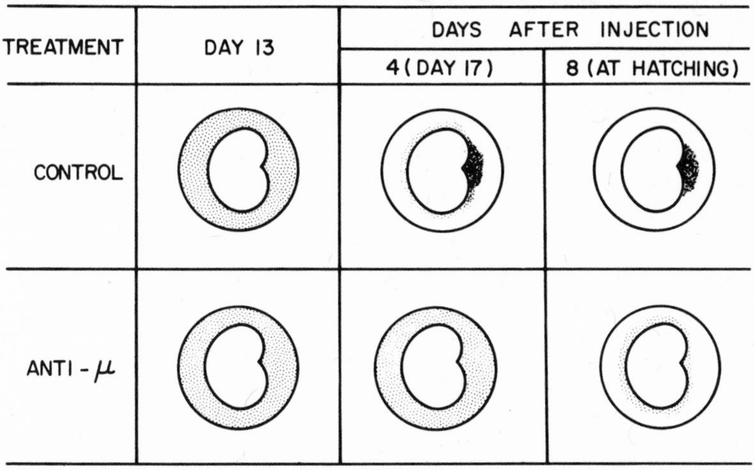

TREATMENT	DAY 13	DAYS AFTER INJECTION	
		4 (DAY 17)	8 (AT HATCHING)
CONTROL			
ANTI - μ			

+ 13 day old chick embryos were injected intravenously
with 2.6 mg of purified goat anti chicken μ antibodies
and sacrificed 4 days later or at hatching.

Elsewhere in this volume, other investigators present compelling evidence for inhibition of B cell differentiation by suppressor T cells. This raises the possibility that the persistent agammaglobulinemia following embryonic treatment with anti-μ plus bursectomy at hatching could result from development of suppressor T cells. This seems very unlikely for two reasons. Our present studies seem to indicate that (1) embryonic anti-μ treatment inhibits B cell differentiation at its inception and (2) cells with characteristics of young B cells are not generated in extrabursal sites.

CONCLUSIONS

Our present studies show in chickens that generation of B cell clones in the bursa can be literally nipped in the bud by early exposure to bivalent antibodies. Quite to the contrary, in mammals stable IgM antibody receptors are a relatively late acquisition in the first stage of differentiation along B cell lines. Consequently, exposure to anti-μ antibodies does not affect the numbers of pre-B cells in mammals, nor does it affect their capa-

bility for subsequent differentiation. This could provide mammals
with a protective mechanism against early "clonal abortion" by
antigens and may thus be important for normal generation of clonal
diversity in mammals. A delay in B cell acquisition of surface
antibodies may not be needed by the chick embryo developing within
its relatively impervious eggshell.

Despite the overall similarities between B cell differentiation in birds and in mammals, there are clear differences present
at the very outset. These differences are interesting and have
significant implications for future experimental analysis of the
mechanisms involved in generation of clonal diversity and in tolerance induction.

ACKNOWLEDGEMENTS

These studies were supported by USPHS grants CA16673 and
CA13148, awarded by the National Cancer Institute, DHEW. We
gratefully acknowledge the editorial and typing assistance of
Mrs. Helen Robison and Mrs. Sharon Garrison.

Dr. Grossi's present address is: Universita de Genova, Istituto di
Anatomia Umana Normale, Viale Benedetto XV, Italy.

Dr. Lydyard's current address is: Department of Immunology, The
Middlesex Hospital Medical School, 40-50 Tottenham Street,
London, W1P 9PG, England.

REFERENCES

1. Cooper, M. D., Cain, W. A., Van Alten, P. J. and Good, R. A.,
    Int. Arch. Allergy Appl. Immunol., 35: 242 (1969).

2. Lydyard, P. M., Grossi, C. E. and Cooper, M. D., J. Exp. Med.,
    144: 79 (1976).

3. Ivanyi, J., Murgatroyd, L. B. and Lydyard, P. M., Immunology,
    23: 107 (1972).

4. Osmond, D. G. and Nossal, G. J. V., Cell. Immunol., 13: 132
    (1974).

5. Ryser, J. -E. and Vassalli, P., J. Immunol., 113: 719 (1974).

6. Melchers, F., Von Boehmer, H. and Phillips, R. A., Transplant.
    Rev., 25: 26 (1975).

7. Owen, J. J. T., Cooper, M. D. and Raff, M. C., Nature (Lond.),
    249: 361 (1974).

8. Raff, M. C., Owen, J. J. T., Cooper, M. D., Lawton, A. R., III,
    Megson, M. and Gathings, W. E., J. Exp. Med., 142: 1052 (1975).

9. Raff, M. C., Megson, M., Owen, J. J. T. and Cooper, M. D.,
    Nature, 259: 224 (1976).

10. Nossal, G. J. V. and Pike, B. L., J. Exp. Med., 141: 904
    (1975).

11. Klinman, N. R., Amer. J. Pathol., 85: 694 (1976).

12. Cooper, M. D., Kearney, J. F., Lydyard, P. M., Grossi, C. E.
    and Lawton, A. R., in Origins of Lymphocyte Diversity, Cold
    Spring Harbor Symposia on Quantitative Biology, Volume XLI
    (Cold Spring Harbor Laboratory of Quantitative Biology,
    Cold Spring Harbor, L.I., New York, 1977). In press.

13. Burrows, P. D., Lawton, A. R. and Cooper, M. D., Fed. Proc.,
    36: 1302 (1977).

14. Hayward, A. R., Simons, M., Lawton, A. R., Cooper, M. D.
    and Mage, R. G., Fed. Proc., 36: 1295 (1977).

15. Owen, J. J. T., Wright, D. E., Habu, S., Raff, M. C. and
    Cooper, M. D., J. Immunol., (1977). In press.

16. Okos, A. J. and Gathings, W. E., Fed. Proc., 36: 1294 (1977).

17. Sidman, C. L. and Unanue, E. R., Nature (Lond.), 257: 149
     (1975).

18. Kearney, J. F., Cooper, M. D. and Lawton, A. R., J. Immunol.,
     117: 1567 (1976).

19. Metcalf, E. S. and Klinman, N. R., J. Exp. Med., 143: 1327
     (1976).

20. Cambier, J. C., Kettman, J. R., Vitetta, E. S. and Uhr, J. W.,
     J. Exp. Med., 144: 293 (1976).

21. Grossi, C. E., Lydyard, P. M. and Cooper, M. D., J. Immunol.,
     (1977). In press.

22. Kincade, P. W., Lawton, A. R., Bockman, D. E. and Cooper,
     M. D., Proc. Natl. Acad. Sci., 67: 1918 (1970).

23. Leslie, G. A. and Martin, L. N., J. Immunol., 110: 959 (1973).

24. Kincade, P. W., Self, K. S. and Cooper, M. D., Cell. Immunol.,
     8: 83 (1973).

ANALYSIS OF IMMUNOGLOBULIN RECEPTORS DURING ANTIGEN-INDUCED MATURATION OF B CELLS

Juraj Ivanyi

The Wellcome Research Laboratories

Beckenham, Kent BR3 3BS, England

In view of the existence of the Bursa of Fabricius in birds, the favourite topic of experimental studies on chicken B cells has been related to their ontogeny and to states of immunoglobulin (Ig) deficiency (1-4). The natural seeding of cells from the bursa to peripheral tissues usually ceases within the first week after hatching but may continue at a later age under special circumstances such as in neonatally induced immunological tolerance. It was demonstrated that the slow escape from tolerance is due to new cells which are recruited from the bursa for several weeks after hatching (5). Nevertheless, the bursa represents a strictly 'primary' lymphoid organ from which cells are seeded to peripheral tissues independently of antigenic stimulation. This view is supported by experiments in which immunization failed to influence the rate of bursal recruitment (6,7). It was demonstrated also that the chicken bone marrow represents a post-bursal, secondary lymphoid tissue (8,9). The physiology of avian peripheral B cells and the nature of the antibody response appear similar to that observed in mammalian species considering the information which is available on the kinetics and antibody class (10,11), histological organisation of splenic germinal centers (12), cytology of antibody producing cells (13), distribution of B cells in various organs (14), co-operation with T cells in antibody formation (15,16) and *in vitro* stimulation by B cell antigens (17). On the other hand chickens seem to differ from mice by: (a) giving strong IgM and Ig antibody responses to a single intravenous injection of soluble heterologous albumins without adjuvants (18,10,11); (b) showing lymphocyte stimulation *in vitro* to fluid anti-Ig sera (19) and, (c) poor capping of surface Ig (sIg) of B cells by single treatment with anti-Ig serum (20). The basis of these differences is not understood, but there is no need to view them as characteristically 'avian' considering the known variations in morphology and functions of the lymphoid system within the mammalian kingdom (21).

The objective of this paper is to review our recent work on mechanisms of antigen-induced maturation of chicken B lymphocytes and to point out that changes in sIg expression are an integral part of this process. We have divided the subject into 3 parts dealing with (1) the distinction between the maturation pathways to antibody producing and memory cells respectively; (2) the relationship between the lymphocyte surface bound and secreted Ig class, and (3) the mechanism of the B cell triggering process.

DISTINCT MATURATION PATHWAYS OF HIGH RECEPTOR DENSITY AND MEMORY B CELLS

During a temporal study of *in vitro* anti-SRBC responses by primed chicken spleen cells we have observed that the IgG response of cells harvested 7-10 days after priming had characteristics which were distinct from the response of cells harvested 14 days or later after immunization (22). The early IgG response at 7-10 days was T cell and macrophage independent and could be stimulated equally well by native or formaldehyde-fixed SRBC. We ascribed this IgG response to B_Y cells, in accordance with the X-Y-Z scheme of Sercarz and Coons and suggested that the intermediate precursors of IgG secreting cells are distinct from long-lived memory (B_M) cells.

It was feasible to assume that B_Y cells display antigen-binding receptors and therefore may be detected as SRBC rosette forming cells (RFC). We examined therefore the peripheral blood lymphocytes (PBL) of chickens at various times after immunization and have observed that there was a temporal relationship between the emergence of RFC and the responsiveness to SRBC in Marbrook cultures (Fig. 1). This response started on the second day, reached a peak between 2-7 days of culture and more than 95% of PFC were of the IgG antibody class. When the suspension of PBL was mixed with SRBC and the formed RFC were removed by centrifugation through a BSA density gradient, the responsiveness to SRBC *in vitro* was abolished (23). The proportion of PFC *in vitro* represented approximately 25% of the RFC count of the initial PBL suspension. It is possible that this is due simply to the unfavourable conditions of our tissue culture. However, calculations from *in vivo* parameters, assuming that the peripheral blood (25% B cells) and spleen (45% B cells) lymphocyte compartments are approximately of the same size (10^9 cells/kg body weight) suggest that there is a 10-fold decrease in the frequency of RFC for splenic (1%) when compared with peripheral blood (10%) B cells, and an even lower frequency of splenic PFC (0.2%). Consequently, even in the spleen

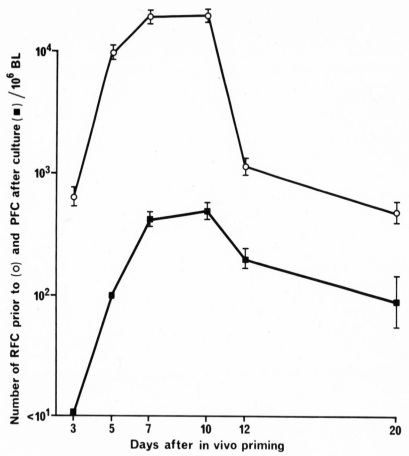

Fig. 1. Response of PBL from SRBC-immunized chickens *in vitro*. 4 day culture with SRBC

which may represent the ideal microenvironment for the maturation of Ab-producing cells, the majority of RFC fail to mature into Ab-secreting cells.

In contrast with the effective suppression of the early B_γ-response by RFC depletion, similar treatment of spleen cells which were harvested later than 14 days after priming failed to inhibit the co-operative memory response *in vitro* (23). This result obviously cannot be due to the lack of receptors on B_M cells but rather to their low surface density. We assume the B_γ^M cells display a high density of receptors which appears more important than the high affinity of receptors on B_M cells for the formation of rosettes *in vitro*.

Table 1. Suppression of IgG, RFC and *in vitro*
response in 3 day BX chickens

BX	HA titre Total ME		RFC per 10^4 PBL	PFC/10^6 spleen cells		4 day *in vitro* 10^7 spleen cells	
				IgM	IgG	IgM	IgG
+	6.3	1.6	1	84	5	<1	<1
−	7.8	6.7	175	88	335	188	381

Assay 1 week after SRBC injection

It had been shown previously that surgical bursectomy (BX) a
few days after hatching severely suppressed IgG responses but not
the IgM antibody response (28). Although there is variation in
the pattern of response to various antigens and in individual
birds, the 'split effect' was achieved in chickens bursectomized
3 days post hatching when immunized with HSA or SRBC (24,25). In
addition to evidence of suppressed IgG but normal IgM response we
have counted the peripheral blood RFC and observed a 100-fold
decrease in RFC numbers when compared with controls (Table 1).

In view of the RFC-dependence of the B_Y response it was not
surprising that spleen cells harvested from BX chickens 1 week
after immunization with SRBC failed to give an antibody response
in Marbrook cultures (Table 1). In contrast to the early suppression, spleen cells harvested 3-4 weeks after immunization
from BX chickens produced both IgM and IgG PFC *in vitro* in numbers
corresponding to those found in the control group (Fig. 2). Thus,
recovery of the *in vitro* memory-type of response (B_M) occurred
despite the preceding severe suppression of the RFC-dependent B_Y
response.

These results, together with previously published data (22)
are interpreted in terms of separate maturation pathways for B_Y
cells having receptors of high density (i.e. RFC precursors of
antibody secreting cells) and of B_M long-lived memory cells with
receptors of high affinity:

$$B_X \rightarrow B_Y \rightarrow B_Z$$
$$B_R \xrightarrow[\text{recruitment}]{\text{selection}} B_M$$

The above scheme implies that new B cells (B_R) are permanently
recruited and that in 3 day BX chickens their pool is less depleted
than that of B_Y cells. This may explain the previously published
in vivo (26,27) and the current *in vitro* results which showed
recovery of normal secondary responses in BX chickens with a
severely suppressed primary IgG response.

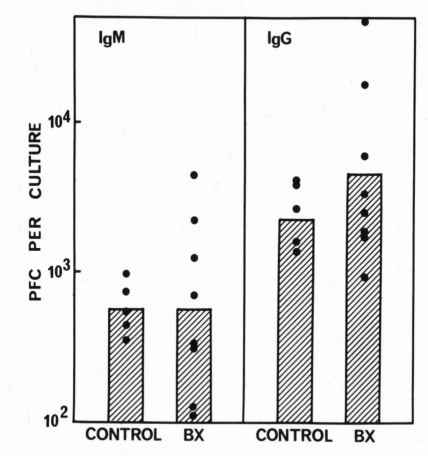

Fig. 2.   Recovery of *in vitro* memory response in 3 day BX chickens. Chickens (8 BX and 5 control) were primed with SRBC at the age of 7 weeks. Spleen cells were harvested 3-4 weeks later and PFC assayed after 4 days of culture.

IgM RECEPTORS ON B CELLS COMMITTED TO IgG ANTIBODY SYNTHESIS

Several reports on the selective suppression of IgG (compared with IgM) were interpreted in terms of sequential seeding from the bursa to peripheral tissues of B cells committed to IgG and IgM antibody responses respectively (28,24,25). These results together with previous demonstrations of distinct requirements of antigen dose for immunity, tolerance and memory of IgM and IgG antibody class respectively (11,29-31) implied the existence of separate cell lines of Ig-class committed peripheral B cells. On the other hand it was demonstrated by sequential stimulation of chicken spleen cells by class-specific rabbit antisera *in vitro*, that anti-γ antibodies stimulated ^{14}C-thymidine incorporation of lymphocytes only

Table 2. Sequential stimulation of chicken spleen[1]
cells with class-specific rabbit antisera

1st culture	2nd culture: 1-3 day		
0-1 day	Normal	anti-μ	anti-γ
Normal	104	1,320	125
anti-μ	22	10,180	1,220
anti-γ	12	825	22

[1] Data from reference no. 32.

[2] DPM-^{14}C-thymidine incorporation

after their preincubation with anti-μ serum (Table 2).

Furthermore it was demonstrated that treatment of memory cells *in vitro* with anti-μ serum abrogated the adoptive transfer of the IgG response (24). The apparent contradiction between the seeding of separate precursors and the evidence for the presence of μ-chain antigens on the surface of IgG-committed cells was reconciled by the hypothesis according to which both of the separate precursors committed to IgM and IgG synthesis respectively express μ-chain determinants in their membrane structure (24). Further support for this view was provided by recent experiments using antisera against the M1 (IgM) and G1 (IgG) allotypes (33). PBL from B14-line chickens (homozygous for various M1 and G1 locus controlled alleles (34)) were taken 1 week after immunization with SRBC and treated *in vitro* with anti-M1 sera. The results showed 90% suppression of RFC with PBL from homozygous birds and approximately 50% suppression with heterozygous PBL (Table 3).

Table 3. Inhibition of PBL RFC with anti-M1 allotype sera

Genotype of PBL donors		% RFC inhibition	
M1	G1	anti-M1[a]	anti-M1[b]
a/a	a/a	89.5	10.5
b/b	e/e	11.7	95.9
a/b	a/e	49.2	59.8

Table 4. Suppression of *in vitro* response
by anti-allotype sera

| PBL genotype | 10% antiserum in culture medium | | | |
	None	anti-M1[a]	anti-G1[a]	anti-M1[b]
M1[a]/M1[a] G1[a]/G1[a]	1,057[1)	20	2	1,010

[1)]PFC per culture

In view of the results which showed that M1 on the surface of heterozygous RFC is subject to allelic exclusion IgM is likely to be an endogenous product of cells rather than cytophilic antibody. The data discussed in the preceding paragraph suggested that RFC from PBL of immunized chickens: (i) are suppressed in BX chickens with selective suppression of IgG (but not of IgM) antibodies, and (ii) result in IgG-PFC responses when cultured *in vitro*. Hence, we interpret the presence of M1 allotype on RFC as evidence for the presence of surface IgM on precursors of IgG antibody producing B cells at an advanced stage of their maturation. We have demonstrated inhibition of RFC by both anti-M1 and anti-G1 antisera (23, 35) but the respective roles of the two classes of receptors is not understood. Inclusion of either of the two antisera in Marbrook cultures effectively inhibited the IgG PFC response (Table 4). Therefore it is likely that both classes of receptors can mediate the stimulation of antibody synthesis.

LIGAND-INDUCED REDISTRIBUTION OF SURFACE Ig RECEPTORS AND ITS
IMPLICATION FOR THE MECHANISM OF B CELL TRIGGERING

RFC in the peripheral blood of SRBC immunized chickens are all B cells with high density of antigen binding Ig receptors and without overlap with antibody secreting cells (36-38). Such a suspension can be used with advantage to study the fate of receptors following interaction with anti-Ig antibodies (38,35). Treatment of immune PBL with rabbit or sheep anti-chicken Ig serum at 0°C blocks rosette formation and we have determined the rate by which RFC receptors recovered following incubation *in vitro* (Table 5).

The recovery is rapid and temperature dependent. Only partial recovery is obtained if PBL were treated with very high (40%) concentration of anti-Ig serum. However, the recovery of such samples can be amplified by the presence of chicken Ig in the medium during recovery-incubation at 37°C (Table 6).

Table 5. Recovery of RFC formation following anti-Ig treatment

Anti-Ig serum concentration	Minutes	Percent of RFC recovery			
		10^0C	20^0C	30^0C	37^0C
40%	10	0	9	18	23
	60	0	18	28	39
2%	10	0	28	66	68
	60	0	70	82	100

RFC were blocked by incubation of immune PBL with sheep anti-Ig serum at 0^0C and washed prior to recovery-incubation.

Table 6. Amplification of RFC recovery by chicken IgG

IgG µg/ml	% RFC recovery
0	31
4	57
20	58
100	84

Recovery incubation for 30 min at 37^0C

Table 7. Prevention of RFC recovery by inhibitors of capping

Drug in medium	% Suppression of RFC recovery
None	0
Sodium Azide, $5 \times 10^{-2}M$	72
α-Methyl-D-mannoside, 0.5M	100
Cycloheximide 50 µg/ml	8

In view of the temperature-dependence of the recovery process we have examined the effect of drugs which are known to inhibit the ligand-induced redistribution ('capping') of membrane bound receptors. The results showed that inhibitors of capping interfered with the RFC recovery whilst an inhibitor protein synthesis (cycloheximide) had little effect (Table 7).

These results suggest that the recovery of RFC receptors is not due to *de novo* synthesis but rather to dissociation of surface Ig-anti-Ig complexes. This interpretation concurs with the fast kinetics and displacing effect of chicken IgG. We assume that RFC receptors are cross-linked by antibody into complexes which aggregate within the membrane into patches by a temperature and energy dependent process. Subsequently antibodies dissociate from patched complexes instead of being capped and stripped by endocytosis and shedding. The data suggest that the stoichiometry of the initial lattice formation determines whether dissociation of the bound antibody or stripping of the complex would ensue.

On the basis of these and other data we have speculated on mechanisms which may play a role in the triggering of B cells (38, 35). The basic assertion rests on the observation that molecules which interact with B cell surface receptors (anti-Ig antibodies and possibly antigen) may dissociate into the medium. It is generally true that mitogen- or antigen-induced stimulation of lymphocytes requires several hours of incubation at $37^{\circ}C$ (19,39). We suggest that the prolonged contact between cells and 'inducer' molecules is necessary to enable their *repeated interaction*. During such a process the inducer molecules would form complexes with receptors which have concurrently changed their distribution pattern within the membrane. It is plausible to assume that such a dynamic 'multiple hit' process would depend on several circumstances such as concentration and physical form of antigen, epitope density, adjuvant and mitogenic properties, antigen handling by accessory cells, T-helper cells, or 'factors' etc. According to this model immune triggering would be determined by the interplay of the circumstances which enable the repeated interaction to occur. On the other hand inhibition or tolerance induction is envisaged as multipoint cross-linking of receptors followed by their effective capping, stripping and failure to resynthesize.

REFERENCES

1.   Glick, B., Chang, T. S. and Jaap, R. G., Poultry Sci., 35: 224 (1956).

2.   Warner, N. L., Folia Biol. (Praha), 13: 1 (1967).

3. Lydyard, P. M., Grossi, C. E. and Cooper, M. D., J. Exp. Med., 144: 79 (1976).

4. Lydyard, P. and Ivanyi, J., Immunology, 28: 1023 (1975).

5. Ivanyi, J. and Salerno, A., Immunology, 22: 247 (1972).

6. Kincade, P. W. and Cooper, M. D., J. Immunol., 106: 371 (1971).

7. Ivanyi, J. and Shand, F. in Phylogenic and Ontogenic Study of the Immune Response and its Contribution to the Immunological Theory (INSERM, Paris, p. 191 1973).

8. Ivanyi, J., Murgatroyd, L. B. and Lydyard, P. M., Immunology, 23: 23 (1972).

9. Eskola, G. and Toivanen, A., Cell. Immunol., 26: 68 (1976).

10. Benedict, A. A., Brown, R. J. and Hersch, R. T., J. Immunol., 90: 339 (1963).

11. Ivanyi, J., Valentova, V. and Cerny, J., Folia Biol. (Praha), 12: 157 (1966).

12. White, R. G., French, V. I. and Stark, J. M., J. Med. Microbiol., 3: 65 (1970).

13. Cerny, J. and Ivanyi, J., Folia Biol. (Praha), 12: 343 (1966).

14. Hudson, L. and Roitt, I. M., Eur. J. Immunol., 3: 63 (1973).

15. Ivanyi, J. and Salerno, A., Eur. J. Immunol., 1: 227 (1971).

16. Rouse, B. T. and Warner, N. L., Nature New Biol., 263: 79 (1972).

17. Weber, W. T., Transplant. Rev., 24: 113 (1975).

18. Wolfe, H. R., Mueller, A. P., Nees, J. and Tempelis, C., J. Immunol., 79: 142 (1957).

19. Ivanyi, J., Skamene, E. and Kurisu, A., Folia Biol. (Praha), 16: 34 (1970).

20. Albini, B. and Wick, G., Int. Arch. Allergy Appl. Immunol., 44: 804 (1973).

21. Sell, S. and Sheppard, H. W., Jr., Science, 182: 586 (1973).

22. Evans, G. and Ivanyi, J., Eur. J. Immunol., 5: 747 (1975).

23. Ivanyi, J. and Evans, G., Eur. J. Immunol. (submitted).

24. Ivanyi, J., Eur. J. Immunol., 3: 789 (1973).

25. Ivanyi, J., Immunology, 28: 1007 (1975).

26. Jankovic, B. D. and Isakovic, K., Nature, 211: 202 (1966).

27. Rose, M. E. and Orlans, E., Nature, 217: 231 (1968).

28. Cooper, M. D., Cain, W. A., van Alten, P. J. and Good, R. A., Int. Arch. Allergy, 35: 242 (1969).

29. Ivanyi, J. and Cerny, J., Current Topics in Microbiol. and Immunol., 49: 114 (1969).

30. Ivanyi, J., Maler, M., Wudl, L. and Sercarz, E., J. Exp. Med., 127: 1149 (1968).

31. Valentova, V., Cerny, J. and Ivanyi, J., Folia Biol. (Praha), 13: 100 (1967).

32. Skamene, E. and Ivanyi, J., Nature, 221: 681 (1969).

33. Ivanyi, J., J. Immunogenetics, 2: 69 (1975).

34. Ivanyi, J. and Lydyard, P. M., Immunogenetics, 2: 285 (1975).

35. Ivanyi, J., in Phylogeny of Thymus and Bone Marrow - Bursa Cells p. 247 (Elsevier/North Holland, Amsterdam, 1976).

36. Crone, M., Koch, C. and Simonsen, M., Transplant. Rev., 10: 36 (1971).

37. Theis, G. A., Weinbaum, F. I. and Thorbecke, G. J., J. Immunol., 111: 457 (1973).

38. Ivanyi, J., Fuensalida, E. and Lydyard, P. M., Eur. J. Immunol., 6: 25 (1976).

39. Pike, B. L. and Nossal, G. J. V., J. Exp. Med., 144: 568 (1976).

Lymphocyte Antigens, Receptors, and Factors

THE PRODUCTION OF A LYMPHOCYTE INHIBITORY FACTOR (LyIF) BY BURSAL AND THYMIC LYMPHOCYTES

D. S. V. Subba Rao and Bruce Glick

Department of Poultry Science
Mississippi State University
Mississippi State, MS 39762

ABSTRACT

In this study the migration and migration inhibition of different lymphoid cell populations from immunized and control birds were evaluated. Bursal, thymic, and splenic cells migrated in a capillary tube with thymic cells forming the characteristic cone of cells within 4 hours of culture. Both thymic and bursal cell populations from birds sensitized by Mycobacterium tuberculosis produced a lymphocyte inhibitory factor (LyIF) when stimulated by specific antigen in vitro. The ability of bursal cells to release LyIF declined subsequent to 10 weeks of age while LyIF was not apparent in thymic lymphocytes until 9 weeks of age and remained high until 27 weeks of age. The active material generated in specifically stimulated cultures from sensitized bursal cells appeared to be antigen dependent whereas thymic cell mediator is antigen independent. The production of LyIF in chickens, while correlating with delayed type hypersensitivity, does not solely reflect T-cell function but B-cell response as well.

INTRODUCTION

Sensitized lymphocytes in the presence of the specific antigen are known to elaborate a spectrum of chemical mediators (1). In this study, migration inhibition of different lymphoid cell populations from immunized and control birds were evaluated using direct and indirect migration inhibition assays. It appears that both thymic and bursal cell populations from sensitized birds produce a lymphocyte inhibitory factor (LyIF) when stimulated by specific antigen in vitro.

MATERIALS AND METHODS

Birds:

A closed flock of New Hampshire, an American breed, maintained by Professor L.J. Dreesen of our poultry department was used during the entire study. Birds were wingbanded, reared either in all metal batteries or on floor pens and fed a basal ration ad libitum.

Antigens:

All birds were sensitized with Freund's complete adjuvant (CFA) (Difco Laboratories, Detroit, MI) fortified with 10 mg/ml killed H 37Ra strain Mycobacterium tuberculosis (CFA-Mt). As a test antigen for immunized animals and also for stimulation in cultures, purified protein derivative (PPD) (Parke Davis and Company, Detroit, MI) was used. PPD was dissolved in saline at a concentration of 100 µg/ml for sensitivity testing and 25 µg/ml for use in culture chambers.

Sensitization:

To induce sensitivity to tuberculin, the birds, 2-3 weeks of age, were inoculated intraperitoneally (IP) with 0.5 ml of CFA-Mt followed by a second 0.5 ml of CFA-Mt at two intramuscular sites within the next 24 hours.

Sensitivity testing:

Approximately three weeks after sensitization each bird was injected intradermally in the wattle with 0.1 ml of PPD solution (10 µg). Two or three days after the PPD injection wattle thickness was measured. Birds were considered sensitized when their wattles experienced an increase of 5-8 mm in thickness (2).

Cell collections:

Peritoneal Exudate cells: Within three days after testing for sensitivity birds were injected IP either with 30 ml of sterile mineral oil (Scientific Products, Marcol 52, Humble Oil and Refining Co., Houston, TX) or with 30-40 ml of 0.5% sterile starch solution (KeeStar, Modified Wheat Starch, MCB Manufacturing Chemists, Norwood, OH) to induce exudates. Three days later the birds were sacrificed by cervicle dislocation and their peritoneal cavities were lavaged with 300 ml of cold Hank's Balanced Salt Solution (BSS) containing heparin (5 units/ml), penicillin (100 units/ml),

and streptomycin (100 μg/ml). After centrifugation, the cells were
pooled and leukocytes were isolated by Ficoll-Hypaque centrifugation (3). These cells were washed three times in Eagle's minimal
essential medium (MEM) (Microbiological Associates, Bethesda, MD)
containing sodium bicarbonate, glutamine and antibiotics. After
final washing the concentrated leukocytes were suspended in MEM
containing 15% heat inactivated normal chicken serum (NCS).

Lymphocytes:

     The bursa, spleen and thymus were removed and placed in cold
Hank's BSS. They were cut into fine pieces and teased (with a
needleless 5 ml syringe) to release cells into the medium. Cell
suspensions were filtered through lens paper. The buffy coat layer
of splenic cell suspensions was collected after centrifugation at
800 x g for 10 min. The spleen cells were resuspended in Hank's
and treated with carbonyl iron for 15 min. at 37°C. to remove the
phagocytic cells (4). Bursal and thymic cells were also washed
twice and suspended in MEM with 15% NCS. Cell viability determined
by trypan blue exclusion was usually greater than 90% for all types.

Cell Migration Chambers:

     Capillary tubes (non-heparinized Fisher Brand 1.25 x 75 mm)
were filled with cell suspension and sealed with tube sealer and
holder (Clay Adams, Parsippary, NJ). The original cell suspension
contained 2 x 10^8 cells/ml. The capillary tubes were centrifuged
at 500 x g for 5 min. The capillary tubes were cut at the cell-
fluid interface and mounted (in duplicate) in Sykes-Moore chambers
(5) with sterile high vacuum stopcock grease (Dow Corning Corp.,
Midland, MI). Cells from the bursa, spleen, thymus and the peritoneal cavity of each bird, normal or sensitized, were incubated
with media containing antigen (25 μg/ml PPD) or no antigen. The
chambers were incubated at 37°C for 16-18 hours and areas of cell
migration were measured at 25 x magnification with ocular micro-
meter. The cell migration area was calculated as the product of
2 diameters of the migration zone. The areas of migration of four
capillaries (duplicate chambers) were averaged and the results expressed as percent migration inhibition.

Preparation of Inhibitory Supernatant Fractions:

     Thymus and bursal cells from normal and sensitized birds were
collected at various ages. Two ml of each cell suspension (2 x 10^8/
ml) was added to 8 ml of serum-free media containing 25 μg/ml PPD.
The suspensions were incubated at 37°C for 16-18 hours in a moist
chamber. The cells were removed by centrifugation at 800 x g for

15 min. The supernatants of each group were pooled (40 ml).

Dialysis:

Pooled supernatants were placed in a cellophane tubing (Union
Carbide Corp., Chicago, IL) and dialysed in normal saline for 6
hours at 4°C. They were then dialysed against serum-free MEM
at 4°C for 18 hours. The supernatants were supplemented with heat
inactivated NCS and pH adjusted to 7.2 with NaHCO₃. They were
divided into small aliquots, quickly frozen, and stored at -25°C
for later use.

Migration in the Presence of the Dialysed Supernatant:

Bursa and thymus cells from normal birds were centrifuged in
capillary tubes and placed in sterile chambers. These were filled
with the appropriate supernatant fluid. After incubation at 37°C
for 18 hours, the area of cell migration was measured and the percentage of inhibition was calculated.

In addition, the following experiment was performed to determine whether antigen in supernatants from stimulated and non-stim-
ulated cells would affect the migration of normal thymic and bursal
cells. Thymic and bursal supernatants from sensitized and non-
sensitized birds (7, 13, and 27 weeks old) were reconstituted with
PPD (10 μg/ml). Thymic and bursal cells from younger birds were
simultaneously incubated with and without the respective supernatants. They were assayed along with the supernatants for inhibitory activity as described above.

RESULTS

We collected bursal, thymic, and splenic cells and observed
that all three populations of cells migrated in a capillary tube
with thymic cells forming the characteristic cone of cells as
early as 4 hours. The addition of PPD to bursal, thymic, or
splenic lymphocytes derived from sensitized birds will markedly
impair their migration (Table 1). No significant differences in
inhibition were observed at concentrations greater than 25 μg PPD.
Therefore, in all subsequent tests 25 μg/ml PPD was chosen as the
antigen concentration for the test media. These data strongly
suggested the release of a lymphocyte inhibitory factor (LyIF) by
bursal and thymic lymphocytes.

Table 1. Mean migration area of bursal, splenic and thymus cells
          from control and sensitized birds at various concentra-
          tions of PPD.

Type cell	PPD Concentration µg/ml	Migration area* SEM	
		Control	Sensitized
Bursal	0	15.78±0.71	17.64±2.03
	10	17.61±0.27	13.71±0.35
	25	17.93±0.40	8.49±0.23
	50	17.54±0.61	8.92±0.34
	100	17.33±0.35	8.31±0.26
Spleen	0	15.89±0.89	16.46±0.65
	10	16.82±0.51	14.62±0.70
	25	17.45±0.28	8.89±0.19
	50	17.04±0.52	8.81±0.40
	100	17.87±0.39	9.42±0.46
Thymus	0	23.08±0.65	22.77±1.14
	10	23.98±0.81	19.48±0.70
	25	22.70±0.74	10.26±0.98
	50	23.07±0.45	14.37±0.66
	100	20.92±1.16	12.48±2.60

*Migration area is the product of the two diameters of the migration
 zone ÷ 10.

Each mean represents 8 observations and is accompanied by Standard
Error of the Mean (SEM).

     Was the ability of bursal and thymic lymphocytes to release an
inhibitory factor age dependent? To answer this question we sampled
sensitized and control birds at various ages beginning at 5 weeks
and ending at 36 weeks. The addition of PPD to bursal lymphocytes
from sensitized birds inhibited up to 80% of cell migration between
5 and 10 weeks of age; thereafter, the ability of bursal cells to
release LyIF declined and approached control values by 22 weeks of
age (Fig. 1). On the other hand, LyIF was not apparent in thymic
lymphocytes until 9 weeks of age and remained high until 27 weeks
(Fig. 1). The addition of PPD to splenic and PE cells from sensitized birds revealed no age dependency for the release of LyIF
(Fig. 2). These results were expected especially since T and B-
cells are present in the spleen.

     We tested the ability of T and B-cells from 1-4 week old birds
to respond to LyIF since it was not possible to produce sensitization at these ages to CFA-Mt. One-week old bursal cells failed to

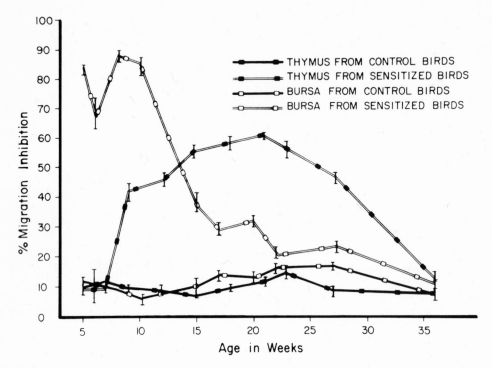

Fig. 1.   Percent migration inhibition of bursal and thymic cells
          from normal and sensitized birds in the presence of PPD.

$$\% \text{ Inhibition} = 1 - \frac{\text{area of migration with PPD}}{\text{area of migration without PPD}} \ X \ 100$$

Each mean (point) represents 8 observations and is
accompanied by SEM.

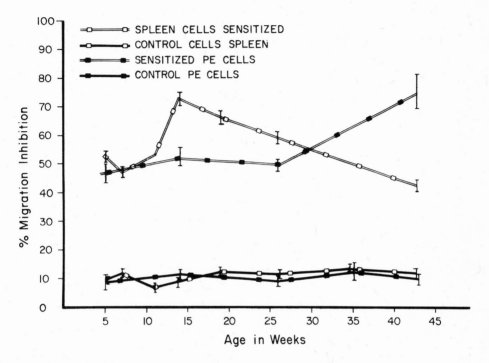

Fig. 2.   Percent migration inhibition of peritoneal exudate cells
           (PEC) and spleen cells from normal and sensitized birds
           in the presence of PPD.

$$\% \text{ Inhibition} = 1 - \frac{\text{area of migration with PPD}}{\text{area of migration without PPD}} \times 100$$

Each mean (point) represents 10 observations and is
accompanied by SEM.

be inhibited in their migration to supernatants from 7 or 27-week
old bursal cells (Table 2). Bursal cells from 2, 3, and 4-week
old birds were inhibited by supernatants from 7 and 13-week bursal
cells but not 27-week old bursal cells. The addition of PPD enhanced the inhibition. These results reconfirm the data of Fig.
1 suggesting a decline in bursal LyIF after 10 weeks and its absence by 22 weeks. The results with 13-week bursal extracts were
intermediate. Thymic cell supernatants derived from 7 and 13-week
old birds possessed LyIF as evidenced by their inhibitory influence
on thymic cells from 3 and 4-week old birds (Table 3). LyIF appeared to be absent from the supernatants of 27-week old thymic
cells. The addition of PPD did not augment the response. Supernatants collected from the bursa and thymus of normal birds did
not cause inhibition. Also, addition of PPD to these extracts
has no influence on the migration pattern of normal bursal and
thymic cells.

DISCUSSION

        It is now well known that sensitized lymphocytes release vari-
ous effector substances when stimulated by specific antigens in
vitro (1). Our observations reveal that both thymic lymphocytes
(T-cells) and bursal lymphocytes (B-cells) were capable of elabor-
ating a lymphokine which impaired their respective mobility. This
lymphokine has been termed a lymphocyte inhibitory factor (LyIF).
LyIF may be identical to MIF since we have unpublished observations
that the supernatant of sensitized T-cells will not only inhibit
T-cell mobility but also the migration of pure populations of throm-
bocytes which are known to be phagocytic (6, 7). Obviously chemical and physical experiments are necessary before one may classify
LyIF and MIF as distinct chemical fractions. A factor inhibiting
lymphocyte proliferation and released by lymphocytes has been reported (8). Our LyIF would appear to act other than on proliferation since the cell cycle for chicken erythroblasts was 13.5 hours
(9) and T and B-cell migration occurred between 4 and 18 hours,
respectively. LyIF production of bursal cells could not be due
to stimulation by a small number of contaminating T-cells since
our findings demonstrate a different threshhold of response for
thymus and bursal cells.

        Bursal cells peaked in LyIF production by 5 weeks (Fig. 1)
whereas the thymus cell production of LyIF at that time was minimal.
Thymus cells did not attain their peak LyIF production until 12
weeks of age and at that time bursal cell LyIF production was declining. Also, thymus cells showed a more prolonged LyIF production. These observations suggest the existence of an age related
response and indicate that the small number of B and T-cells which
may reside in the thymus and bursa, respectively (10), are not
significantly influencing our results.

Table 2. Percent inhibition of the migration area of normal bursal cells in the presence of supernatant (S) fluid derived from sensitized bursal cells on incubation with PPD

Donor age[1]	Age of the birds when normal bursal cells were collected							
	1 wk		2 wk		3 wk		4 wk	
	S*only	S+PPD**	S only	S+PPD	S only	S+PPD	S only	S+PPD
7th week	-2.83 ±3.73	0.26 ±2.65	11.80 ±1.37	40.89 ±0.67	14.52 ±1.56	49.46 ±2.70	20.47 ±1.66	54.26 ±1.19
13th week			9.32 ±2.89	25.48 ±3.17	13.01 ±1.64	18.41 ±1.46	6.38 ±1.78	11.80 ±2.69
27th week	-5.62 ±8.53	-7.67 ±14.71			2.01 ±5.58	11.20 ±6.39	0.14 ±7.37	1.38 ±8.02

[1]Age of sensitized birds contributing bursal supernatant.

Each mean represents 12 observations and is accompanied by SEM.

*1 - $\dfrac{\text{area of migration with Supernatant}}{\text{area of migration without Supernatant}}$ X 100

**1 - $\dfrac{\text{area of migration with Supernatant + PPD}}{\text{area of migration without Supernatant}}$ X 100

Table 3. Percent inhibition of the migration area of normal thymic cells in the presence of supernatant (S) fluid derived from sensitized thymus cells on incubation with PPD

Donor age [1]	Age of the birds when normal thymus cells were collected							
	1 wk		2 wk		3 wk		4 wk	
	S*only	S+PPD**	S only	S+PPD	S only	S+PPD	S only	S+PPD
7th week	-1.90 ±9.86	3.42 ±6.60	-5.28 ±7.85	-3.39 ±7.21	10.12 ±1.25	10.14 ±0.33	8.68 ±0.97	7.60 ±1.53
13th week	12.05 ±1.39	13.00 ±1.75	19.41 ±1.82	20.43 ±1.40	39.61 ±0.71	37.61 ±1.10	51.33 ±2.47	51.55 ±2.32
27th week			1.85 ±1.21	0.04 ±1.40	-2.35 ±1.58	0.87 ±1.45	1.32 ±1.20	1.21 ±1.20

[1]Age of sensitized birds contributing bursal supernatant.

Each mean represents 12 observations and is accompanied by SEM.

*] - $\dfrac{\text{area of migration with Supernatant}}{\text{area of migration without Supernatant}}$ X 100

**] - $\dfrac{\text{area of migration with Supernatant + PPD}}{\text{area of migration without Supernatant}}$ X 100

The LyIF produced by bursal cells in vitro depends on antigen for its activity response whereas thymic LyIF was antigen independent. This observation may be used in the avian system as a tool for differentiating T and B-cell populations. Furthermore, an antigen dependent lymphocyte mediator in B-cells might function as a receptor for antigens or as a communicating system between lymphocytes and phagocytic cells (11, 12).

Since both thymus and bursal cells produce LyIF, it cannot be considered as an assay for T-cell function in chickens. It should be emphasized that only lymphocytes obtained from birds exhibiting delayed wattle reaction to the antigen were capable of producing LyIF. Thus in one way LyIF production is associated with the presence of delayed hypersensitivity but not with a particular cell type. These observations lend further support to the concept that lymphokine production is a general biologic phenomena (13) in addition to being a measure of cell mediated immunity.

ACKNOWLEDGEMENT

We thank Karen Anderson for typing this manuscript and Doris Thompson and Dr. John M. Barnett for their assistance.

Supported, in part, by USPHS grant AI 11894 from the National Institute of Allergy and Infectious Diseases.

Journal article number 3507 from the Mississippi Agricultural and Forestry Experiment Station.

REFERENCES

1. Bloom, B.R., Adv. Immunol., 13: 101 (1971).

2. Zwelling, B.S., Barrett, J.T. and Breitenbach, R.P., Cellular Immunol., 4: 20 (1972).

3. Boyum, A., Scand. J. Clin. and Lab. Invest. (Suppl.) 99 (1968).

4. Schlossman, S.F. and Hudson, L., J. Immunol., 110: 313 (1973).

5. Sykes, J.A. and Moore, E.B., Proc. Soc. Exp. Biol. and Med., 100: 125 (1959).

6. Glick, B., Sato, K. and Cohenour, F., J. Reticuloendothelial Soc., 1: 442 (1964).

7. Carlson, H.C., Sweeney, P.R. and Tokaryk, J.M., Avian Dis., 12: 700 (1968).

8. Florentin, I., Kiger, N. and Mathe, G., Cellular Immunol., 23: 1 (1976).

9. Grosset, L. and Odartchenko, N., Cell Tissue Kinet., 8: 81 (1975).

10. Glick, B., Int. Rev. Cytology, 48: 342 (1977).

11. Feldman, M., Cone, R.E. and Marchalonis, J.J., Cellular Immunol., 9: 1 (1973).

12. Lachmann, P.J., Proc. Royal Soc., 1976: 425 (1971).

13. Yoshida, T., Sonozaki, H. and Cohen, S., J. Exp. Med., 138: 784 (1973).

DETERGENT SOLUBILIZATION OF B-LYMPHOCYTE IMMUNOGLOBULIN*

John Lifter and Yong Sung Choi

Memorial Sloan-Kettering Cancer Center

Walker Laboratory, Rye, NY   10580

EXPERIMENTAL

We recently completed a study of the ability of bursal and splenic lymphocytes to synthesize and release immunoglobulin (1). We had asked the question whether the capacity to synthesize immunoglobulin changes during differentiation. The bursae of newly hatched chicks were used as a source of immature B lympho- cytes uncontaminated by plasma cells (2), and mature lymphocytes were isolated from the spleens of 3-month-old birds. Cell sus- pensions were fractionated by sedimentation velocity as a means to separate the lymphocytes, on the basis of size, into subpopulations (3,4).

The synthetic capabilities of the large (sedimentation rate >3.5 mm/hr) and small (sedimentation rate 2.3 mm/hr) cells from the bursa and spleen were compared by culturing cells in the presence of ^{3}H-leucine and quantitatively isolating the newly synthesized immunoglobulin by serologic precipitation (1,5). Since much of the B-cell immunoglobulin would be membrane bound, the labeled cells were lysed and the membrane proteins solubilized by treatment with the nonionic detergent Nonidet-P40 (NP-40) (6).

The results of these experiments are summarized in Table I. The splenic and bursal lymphocytes were fractionated into rapidly

*Supported by grants from the National Cancer Institute (CA-17049 and CA-17404) and the American Cancer Society (IM-28). J.L. is the recipient of a research fellowship from the National Institutes of Health (AI-05162).

Table I

Synthesis of Ig by splenic and bursal lymphocyte subpopulations
Summary of typical experiments on adult spleen and two-day-old bursa

	# of cells cultured	Total Ig synthesized per 10^6 Ig+ cells cpm	Relative rate of Ig synthesis	Total Ig released per 10^6 Ig+ cells cpm	Relative rate of Ig release
Spleen					
Rapidly Sedimenting	1.03×10^7	9.82×10^5	900	4.72×10^5	3700
Slowly Sedimenting	1.03×10^7	1.09×10^3	1	1.29×10^2	1
Bursa					
Rapidly Sedimenting	3.58×10^7	2.09×10^3	2	6.24×10^2	5
Slowly Sedimenting	3.58×10^7	1.15×10^3	1	2.62×10^2	2

and slowly sedimenting subpopulations. The rapidly sedimenting spleen cell subpopulation contained the plasma cells as demonstrated by intracellular immunofluorescent staining with fluorescein labeled anti-light chain. The slowly sedimenting spleen cells and both sub-populations of bursal cells were identified as B-lymphocytes since they were positive for surface immunoglobulin. The number of immunoglobulin positive cells, either intracellular or surface, in each fraction was determined and the amount of immunoglobulin syn-thesized by each subpopulation was normalized to the number of immunoglobulin positive cells. Plasma cells synthesized immuno-globulin at a rate 900-times greater than the B-lymphocytes and re-leased immunoglobulin into the culture media at a rate 3700-times greater. Splenic and bursal B lymphocytes synthesized and released immunoglobulin at identical rates demonstrating that these subpop-ulations were indistinguishable by this criterion and suggesting that it is unlikely that the capacity to synthesize immunoglobulin changes as the B-lymphocytes mature.

It has been previously reported that plasma cells synthesize 10 to 100-times as much immunoglobulin as the B-lymphocytes (7,8,9). In these experiments, attempts were not made to determine the actual number or type of cells contributing to the synthesis of immunoglobu-lin. Accumulation of immunoglobulin in the culture media could be due to a small number of plasma cells or larger numbers of B-lympho-cytes. We determined the number of plasma cells or B-lymphocytes in each cell fraction by counting cells stained with fluorescent anti-light chain. The amount of immunoglobulin synthesized or released was normalized to the number of immunoglobulin positive cells, per-mitting a more accurate estimation of the immunoglobulin synthetic capacities to be made.

During the course of this work we realized that the procedures used for detergent solubilization of membrane proteins may affect the experimental results. NP-40 has been used to lyse cells since it is known not to interfere with the subsequent isolation of cellu-lar proteins by serologic precipitation. Because NP-40 does not dis-rupt some protein-protein interactions, it is possible that cellular proteins will remain associated in the presence of detergent and the serologic precipitates may be contaminated by co-precipitating pro-teins antigenically unrelated to the molecule of interest.

The material isolated by serologic precipitation can be further studied by sodium dodecyl sulfate-polyacrylamide gel electrophoresis (SDS-PAGE), and changes in the gel profile could be used to demon-strate the presence of contaminates in the specific serologic pre-cipitate. If nonimmunoglobulin material can co-precipitate during serologic precipitation with anti-immunoglobulin, it would be impor-tant to determine whether the conditions under which the precipi-tations were carried out could affect the gel patterns of the isolated

material; i.e., whether the association of the co-precipitating
protein with the immunoglobulin isolated from chicken B-lymphocytes
results from the incomplete solubilization of the B-lymphocyte
immunoglobulin by NP-40, and whether the co-precipitating proteins
are antigenically related to the immunoglobulin chains.

Cells isolated from the bursae of 5-day-old chicks (strain SC,
Hy-Line Poultry Farm, Johnston, Iowa) were cultured in the presence
of L-(4,5,6)-^{3}H-leucine (100 Ci/mM, New England Nuclear) according
to previously published methods (1,5). Radiolabeled cells were
lysed by suspension, at 5×10^8 cells/ml, in 0.5-1.0% NP-40, 15 minutes, 0°C, and the nuclei pelleted by centrifugation at 5000 x g
for 10 minutes. This initial lysis by NP-40 was necessary to separate intact nuclei from the cytoplasm. The supernatant was then
divided into two aliquots. One was further solubilized by adding
20% (w/v) deoxycholate (DOC) to a final concentration of 2%, maintained at 0°C for 30 minutes, and centrifuged at 150,000 x g for 60
minutes at 4°C in order to sediment ribosomes. The concentration of
DOC in the supernatant was decreased from 2% to 0.5% by adding 3
volumes of phosphate buffered saline (PBS), and dialyzed against
0.1% DOC in PBS overnight at 4°C.

The second aliquot of the NP-40 lysate was not treated with DOC.
Ribosomes were removed by centrifugation and the volume increased to
the same extent as the DOC treated aliquot by adding 0.5% NP-40 in
PBS. The aliquot was dialyzed against 0.1% NP-40 in PBS overnight
at 4°C.

To check for possible proteolysis (10), purified ^{14}C-labeled
chicken IgG, 7000 cpm (9), was added to both samples before dialysis
as an internal control.

Radiolabeled immunoglobulin was isolated from both samples by
serologic precipitation with a goat antiserum containing anti-γ, μ,
and light chain antibodies and the precipitates were further studied
by SDS-PAGE (5).

As shown in Table II, all the ^{14}C-immunoglobulin added initially
was recovered in specific serologic precipitates, thus excluding proteolysis of the immunoglobulin. Under such conditions, the radioactivity isolated from the NP-40 treated aliquot (54,840 cpm) was
always greater than that from the 2% DOC treated aliquot (42,360 cpm).

That the radiolabeled material in specific precipitates included immunoglobulin was confirmed by SDS-PAGE of equivalent aliquots from the precipitates (Figure 1). The SDS-PAGE profile of the
material isolated from the aliquot treated only with NP-40 (Figure
1a) shows that a significant percentage of the radioactivity was associated with a protein(s) (approximate molecular weight 50,000

Table II

^{3}H-Radioactivity in the serologic precipitates from 10 B-lymphocytes cultured for four hours with ^{3}H-leucine

Detergent		cpm		
		Specific*	Nonspecific*	Ig**
0.5% NP-40 + 2% DOC	^{3}H	60,920	18,560	42,360
	^{14}C	7,680	280	7,400
0.5% NP-40	^{3}H	78,620	23,780	54,840
	^{14}C	7,340	190	7,150

*Direct serologic precipitation: specific, 200 µl goat antichicken-Ig with 50 µg chicken IgG; nonspecific, 200 µl goat antihuman-IgG with 50 µg human IgG.
**Specific cpm - nonspecific cpm

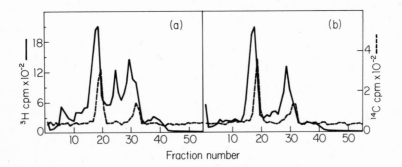

Figure 1

SDS-PAGE of specific serologic precipitates. Intracellular proteins
of B-lymphocytes were labeled with ^{3}H-leucine and the cells solubilized by detergents as described: (a) 0.5% NP-40; (b) 0.5% NP-40 plus
2% DOC. The detergent-soluble fraction of the cells was subjected to
serologic precipitation and analyzed by SDS-PAGE after being fully
reduced and alkylated. (———), ^{3}H-labeled Ig of B-lymphocytes;
(---), ^{14}C-labeled chicken IgG added as an internal standard.

daltons) which migrated between the heavy and light chains. However, this protein could be virtually eliminated by treating the NP-40 lysate with 2% DOC before serologic precipitation in the presence of 0.1-0.5% DOC (Figure 1b). Since all the ^{14}C-immunoglobulin, added as an internal standard, was recovered as heavy and light chain peaks on SDS-PAGE, it is not likely that the 50,000 dalton co-precipitating protein is a degradation product of radiolabeled heavy chains. The radioactivity associated with the co-precipitating protein may account for the quantitative difference in radioactivity between specific precipitates of the NP-40 and DOC treated aliquots (Table II). The fact that the chicken co-precipitating protein was not found in the anti-immunoglobulin serologic precipitate of the DOC treated aliquot suggests that it does not share the immunoglobulin class or subgroup antigenic determinants with the heavy and light chains and that it is not covalently linked to the B-cell immunoglobulin.

The use of DOC in the purification of immunoglobulin from lymphoid cells has been described previously (11,12), but in these studies either low concentrations of deoxycholate were not maintained during the serologic precipitation (11) or the immunoglobulin precipitating in the presence of deoxycholate was not compared to immunoglobulin isolated under different conditions (12). The experiments described here clearly demonstrate that the continued presence of DOC affects the nature of the material isolated by serologic precipitation.

DISCUSSION

Immunoglobulins of B-lymphocytes can be classified as integral proteins of the plasma membrane (13) since they: (a) require detergents or 8 M urea for extraction (6); (b) are primarily localized at the cell surface as demonstrated by staining with fluorescent anti-immunoglobulin (14); and (c) comprise a metabolically stable constituent which is not rapidly secreted by the cell (1,7,9,15).

In previous studies, a protein with molecular weight of 35,000 to 50,000 daltons has been reported to be associated with anti-immunoglobulin serologic precipitates obtained from NP-40 lysates of chicken bursal cells (5), murine B-lymphocytes (7) and human lymphoid cells bearing surface IgM (11). However, in NP-40 lysates of unfractionated spleen cells (a mixture of both B-lymphocytes and plasma cells), the association of co-precipitating proteins with cellular immunoglobulin was not observed (5,6). Since plasma cells in chickens synthesize immunoglobulin at a rate 900-fold greater than the B-lymphocytes (1), it is likely that in biosynthetic experiments with mixtures of B-lymphocytes and plasma cells, the greater part of the detectable immunoglobulin has its origin in the plasma cells.

The presence of low levels of co-precipitating proteins which may be associated with this serologic precipitate would be masked (i.e., suppressed into the background level of radioactivity) when examined by SDS-PAGE. Co-precipitating protein has not been observed in NP-40 lysates of plasma cells (7). These results are consistent with two possible interpretations. The co-precipitating protein(s) may be uniquely associated with the membrane bound immunoglobulin of B-lymphocytes, or the proteins may be other cellular proteins which contaminate the serologic precipitate.

Our results suggest that the co-precipitating protein is associated with the immunoglobulin by a type of bond which is unaffected by the nonionic detergent NP-40. Since 0.5-1.0% NP-40 is known not to disrupt some protein-protein interactions (e.g., the antibody-antigen binding which occurs in a serologic precipitation), it was not unexpected to find that the co-precipitating protein and immunoglobulin remained associated after NP-40 lysis. The weakly ionic detergent DOC was, however, able to disrupt the noncovalent interaction between immunoglobulin and the co-precipitating protein. In an analogous situation, the Thy-1 antigen remains associated with other membrane constituents after NP-40 solubilization, but is isolated in a pure form by treatment with 2% DOC (16).

The stability of the bond between immunoglobulin molecules and the co-precipitating protein to nonionic detergent, but its susceptibility to ionic detergent, suggest that the 50,000 dalton co-precipitating protein contains hydrophobic and hydrophilic regions and supports the interpretation that it may be responsible for holding immunoglobulin in the membrane. The co-precipitating protein may, therefore, be equivalent to the "proreceptor" proposed by Ramasamy (17).

The interaction of B-lymphocyte immunoglobulin with a "proreceptor" in the membrane may indicate structural differences between membrane bound and secreted immunoglobulin. Melcher et al. (18) showed that membrane bound immunoglobulin aggregated in the absence of detergent while secreted immunoglobulin remained soluble, prompting them to suggest structural differences between these immunoglobulin molecules. Alternatively, the insolubility of membrane bound immunoglobulin may be due to its association with the hydrophobic "proreceptor."

We wish to emphasize the point that membrane bound antigens, and possibly intracellular protein, may remain associated with other molecules in the presence of mild detergents, and that the material isolated by specific serologic precipitation may be contaminated with other antigenically unrelated proteins. Since serologic precipitation is being used to isolate many of the antigenic markers present on the surface of cells, precautions should be taken to insure that the material in a precipitate is specifically bound by the antisera and not present as a result of noncovalent association with either the molecule of interest or the antisera added to form the precipitate.

REFERENCES

1. Lifter, J., Kincade, P.W. and Choi, Y.S., J. Immunol., 117: 2220 (1976).
2. Kincade, P.W. and Cooper, M.D., J. Immunol., 106:371 (1971).
3. Miller, R.G. and Phillips, R.A., J. Cell. Physiol., 73:191 (1969).
4. Miller, R.G. in New Techniques in Biophysics and Cell Biology, Vol. 1 (R. Pain and B. Smits, Eds.) (John Wiley and Sons, London, 1973).
5. Choi, Y.S. and Good, R.A., J. Exp. Med., 135: 1133 (1972).
6. Vitetta, E.S., Baur, S. and Uhr, J.W., J. Exp. Med. 134:242 (1971).
7. Andersson, J., Lafleur, L. and Melchers, F., Eur. J. Immunol., 4: 170 (1974).
8. Melchers, F., Cone, R.E., von Boehmer, H. and Sprent, J., Eur. J. Immunol., 5: 382 (1975).
9. Choi, Y.S., Biochemistry, 15: 1037 (1976).
10. Melchers, F., von Boehmer, H. and Phillips, R.A., Transplant. Rev., 25: 26 (1975).
11. Premkumar, E., Singer, P.A. and Williamson, A.R., Cell, 5: 87 (1975).
12. Askonas, B.A., Roelants, G.E., Mayor-Withey, K.S. and Welstead, J.L., Eur. J. Immunol., 6: 250 (1976).
13. Singer, S.J. and Nicolson, G.L., Science, 175: 720 (1972).
14. Raff, M.C., Sternberg, M. and Taylor, R.B., Nature, 225: 553 (1970).
15. Melchers, F. and Cone, R.E., Eur. J. Immunol., 5: 234 (1975).
16. Letarte-Muirhead, M., Acton, P.T. and Williams, A.F., Biochem. J., 143: 51(1974).
17. Ramasamy, R., Immunochemistry, 13: 705 (1976).
18. Melcher, U., Eidels, L. and Uhr, J.W., Nature, 258: 434 (1975).

ASSOCIATION OF LYMPHOCYTE ALLOANTIGEN GENOTYPES WITH LEVELS OF IMMUNE RESPONSES

D.G. Gilmour*, M.A. Palladino*, A.R. Scafuri*,

L.W. Pollard† and A.A. Benedict†

*New York Univ. School of Medicine, New York, N.Y. 10016. †University of Hawaii, Honolulu, Hawaii 96822

The association of specific immunological unresponsiveness with genes coding within the major histocompatibility complex (MHC) in mammals has been known for some time (1, 2), and was reported more recently in chickens (3, 4). It was presumed that MHC-determined surface antigens on lymphocytes, and perhaps on other immunological effectors such as macrophages, must play a major role in the mechanism of these associations (2, 5). However, direct information on the mode of action, in this context, of MHC antigens such as Ia, H-2D or H-2K has been forthcoming only in the last year or so (6, 7). The question of the genetic determination of differing levels of immune response among responders was extensively discussed at a meeting in 1972 (8), but this issue has not been widely followed up. We became interested in this question because of our work with two inbred lines of chickens which are identical at the B MHC, and yet exhibit marked differences in resistance to oncogenesis of lymphoid cells by exogenous viruses subsequent to the initiation of systemic infection. Chickens from East Lansing inbred line 6 (EL6) develop only a very low incidence of Marek's disease (MD) or of Lymphoid Leukosis (LL) following exposure to the appropriate virus by inoculation or contact (9, 10). In contrast, line 7 (EL7) chickens are highly susceptible to the development of MD following exposure to MD virus (9). These EL7 chickens cannot be directly tested for LL susceptibility, because they are homozygous for recessive resistance to initial infection by leukosis-sarcoma viruses of subgroups A and B (11).

However, it can be inferred that they carry dominant genes for postinfection susceptibility to LL, since F_1 chickens from lines 6 and 7 are highly susceptible (10).

In MD it is likely that only T cells undergo malignant transformation (12, 13), while in LL it is established that only B cells are transformed (14, 15). It is possible that the differences between lines EL6 and EL7 in resistance to oncogenesis involving T or B cells are directly related to surface properties of these cells. Such properties, potentially detectable as alloantigens, might, for example, influence cell accessibility to transformation by virus. Alternatively, resistance might operate as a restraint on progressive growth of already transformed cells, involving some form of specific immune responsiveness. This is likely to be mediated by surface structures on immunological effector cells, in particular the lymphocytes themselves, which would be potentially detectable as alloantigens. We tested these suppositions by making reciprocal immunizations between these lines with bursal or thymic cells. The resultant antisera were used to establish two independent autosomal loci, Bu-1 and Th-1, determining alloantigens of B or T lymphocytes respectively (16). Meanwhile, we and others identified some immune responses in which the lines differ (Table 1), including previously published data (17, 18), and the new finding that EL7 shows consistently higher antibody responses than EL6 to the synthetic aminoacid co-polymer GAT[10], as determined by previously published methods (4). The differences listed were usually quantitative rather than response versus nonresponse (17). It can be seen from Table 1 that EL6 is the high responder to some antigens, with delayed hypersensitivity and antibody responses running in parallel. In contrast, EL7 is the high responder to two other antigens, without corresponding differences in DH responses, and is a high graft-versus-host responder.

We have made three different tests of association of lymphocyte alloantigen genotypes with immune response differences. In each test an F_2 population was raised, derived from crosses of EL6 x EL7, and was typed for Bu-1 and Th-1 antigens as in (16). By measuring the immune response levels of chickens of the 9 possible combined Bu-1 and Th-1 genotypes, it was possible to test association of response levels with genotypes at both loci by analyses of variance, and to examine modes of genetic action.

Table 1. Differences between inbred lines EL6 and EL7 in levels
of immune response.

	EL6	EL7
Antibody to Ferritin, BSA, and Dodecanoic-BSA	High	Low
Antibody to DNP, GAT^{10} [a]	Low	High
Delayed Hypersensitivity to BSA, Ferritin, Oxazolone	High	Low
GVH (Splenomegaly or CAM) Reaction to $\underline{\underline{B}}$ Antigen [b]	Low	High

Data from Palladino et al. 1977 (17), except [a] this study, [b] Pazderka
et al. 1975 (18).

ASSOCIATION WITH DELAYED HYPERSENSITIVITY

In the first experiment, 54 chickens (27 males, 27 females)
were immunized at 38 weeks of age with dodecanoic-acid-conjugated
BSA in Freund's complete adjuvant, and 14 days later were bled for
primary antibody response and skin tested for delayed hypersensitivity, as in (17). The results from males and females were pooled
because preliminary analyses showed no effect of sex on the levels
of response. The 3 x 3 analyses of variance by Bu-1 and Th-1
genotypes were performed by fitting constants as in (19). For
delayed hypersensitivity (Table 2), the analysis showed a tendency
to association with Bu-1 genotypes ($p < 0.10$). This analysis
primarily tests for linearity, which may indicate additive genetic
action if the heterozygote mean is intermediate. This is not so
(Table 2). However, we had postulated that the superiority of
EL6 over EL7, hence possibly of the a allele over b, might be
dominant, because this mode of genetic action frequently occurs
in immune response differences. We tested this hypothesis
by making another variance analysis in which the data for the
a/a and a/b genotypes at Bu-1 were pooled, and compared with
b/b. In this test the p value was < 0.05, equivalent to a significance level of < 0.025 for the one-tail test for dominance of
Bu-1^a over Bu-1^b for high response. In fact, inspection of the

Table 2. Delayed hypersensitivity responses to dodecanoic-BSA by F_2 chickens classified by Bu-1 and Th-1 genotypes.

		Bu-1			Least squares means
		a/a	a/b	b/b	
Th-1	a/a	3.17[a] (3)	3.84 (8)	3.40 (3)	3.39 (14)
	a/b	3.02 (8)	3.36 (8)	2.02 (6)	2.81 (22)
	b/b	2.90 (6)	3.63 (9)	1.87 (3)	2.89 (18)
Least squares means		3.09 (17)	3.62 (25)	2.38 (12)	3.03 (54)

[a]Mean of 24-hour increases in wattle thickness, mm (Number in group).
Analysis of variance, 3 x 3
Bu-1, $p < 0.10$; Th-1, NS; Interaction, NS.

Table 3. Primary antibody responses to dodecanoic-BSA by F_2 chickens classified by Bu-1 and Th-1 genotypes.

		Bu-1			Least squares means
		a/a	a/b	b/b	
Th-1	a/a	570[a] (3)	160 (6)	160 (3)	202 (12)
	a/b	113 (3)	254 (6)	180 (6)	181 (15)
	b/b	57 (4)	320 (7)	101 (3)	140 (14)
Least squares means		142 (10)	242 (19)	149 (12)	172 (41)

[a]Geometric mean of endpoint titres (Number in group).

Analysis of Variance, 3 x 3
Bu-1, NS; Th-1, NS; Interaction, $p < 0.10$.

Table 4. Secondary antibody responses to GAT^{10} by F_2 chickens classified by <u>Bu-1</u> and <u>Th-1</u> genotypes.

| | | Bu-1 | | | |
		a/a	a/b	b/b	Least squares means
	a/a	1328[a]	771	1105	991
		(5)	(12)	(7)	(24)
<u>Th-1</u>	a/b	1759	1617	1711	1721
		(9)	(18)	(13)	(40)
	b/b	1256	1079	888	1145
		(3)	(16)	(3)	(22)
Least squares means		1401	1119	1245	1250
		(17)	(46)	(23)	(86)

[a]Geometric mean of titres for 50% antigen binding (Number in group).
Analysis of Variance, 3 x 3
<u>Bu-1</u>, NS; <u>Th-1</u>, p < 0.05; Interaction, NS.

data suggests overdominance (heterozygote superiority), since the value for <u>a/b</u> is higher than for either homozygote. However, since we had not postulated this type of genetic action in advance, we did not test for it. The variance analysis of the primary antibody responses to dodecanoic-BSA was made on the logs of the endpoint titres, although the means in Table 3 are given as antilogs, i.e., geometric means. There is no evidence for association of antigen genotypes with level of response, although inspection shows a tendency to overdominance at <u>Bu-1</u>, thus paralleling the DH results.

ASSOCIATION WITH SECONDARY ANTIBODY RESPONSE TO GAT^{10}

For the second test, a much larger F_2 generation was raised, and only females were tested. A total of 86 females were immunized with 0.5 mg GAT^{10} in Freund's complete adjuvant at 16 weeks old, were boosted 4 weeks later with 0.25 mg in Freund's incomplete adjuvant (oil alone), and were bled for secondary antibody 10 and 20 days later. The variance analyses given in Table 4 and below refer to the 20-day secondary bleeds, and were performed on logs of the reciprocal dilution for 50% antigen binding, as in (4). Because of the indication of overdominance in the first test, we postulated in advance three possibilities for the mode of genetic action of any association with GAT^{10} antibody response: additive, dominant, or overdominant. The first 3 x 3 variance analysis by fitting constants (19) showed significant association of Th-1 genotypes with level of response ($p < 0.05$), but this was clearly not additive genetic action (Table 4). Further analyses were made using pooling of b/b with a/b as a test of dominant superiority of b over a, or pooling of homozygotes as a test of overdominance. The p values were < 0.05 and < 0.01 respectively, corresponding to significance levels for one-tail tests of < 0.025 for dominance and < 0.005 for overdominance. Clearly the over-dominant effect (heterozygote advantage) is the major one.

ASSOCIATION WITH GRAFT-VERSUS-HOST RESPONSIVENESS

In the third series of experiments, a total of 30 F_2 chickens (5 males, 25 females) were used as donors of leukocytes to induce splenomegaly in unrelated F_1 embryos (type FP, major histocompatibility genotype B^{15}/B^{21}, from Hy-Line International, Des Moines, Iowa). Lines EL6 and EL7 have identical erythrocyte and leukocyte antigens determined by the B major histocompatibility complex (MHC), as shown by a number of serological and functional tests (17, 18). In particular, lymphocytes from EL6, EL7, or B^2/B^2 reference chickens do not induce a strong graft-versus-host GVH reaction in embryos from any of these sources, as determined by the complete absence of B-type large pocks on the chorio-allantoic membrane (18). Thus, all F_2 progeny derived from EL6 x EL7 must have the MHC genotype B^2/B^2. Genetic variation between F_2 donors in the intensity of induction of GVH reaction cannot therefore be ascribed to MHC antigen differences, through the mechanism of varying "antigenic distance" between donor and host, but may instead be associated with segregation of non-MHC genes determining the difference between the lines. These genes are presumably those which determine that EL7 leukocytes induce much larger GVH reactions in unrelated embryos than EL6 leukocytes (18).

The F_2 donors were 32 weeks old at the start of 8 separate experiments spread over 3 months. Although representatives of all 9 combined Bu-1 and Th-1 genotypes were tested, it was not

Table 5. Intensity of splenomegaly induced by leukocytes from
F$_2$ chickens classified by <u>Bu-1</u> and <u>Th-1</u> genotypes.

		Bu-1 a/a	a/b	b/b	Unweighted geometric means
Th-1	a/a	173[a] (1)	192 (5)	179 (5)	181 (11)
	a/b	150 (5)	194 (3)	200 (5)	180 (13)
	b/b	148 (4)	144 (8)	200 (7)	161 (19)
Unweighted geometric means		157 (10)	174 (16)	192 (17)	174 (43)

[a] Geometric mean of embryo spleen weights, mg (Number
of donors + replicates).
Nested Analysis of Variance, 3 x 3
Genotypes: <u>Bu-1</u>, p < 0.02; <u>Th-1</u>, p < 0.10; Interaction, p < 0.02.
Donors + Replicates: p < 0.002.

possible to include all 9 in each test. An average of 5 (range 4 - 7)
genotypes were compared on each occasion. Using methods as in
(20), embryos at 13 days of incubation were injected intravenously
with 2.5 x 10^5 viable lymphocytes, 15 embryos per donor. Spleen
and body weights were recorded at 19 days. Two adjustments were
made to the data. First, within occasions each spleen weight was
adjusted to the modal body weight by multiplying it by modal body
weight/individual body weight. This reduced the variance between
embryos while retaining the data in weight units. The overall
mean of log spleen weights from all 8 tests was then calculated,
and adjustments were made so that the overall mean per occasion
was identical, and equal to the overall mean of 8 tests. This ad-
justment reduced between-occasion variance and allowed pooling
of data for each genotype over occasions.

Because of restricted availability, some donors had to be
used more than once, so that variance between groups of embryos
included variance between donors and replicates of donors. A preliminary nested analysis of variance (21) by genotypes, by donors
+ replicates, and by embryos showed significant variance between

donors + replicates ($p < 0.002$). Consequently, in the 3 x 3 variance analyses the genotype effects were tested against the mean
square for donors + replicates, derived from the nested analysis.
In the variance analysis by fitting constants (19) the Bu-1 x Th-1
interaction was significant ($P < 0.02$), and so it was necessary to
test main effects in a further analysis by the method of weighted
squares of means (19). In this analysis, significance was seen
for association with Bu-1 genotypes ($p < 0.02$), which was valid
despite the significant interaction. Inspection of Table 5 shows
that the Bu-1 effect was genetically additive, with b superior to a
as might be expected from the line differences. The Th-1 effect
was near-significant ($p < 0.10$), and inspection of the values in
Table 5 suggests possible dominant superiority of a over b. This
finding had not been anticipated, so that it was not valid to make a
further analysis with pooling of data for a/a + a/b as a direct test
of dominance.

DISCUSSION

Inbred lines EL6 and EL7 show quantitative differences in
levels of immune response to several types of antigenic stimulation, with sometimes one line higher and sometimes the other
(Table 1). We have tested some of these responses for association with Bu-1 and Th-1 genotypes in F_2 progeny from these lines,
with results summarized in Table 6. The higher delayed hypersensitivity response to lipid-BSA was associated with dominant
(perhaps overdominant) expression of the Bu-1^a gene. This gene
is homozygous in EL6, the line giving the higher response in the
line comparisons. Our data on F_2 chickens were not adequate to
confirm the parallelism between primary antibody and DH responses seen for BSA, lipid-BSA, and ferritin in our previous line
comparisons (17). The lower GVH response to MHC antigens was
associated with additive expression of Bu-1 , and this also agreed
with the lower GVH inducing ability of EL6 leukocytes. Both DH
and GVH responses are thought to be primarily T cell functions,
and it appears that Bu-1^a was associated with the higher activity
in the first of these and the lower activity in the second. The
involvement of a gene determining a B cell antigen with two different T cell functions suggests either that the Bu-1 antigens, like
Ia, are detectable easily on B cells but only with difficulty on T
cells although they are functional mainly on T cells; or that
there is B cell modulation of T function, as reported for DH in
guinea pigs (22).

Table 6. Association of immune response levels with inbred lines and F_2 alloantigen genotypes: Summary.

| Response | Antigen | High Responder | | p[a] | Gene action[b] |
		Line	F_2 genotype		
DH	Lipid-BSA	EL6	Bu-1 a/a, a/b	< 0.025	Dominant
1° antibody	Lipid-BSA	EL6	Bu-1 a/b	NS	(Overdominant)
2° antibody	GAT[10]	EL7	Th-1 a/b	< 0.005	Overdominant
GVH	MHC	EL7	Bu -1 b/b	< 0.02	Additive
			Th-1 a/a, a/b	< 0.10	(Dominant)

[a] Significance level for association of F_2 genotypes with response difference.

[b] Tentative conclusion for effect of the locus in F_2 generation.

The Th-1 locus showed marked association with the levels of 20-day secondary antibody response to GAT[10], and this took the form of overdominant genetic action (geometric mean titres: heterozygotes, 1971; homozygotes, 1059). This specific one-locus heterosis was additional to the general heterosis associated with release from inbreeding depression, as shown by our finding of 195 and 356 as the corresponding GM titres for EL6 and EL7 respectively, compared with an overall mean of 1250 (range 23-4672) in F_2. Our values for inbreds are similar to the GM values of 271, 120, and 81 for responder lines UCD2, UCD3, and UCD22 respectively (calculated from data in ref. 4), and contrast with the near-zero response of the non-responder line UCD7 (geometric mean, 1), which was associated in F_2 tests with a particular B MHC allele (4). We appear to have identified a non-MHC locus with a marked effect on the level of response to GAT[10]. In mice, MHC-associated nonresponse to GAT[10] has been extensively studied, but in addition non-MHC-associated variation in the levels of response among responders has been reported (23). It was concluded that this variation was under multigenic control, but that one locus involved determined an IgG H chain allotypic marker (23). This suggests a possible relation between Th-1 antigens and H chain allotypes, which we plan to investigate.

Our finding of associations between two lymphocyte alloantigen loci and levels of immune responses suggests a direct function of the antigens in controlling the levels. The alternative possibility, of linkage between separate loci determining antigens and functions, seems less likely now in view of recent knowledge on the functions of Ia and other MHC antigens (6, 7). This is not to suggest that the function of our antigens is necessarily analogous to that of MHC antigens. A recent publication (24) described a search for new lymphocyte alloantigens in mice, based on reasoning similar to ours. Immunizations were made between F_1 mice differing in their X-chromosome with respect to X-linked immune responsiveness to so-called thymus-independent antigens such as type III pneumococcal polysaccharide, poly (I).poly (C), and denatured DNA. The resultant alloantisera detected three LyX antigens present on a subset of T cells. Since their characteristic distribution between inbred lines paralleled that of X-linked histocompatibility differences, these authors suggested that the LyX antigens might be similar to Ia antigens (24).

ACKNOWLEDGMENTS

We should like to thank Melvin Bell for excellent technical assistance, Dr. J.R. Morton for advice on statistical analyses, and Dr. Paul Maurer for generously supplying GAT[10]. This work was supported by U.S. Public Health Service Grant CA-14061 from the National Cancer Institute, U.S.P.H.S. predoctoral training grant GM-00127 (to M.A.P.) from the National Institute of General Medical Sciences, and U.S. Public Health Service Grant AI-05660.

REFERENCES

1.   McDevitt, H.O. and Benacerraf, B., in Advances in Immunol., Vol. 11, pp 31-74 (Academic Press, New York, 1969).

2.   Benacerraf, B. and Katz, D.H., in Advances in Cancer Research, Vol. 21, pp 121-173 (Academic Press, New York, 1975).

3.   Karakoz, I., Krejci, J., Hala, K., Blaszczyk, B., Hraba, T. and Pekarek, J., Europ. J. Immunol., 4: 545 (1974).

4.   Benedict, A.A, Pollard, L.W., Morrow, P.R., Abplanalp, H.A., Maurer, P.H. and Briles, W.E., Immunogenetics, 2: 313 (1975).

5.   McDevitt, H.O., in The Role of Products of the Histocompatibility Gene Complex in Immune Responses, pp 257-275 (D.H. Katz and B. Benacerraf, Eds.) (Academic Press, New York, 1976).

6.   Raff, M., Nature, 263: 10 (1976).

7.   Munro, A. and Bright, S., Nature, 264: 145 (1976).

8.   McDevitt, H.O. and Landy, M. (Eds.), Genetic Control of Immune Responsiveness, 469 pp (Academic Press, New York, 1972).

9.   Crittenden, L.B., Muhm, R.L. and Burmester, B.R., Poultry Sci., 51: 261 (1972).

10. Crittenden, L.B., Purchase, H.G., Solomon, J.J., Okazaki, W. and Burmester, B.R., Poultry Sci., 51: 242 (1972).

11. Crittenden, L.B., Stone, H.A., Reamer, R.H. and Okazaki, W., J. Virology, 1: 898 (1967).

12. Powell, P.C., Payne, L.N., Frazier, J.A. and Rennie, M., Nature, 251: 69 (1974).

13. Nazerian, K. and Sharma, J.M., J. Nat. Cancer Inst., 54: 277 (1975).

14. Peterson, R.D.A., Purchase, H.G., Burmester, B.R., Cooper, M.D. and Good, R.A., J. Nat. Cancer Inst., 36: 585 (1966).

15. Purchase, H.G. and Gilmour, D.G., J. Nat. Cancer Inst., 55: 851 (1975).

16.   Gilmour, D.G., Brand, A., Donnelly, N. and Stone, H.A.,
       Immunogenetics, 3: 549 (1976).

17.   Palladino, M.A., Gilmour, D.G., Scafuri, A.R., Stone,
       H.A. and Thorbecke, G.J., Immunogenetics, in press
       (1977).

18.   Pazderka, F., Longenecker, B.M., Law, G.R.J., Stone,
       H.A. and Ruth, R.F., Immunogenetics, 2: 93 (1975).

19.   Steel, R.G.D. and Torrie, J.H., Principles and Procedures
       of Statistics, 481 pp (McGraw-Hill, New York, 1960).

20.   Lydyard, P. and Ivanyi, J., Transplantation, 12: 493
       (1971).

21.   Sokal, R.R. and Rohlf, F.J., Biometry, 776 pp (Freeman,
       San Francisco, 1969).

22.   Neta, R. and Salvin S.B., J. Immunol., 117: 2014 (1976).

23.   Dorf, M.E., Dunham, E.K., Johnson, J.P. and Benacerraf,
       B., J. Immunol., 112: 1329 (1974).

24.   Zeicher, M., Mozes, E. and Lonai, P., Proc. Nat. Acad.
       Sci., 74: 721 (1977).

ROSETTE FORMATION IN CHICKS: WITH SPECIAL REFERENCE TO QRBC-ROSETTES

Koji Sato and Makoto Itoh

Department of Animal Physiology

Nagoya University, Nagoya, 464, Japan

The significance of rosette forming cells (RFC) has been well documented in the basic and clinical fields of immunology. In general, sheep red blood cells (SRBC) are extensively used as an indicator of the cells. It was reported, however, that lymphoid cells of chicks formed spontaneous rosettes more efficiently with RBCs of several species of birds as compared with any of the RBCs including those from carp, bull frogs, snakes and some mammals examined [1]. Among the RBCs of birds, Japanese quail RBC (QRBC) formed the highest number of rosettes (QRBC-rosettes) in the bone marrow and spleen. On the other hand, it was difficult to detect them in the thymus and peripheral blood lymphocytes (PBL).

Recently, it has been found that QRBC-rosettes in the thymus and PBL are mechanically fragile, and they easily release QRBC from the RFC by shaking after centrifugation in a rosette assay routinely used. There might be two types of RFC concerning QRBC-rosettes, which are loosely (L-RFC) or firmly (F-RFC) bound QRBC. Data presented here suggest that L-RFC and F-RFC might be separable subpopulations of lymphoid cells in chicks.

MATERIALS AND METHODS

Materials

An Anthony strain of chicks was used throughout the experiments and Hy-line chicks were used in part. The bursa of Fabricius was surgically removed at hatch and 3 mg/day of cyclophosphamide (Endoxan) was intramuscularly injected until 3 days of age.

121

Thymectomy was carried out either at the time of hatching or at 3 weeks of age under Somnopentyl anesthesia. A few days later, both the operated and intact group of chicks were irradiated at 20 r/min. for 30 minutes.

In another trial, a dose of 10 mg/kg of cortisone acetate was intramuscularly injected into chicks of 8 to 10 weeks of age.

As a source of QRBC, the wild-type plumage stock of Japanese quail (<u>Coturnix</u> <u>coturnix</u> <u>japonica</u>) was used. There is some strain or individual difference of QRBC, which affects the rosette formation. In each of the experiments, it was tried to obtain the RBC, if possible, from a single male quail. The blood was taken with a heparinized syringe and washed 3 times with Hanks' balanced salt solution (HBSS) by a subsequent centrifugation. The QRBC secured was used within 3 days after taking the blood.

Cyto-kinetic chemicals, enzymes and anti-sera were used for treatment of the cells to clarify interaction between the cells and QRBC. Materials and amounts of them used are as follows: Cytochalasin B (Aldrich) 2.5-20.0 µg, Vinblastine sulfate (Sigma) 10^{-5}M -10^{-4}M, Colchitin (Merck) 10^{-4}M -10^{-3}M, Pronase (Kaken) 200-400 µg, Trypsin (Difco, 1:250) 200 µg, Neuraminidase (Cl. perfringens, Sigma) 0.1 unit and Hyaluronidase (Boeringer) 50 units.

Anti H_μ and anti-L chain rabbit sera were obtained by the courtesy of Dr. Oki of the National Institute of Animal Health, Kodaira. Anti H_γ and anti-thymic sera were prepared in rabbits as reported elsewhere [2].

Preparation of lymphoid cell suspension

The bone marrow, spleen and thymus were removed and teased with forceps and scissors in cold HBSS. After centrifugation of the tissue-HBSS suspension at 40 g for 10 minutes in order to remove coarse particles, the cell pellet was obtained by centrifugation at 300 g for 10 minutes. Subsequently, the pellet was suspended in 4 ml of HBSS and layered on top of 3 ml of Lymphoprep (Nyegaard & Co.). After centrifugation at 400 g for 30 minutes, the cells in the intermediate layer were secured and washed 3 times with HBSS and underwent the subsequent centrifugation. Similarly, the PBL was isolated from heparinized blood by using Lymphoprep. Thus HBSS was added to the washed cells and the concentration of the cells was adjusted to around 5-10 X 10^7/ml.

Rosette forming cell assay

The assay previously described [3] was used with a minor

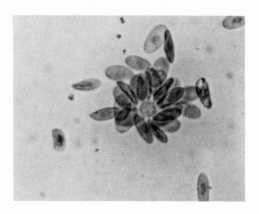

Fig. 1. A representative example of QRBC-rosettes in the PBL
(500 X).

modification. Two-tenths ml of the cell suspension was incubated
with 0.2 ml of a 3% QRBC suspension at 37°C for 60 minutes shaking
at 78/min. In place of the RBC suspension, 0.2 ml of HBSS was
added and run as a control procedure in parallel with the test
mixture. After incubation, the first sample for the counting of
total RFC was taken from the test mixture, which was still being
shaken. Following this, the mixture was centrifuged at 300 g for
5 minutes, and resuspended by a gentle shaking. The second sample
for the counting of F-RFC was taken. The number of L-RFC was
calculated by a subtraction of the second counting from the first
counting.

Counting of the rosettes

The test mixture was 10 times diluted with 0.1% eosin-HBSS and
placed in a hemocytometer. At least 1–5 X 10^3 lymphoid cells were
scanned. The rosettes bearing 5 QRBC or more were counted (Fig. 1).
The results were expressed as the number of RFC per 10^3 viable
lymphoid cells.

Treatments of the cells with chemicals, enzymes and anti-sera

Two-tenths ml each of chemicals, enzymes and anti-sera, were
added to 0.2 ml of the cell suspension and incubated at 37°C for
30 minutes. The mixture was centrifuged at 300 g for 5 minutes,
and the supernatant was discarded. Then 0.2 ml of HBSS was added
to the cell pellet and the rosette assay was carried out, as

already mentioned. Viability of the cells was examined in each
case of treatments.

In one of the experiments, the cells were incubated with undiluted anti-QRBC chick's serum for 30 minutes in ice water (3°C).
The cells were washed 3 times with HBSS and underwent centrifugation.
Subsequently, 0.2 ml of HBSS was added and the incubation for the
rosette assay with 3% QRBC suspension was divided two ways. They
were incubated at 37°C and 3°C, respectively, and the QRBC-rosettes
were counted 60 minutes after incubation.

RESULTS

Distribution and ontogenetic developments of RFCs

The number of RFCs in several lymphoid organs of chicks of 8
to 10 weeks of age are shown in Table 1. It is evident that the
distribution of L-RFC and F-RFC in the PBL and thymus is different
from those in the bone marrow, spleen and bursa of Fabricius. The
PBL and thymus contained significant number of L-RFC, but most of
their QRBC-rosettes were disrupted by mechanical shaking after
centrifugation. The number of both of the RFCs was rather stable
in the bone marrow, while those in the spleen and bursa of
Fabricius were highly variable.

Occasionally, a different type of QRBC-rosettes was found in
the bone marrow and spleen. They were easily discriminated from
the shape of the rosettes and from the morphological features of
the cells, possibly granulocytes, and were excluded from the
counting.

There are several factors which influence the number of QRBC-
rosettes. One factor is the age of the chicks, as shown in Figure
2. L-RFC in the PBL already appeared in the embryo one day before
hatch. After hatch, the number of L-RFC increased until 4 weeks of
age, and then decreased to approximately the level of L-RFC in adult
chicks.

Following the decrease of L-RFC, the number of F-RFC in the
bone marrow, spleen and bursa of Fabricius increased after around
10 weeks of age. A small number of F-RFC was counted 1 to $2/10^3$
in the PBL and thymus after 13 weeks of age. It may be suggested
that L-RFC and F-RFC are interrelated in the maturation process of
the lymphoid system in chicks.

Differences in the breed or strain of the chicks is also an
important factor in the modification of rosette formation. Recently,
Itoh [4] described that the number of L-RFC of the PBL in two of the

Table 1. Distribution of L-RFC and F-RFC in several lymphoid organs of chicks at 8 to 10 weeks of age. A range of the number of RFCs/10^3 is shown.

Source of cells	L-RFC/10^3	F-RFC/10^3
PBL	80 – 120	0.01
Thymus	9 – 40	0.01
Bone marrow	20 – 90	9 – 30
Bursa of Fabricius	9 – 90	1 – 15
Spleen	6 – 95	2 – 15

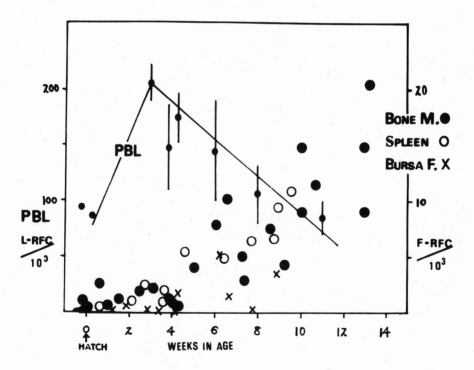

Fig. 2. Ontogenetic developments of L-RFC in the PBL and F-RFC in the bone marrow, spleen and bursa of Fabricius. Mean ± SE with bar in L-RFC.

inbred strains, WL-G and BM-C, was several times higher than those
in the NG-N and NH-H strains of chicks. Generally, the Anthony
strain of chicks showed a higher number of L-RFC in the PBL as
compared with those in Hy-line chicks, which is shown in Figs. 2
and 3.

Nature of the receptor site of the cells for QRBC

Technically, it is known that incubation of cells in chilled
conditions and the packing of the cells and of RBC by centrifugation
increase the number of rosettes. Table 2 shows that the temperature
of incubation significantly affects the QRBC-rosette formation in
the opposite way. When the cells were incubated at 3°C, neither
L-RFC nor F-RFC developed the rosettes. On the other hand, the
significant number of QRBC-rosettes, either by L-RFC or by F-RFC,
were counted at 37°C for incubation. Therefore QRBC-rosettes
might be formed in active process, which is an energy-requirement.

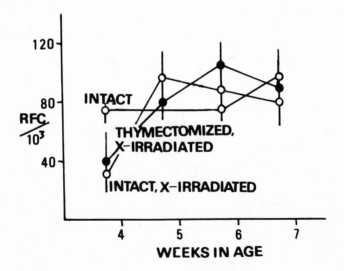

Fig. 3. Effects of thymectomy and additional x-irradiation on the
number of L-RFC in the PBL. Chicks were thymectomized at 3 weeks
of age, and x-irradiated on the following day. In this experiment,
Hy-line chicks were used. Mean ± SE with bar, 7 to 8 chicks each.

Table 2. Effects of the temperature of incubation on the rosette formation.

| | No. of RFCs/10^3 | | | |
| | L-RFC | | F-RFC | |
	3°C	37°C	3°C	37°C
PBL	0	63.10	1.16	2.32
	0	278.01	0	0.21
Thymus	0	10.33	0	0
	0	168.78	0	0.29
Bursa F.	0	33.86	0	16.91
Spleen	0	26.77	0	19.83
	0	175.01	0	32.02
Bone M.	0	68.88	0	7.65

The experiments, shown in Table 3, were undertaken in order to clarify the possible role of the cytophilic antibody on the rosette formation. It has been reported that T cells in chicks require the cytophilic antibody to form rosettes with SRBC [5, 6].

Table 3. Effects of sensitization of the cells with anti-QRBC on the rosette formation.

| | L-RFC/10^3 | | F-RFC/10^3 | |
	3°C	37°C	3°C	37°C
Thymus				
with Ab*	0	32.41	11.81	0
control	0	168.78	0	2.91
with Ab	1.19	9.20	1.78	0
control	0	10.33	0	0
Bursa F.				
with Ab	0.30	220.81	124.21	56.50
control	0	338.61	0	169.10
PBL				
with Ab	0	82.41	17.31	30.81
control	0	278.01	0	0.21

*Cell suspension 0.2 ml, Anti-QRBC, Titer ($\log_2$) 10, 0.2 ml, incubated at 3°C for 30 min.

This is also the case with QRBC-rosettes, in which the sensitized cells were incubated with QRBC. After centrifugation, a
relatively large number of RFC was counted in the cells sensitized
with anti-QRBC, though none of F-RFC was detected in control without
sensitization, if incubated at 3°C.   In presence of anti-QRBC for
sensitization, however, incubation at 37°C reduced the number of
both RFCs, as compared with those in control. Evidently, anti-QRBC
does not work well in the rosette formation with QRBC at 37°C.

Table 4 summarizes the effects of cyto-kinetic chemicals,
enzymes and anti-sera against chick's immunoglobulin (Ig) on the
rosette formation. Amounts of them added into medium for treatment
were limited to the range of tolerance which did not significantly
affect viability of the cells. Maximum percent of inhibition obtained in each treatment is preferentially shown with a mark.

Table 4. Effects of cyto-kinetic chemicals, enzymes and anti-Ig
sera on the rosette formation.

| Treatment | Thymus | Bone marrow | |
	L-RFC	L-RFC	F-RFC
Cytochalasin B	+++ *	+++	+++
Vinblastine sulfate	−	−	−
Colchitin	+	−	−
Pronase	+++	+++	+++
Trypsin	+++	+++	+++
Hyalurodinase	−	−	−
Neuraminidase **	++	++	−
Anti-Hγ	+	+	+
Anti Hμ	++	++	++
Anti-L	++	+	+++

* Percent Inhibition: more than 50%, +++; more than
20%, ++; less than 20%, +; no inhibition, −.
** Slightly hemolyzed QRBC.

Inhibitory activity of the materials used, if it occurred, was almost equal in L-RFC and F-RFC. Among those examined, cytochalasin B completely inhibited the rosette formation. It appears that process of the rosette formation might be confined through the mechanism of the microfilaments in surface of the RFCs.

Further, the data suggest that the receptor site specific to QRBC might be composed of protein, possibly Ig-like protein. Anti-L chain serum most effectively inhibited the rosette formation.

Source and origin of QRBC-RFC

Table 5 shows that cortisone significantly reduced the number of both of the RFCs 48 to 72 hours after injection. In this connection, L-RFC and F-RFC were sensitive to x-irradiation, as shown in Figure 3 and in our previous report [3]. These responses of the cells to cortisone and x-irradiation are physiologically characteristic of lymphoid cells.

In Table 6, surgical bursectomy at hatch and additional treatment of cyclophosphamide had no influence on the number of L-RFC in the PBL. A failure of the bursectomy on the rosette formation by F-RFC has already been reported [1, 3].

Table 5. Effects of cortisone on the number of L-RFC and F-RFC in the thymus and bone marrow (Mean ± SE).

	Thymus	Bone marrow	
	L-RFC	L-RFC	F-RFC
Cortisone (7)*	2.32 ± 0.96**	7.18 ± 2.57	4.60 ± 1.26**
No injection (7)	25.53 ± 7.72	42.84 ±10.13	14.63 ± 3.36

* No. of chicks   ** P $\leqslant$ 0.01

Table 6. Effects of bursectomy on the number of L-RFC in the PBL (Mean ± SE).

	L-RFC, weeks of age	
Treatments	3	4
Bursectomized, Cyclophosphamide (7)*	254.7 ± 23.7	203.7 ± 18.0
Bursectomized (4)	161.7 ± 23.9	178.7 ± 20.3
Cyclophosphamide (8)	173.1 ± 29.1	119.1 ± 45.3
Control, Intact (7)	155.1 ± 28.6	149.5 ± 21.5

* No. of chicks

Table 7. Effects of thymectomy on the number of L-RFC and F-RFC in the bone marrow (Mean ± SE).

	L-RFC	F-RFC
Thymectomized (7)[*]	32.06 ± 9.57	4.24 ± 1.46[**]
Intact or Sham (7)	42.84 ± 10.13	14.63 ± 3.36

[*] No. of chicks.   [**] $P < 0.05$.
1) Thymectomized at hatch with additional x-irradiation.
2) Estimation of RFCs at 8 to 10 weeks of age.

In our previous report [3], the number of F-RFC in the bone marrow and spleen was not restored to their original level in the thymectomized chicks 14 to 21 days after x-irradiation. This is compatible with the results shown in Table 7, where selective reduction in the number of QRBC-rosettes by thymectomy does occur. Obviously, the thymus plays a significant role in the genesis of QRBC-rosettes, especially concerning F-RFC.

Anti-thymic serum inhibited the rosette formation of lymphoid cells against QRBC in vitro, even in the absence of complement [3], (Fig. 4). This inhibition might be ascribed to steric interference with the receptor sites for QRBC. As shown in Fig. 4, it is observed that the inhibitory activity of the anti-serum is more prominent in F-RFC.

Addition of complement to the test mixture enhanced the inhibitory activity of the anti-serum. For example, percent inhibition in L-RFC of the thymic cells by the anti-serum (1:10) increased from 33.0% to 84.2% in the presence of guinea pig complement. Viability of the cells decreased from 88.2% to 41.8%. At times, a drastic increase of cytotoxic death of the cells resulted in difficulty in counting of the rosettes. Probably, one more step to remove the dead cells would be required before the rosette assay.

DISCUSSION

Most of QRBC-rosettes examined here are mechanically unstable. It is known that some of SRBC-rosettes in human T cells are sensitive to mechanical trauma [7, 8]. There might be two types of RFC, depending upon the strength of binding for RBC. They might be seperable subpopulations of lymphoid cells in reference to the thymus dependency.

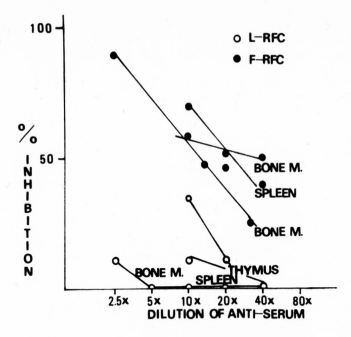

Fig. 4.   Effects of anti-thymic serum on the rosette formation.

F-RFC should be T cells, which is concluded from the experiments in thymectomized chicks and inhibition due to anti-thymic serum.   Further, it was proved that anti-bursal serum failed to block the rosette formation by F-RFC [3].

In contrast, the number of L-RFC was not changed even 8 to 10 weeks after thymectomy, though temporarily decreased by x-irradiation.   If all of T cells were effectively exhausted in thymectomized chicks, they might not be T cells.   It has been realized, however, that the life span of peripheral T cells is long, and usually longer than 1 year [9].   Relative to the inhibition in F-RFC, anti-thymic serum insufficiently inhibited the rosette formation in L-RFC, especially in the bone marrow and spleen.   It might be explained by the possibility of L-RFC carrying a lower density of T-specific antigen.   Cytotoxic death of the thymic cells resulted in a reduction in the number of L-RFC.   It seems to be that L-RFC is also T cells, but a further confirmation along this line may be required.

Interrelations between L-RFC and F-RFC are suggested from the results based upon the ontogenetic correlations and the similarity in their nature of the receptor.

It is already suggested that the thymus exerts an influence on the genesis of F-RFC through a humoral mechanism [3]. There might be two possible processes involving a differentiation of RFC and in the gaining of binding capacity, quantitatively or qualitatively, of the receptor for QRBC. One question still arises; that is, why the thymus contains a large number of L-RFC and a small, almost undetectable, number of F-RFC, even though the thymic humoral factor might be responsible for controlling either or both of the processes. The humoral factor inside of the thymus may be an inactive form and/or requires some microenvironment other than the thymus for performing their role. A type of cell transfer experiment which will provide an answer to this question is now being planned.

Recently, Isakoviç, et al. [10] detected the spontaneous rosettes using guinea pig RBC in the bone marrow, spleen and bursa of Fabricius in chicks. One-half to one-third of their rosettes were reduced by thymectomy. Rabbit RBC was also able to form the spontaneous rosettes [1, 11]. The RBCs of mammalian origin form the rosettes with lymphoid cells in chicks, but the number of them detected is quite low as compared with those of QRBC-rosettes [1]. Ivanyi [6] amplified the number of SRBC-rosettes by using formali-nized SRBC. It appears that QRBC-rosettes are different from SRBC-rosettes in the nature of interaction, as cytophilic antibody does not work on the rosette formation by QRBC.

Early in the immune response to QRBC, L-RFC and F-RFC transi-ently decreased. Cytodynamic studies concerning QRBC-RFC in the process of immunization may disclose the possible role of the RFC.

SUMMARY AND CONCLUSIONS

There are two types of RFC in lymphoid cells of normal un-immunized chicks, which form rosettes with QRBC. They might be separable subpopulations of lymphoid cells in reference to the thymus dependency.

Ontogenetic developments of both of the RFCs suggest the presence of their interrelations in the maturation process of the lymphoid system in chicks.

The nature of the receptor site for QRBC and the source or origin of RFCs are discussed.

REFERENCES

1. Sato, K., Proc. Jap. Soc. Immunol., 5, 135 (1975).

2. Sato, K., and Abe, S., Jap. J. Vet. Sci., 34, supplement, 143 (1972).

3. Sato, K., Immunology, 32, 2 (1977).

4. Itoh, M., Thesis, Master of Sci., Nagoya University (1977).

5. Webb, S. R., and Cooper, M. D., J. Immunol., 111, 275 (1973).

6. Ivanyi, J., Cellular Immunol., in press.

7. Steel, C. M., Evans, J. and Smith, M. A., Brit. J. Haematol., 28, 245 (1974).

8. Heier, H. E., Scand. J. Immunol., 3, 677 (1974).

9. Elves, M. W., The Lymphocytes, 59 pp. (Lloyd-Luke, Ltd., London, 1972).

10. Isakovič, K., Petrovič, S., Markovič, B. M., and Jankovič, B. D., Experientia, 15, 1204 (1974).

11. Tufveson, G., Bäck, R., and Alm, G. V., Int. Arch. Allergy, 46, 393 (1974).

Regulation of the Immune Response

PROTEIN-INDUCED NEONATAL SPECIFIC AND NON-SPECIFIC IMMUNOSUPPRESSION

Mary Lofy Rodrick and Constantine H. Tempelis

Department of Biomedical and Environmental Health

Sciences, School of Public Health, University of

California, Berkeley, California 94720

INTRODUCTION

Experimentally produced neonatal tolerance to a protein antigen can be induced by injection of a single large dose of tolerogen at or near birth (1). This tolerant state is finite and animals originally tolerant eventually return to full responsiveness to the tolerogen. Studies reported here indicate that there is not only a specific suppression of immune response to the tolerizing antigen following neonatal tolerance induction in chickens, but the development of hypogammaglobulinemia and a non-specific immunosuppression as well.

METHODS AND RESULTS

In the first experiment tolerance was induced in neonatal chickens (strain K 745, Kimber Farms, Niles, California) by intra-peritoneal injection of either: a) 25 mg goose gamma globulin (GGG), b) 25 mg GGG which had been deaggregated by centrifugation at 100,000 x G for 90 minutes, c) 50 mg bovine serum albumin (BSA) (Sigma Chemical, St. Louis, Mo.), or d) 50 mg deaggregated BSA. These dosages corresponded to 625 mg per kg body weight (KBW) and 1250 mg/KBW respectively. Uninjected animals were kept as controls. All animals were bled weekly and serum samples analyzed by several methods presented below.

No evidence of a primary antibody response to the tolerogen was shown in any animals for the first six weeks when sera were tested by passive hemagglutination of tolerogen-coated cells coupled by the bis-diazotized benzidine (BDB) method (2), but animals challenged at 6 weeks with BSA did respond, indicating that the once tolerant animals were responsive as had been shown previously (3).

Pools of serum from tolerant and control animals 10 days after hatching were analyzed by column chromatography on Bio-Gel A-5m (Bio-Rad Laboratories, Richmond, California), exclusion limit 5 x 10^6 daltons, eluting with 0.5M NaCl in borate buffer pH 8.2. A representative chromatogram is shown in Figure 1. Three major peaks of molecular sizes corresponding to: a) more than 5 x 10^6, b) between 5 x 10^6 and 2.5 x 10^4, and c) 2.5 x 10^4 and less. Serum pools from animals made tolerant to any of the four tolerogens showed a significantly smaller peak of protein in the middle fraction (b) which would contain the major immunoglobulins and other serum proteins.

The appearance of the reduced peaks in tolerant animals prompted us to analyze the individual sera from bleedings during the first six weeks after tolerance induction by single radial immunodiffusion (4) in 1% agarose using an antiserum which detected all immunoglobulins of chickens. Levels of immunoglobulin were determined using a standard chicken immunoglobulin from normal adult chicken serum prepared by sodium sulfate precipitation (5). Results are presented in Figure 2, and confirm the apparently decreased levels of immunoglobulin observed by gel chromatography. Testing with monospecific antisera to IgG and IgM (the kind gift of A.A. Benedict) indicated that the reduced immunoglobulin levels were due to a reduction in IgG. Differences in immunoglobulin levels were significantly different from those of control animals by Mann-Whitney and Wilcoxon Signed Rank test at p = 0.001 - 0.05. It can be seen that in animals tolerized with either BSA or GGG serum immunoglobulin levels were decreased from controls for the first 5 weeks after tolerization. Since this decrease did not seem to be attributable to the decrease in response to any single antigen such as the tolerogen, sera were further analyzed for development of natural agglutinins.

The development of natural hemagglutinins has been used to indicate development and depression of immune response (6,7). We tested the same sera analyzed above by radial immunodiffusion for natural hemagglutinins of rabbit red blood cells. Hemagglutination assays were carried out in phosphate buffered 0.15M saline using Microtiter apparatus (Cooke Laboratory Products, Alexander, Virginia) and results expressed in $\log_2$ titers. Figure 3 illustrates the results and shows that there is a delay in development of natural rabbit hemagglutinins in tolerant animals compared with controls. The differences were statistically significant only in weeks 4,5, and 6.

Results of the studies of serum from animals tolerized with either GGG or BSA indicated that there was a suppression of not only the immune response to the tolerogen, but some type of non-specific suppression as well.

In order to confirm and extend the above results a second experiment was carried out. Neonatal chicks (Frazer strain) were tolerized as above with BSA (Armour Co., Los Angeles, California) and blood samples were taken weekly. Each week following hatching five tolerant animals and five control animals were challenged with 1 mg per KBW BSA and the same number of each group with 2 x 10^9 sheep erythrocytes (SE) by intravenous injection. Four days later spleens from all challenged animals and controls of unchallenged animals from each group were assayed for plaque-forming cells by a modified Jerne plaque technique (8,9). Plaque-forming cells (PFC) per spleen were calculated and mean values compared with those of control animals. No evidence of cross-reaction between SE and BSA was found in any animals, and chickens produced few if any background plaques to SE in this test. All SE plaques were determined by the direct method which shows primarily IgM responses which in previous experiments was shown to be the expected type of response. PFC specific for BSA were determined using SE coated with BSA by the BDB method and developed with rabbit anti-chicken gamma globulin serum. Results of these assays are presented in Figure 4. The data show that tolerant chickens responded to challenge with the tolerogen, BSA, corresponding to 8% of the control animals in the first week following hatch, decreasing to 0% at week 2, increasing gradually thereafter to 125% of control by week 12. The tolerant chickens were also suppressed in their ability to respond to the unrelated antigen, SE, although the suppresssion was not as marked as that to the tolerogen. Response to SE gradually increased from 34% of control values in week 1 to 129% in week 5.

Serum samples from the experiment just described were also analyzed by radial immunodiffusion for serum immunoglobulin and again showed decreased levels of immunoglobulin which were statistically significantly different from control levels (data not shown). Serum pools from bleedings taken from these chicks at 2

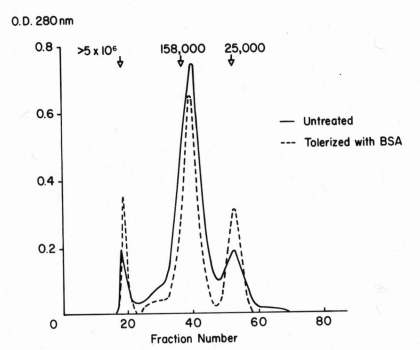

Figure 1. Gel chromatography of serum from chicks untreated or
           tolerized at hatch with bovine serum albumin. Serum
           from chicks 10 days after hatching; chromatography on
           Bio-Gel A-5m, exclusion limit 5×10^6 daltons.

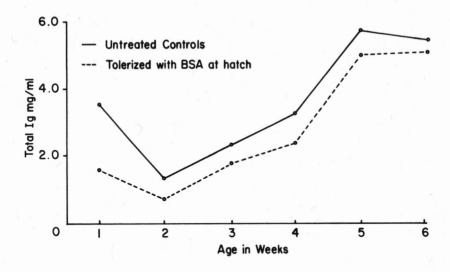

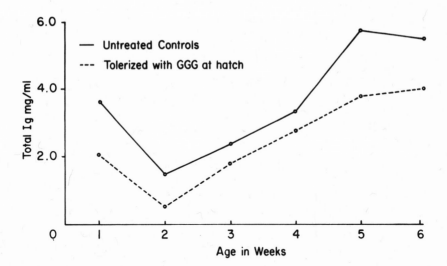

Figure 2. Effect of induction of tolerance in neonatal chickens on total serum immunoglobulin levels. Determined by single radial immunodiffusion.

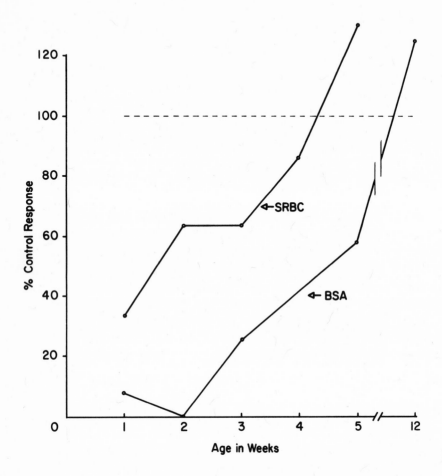

Figure 3. Effects of induction of tolerance in neonatal chicks
           on antibody-forming cell response to the tolerogen
           and a heterologous antigen. Chicks were immunized
           at weekly intervals and spleen removed and assayed
           for plaque-forming cells 4 days later.

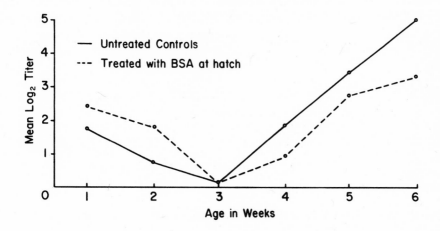

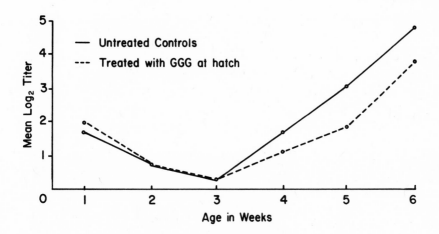

Figure 4.   Effect of induction of tolerance in neonatal chicks
on development of natural rabbit hemagglutinins.
Mean $\log_2$ titers of antibody and rabbit red blood
cells by microtiter assay.

weeks after hatching were analyzed by analytical ultracentrifu-
gation and found to have the 23S component described by Eardley
and Tempelis (3) in sera from tolerant animals and not control
animals.

DISCUSSION

The results presented here indicate that there is a non-
specific suppression of immune response as a result of neonatal
tolerance induction in chickens with a large dose of protein
antigen. This suppression was evidenced by a hypogammaglobulinemia, delay in development of natural hemagglutinins and by
suppression of ability to respond to an unrelated antigen measured
by the sensitive Jerne plaque method. Hirata and Schechtman (10)
showed that chicks tolerized with human gamma globulin (HGG) were
suppressed in their ability to respond to BSA 45 days after
hatching, but the effect was not reciprocal. Timourian and
Schectman (11) further showed depression of response to HGG and
BSA following neonatal tolerance induction with bovine gamma
globulin in rabbits and attributed the phenomenon to "cross-
tolerance." However, the level of antigenic cross-reactivity was
only 3-6%, whereas the cross-tolerance was 70-90%. The hypogammaglobulinemia observed in our results is similar to that seen in
thymectomized or irradiated chicks (6,12), and delay in development of natural hemagglutinins resembles that observed in bursectomized chicks (7). Their similarities suggest a non-specific
suppression rather than a cross-tolerance, or perhaps they are
actually one and the same. If this is in fact a non-specific
supression of immune response, the question remains as to what
mechanism is involved.

Eardley and Tempelis (3) showed that chickens neonatally
tolerized to BSA had immune complexes, consisting of the tolerogen and antibody, circulating in their serum during the time
the animals remained tolerant. They suggested that the antigen-
antibody complex produced a "turn-off" of antibody forming cells
which was transient and probably depended on the particular
structure of the complex. Although the radioimmunoassay for
specific immune complexes reported by Eardley and Tempelis (3)
was not carried out in these experiments, presumptive evidence
was found by ultracentrifugal analysis and is reported elsewhere
in this symposium by Morgan and Tempelis in inbred chickens
tolerized in the same manner. If the supresion is non-specific
as well as specific, the cells which are turned off must have a
more ubiquitous receptor than the antigen receptor, such as the
Fc receptor and/or possibly the complement receptor. Since many
cells of the immune system possess these receptors and the immune

complex is composed of immunoglobulin with Fc and very likely complement as well as antigen, binding to many cells could certainly occur. Other possibilities are that non-specific suppressor cells are activated (13, 14), or that antigenic competition plays a role (15). Studies of the mechanism of both the specific tolerance and the non-specific immunosuppresssion observed here are in progress to deduce the nature of the cells affected and responsible, the molecular nature of the immune complex observed and its role. Immune complexes have been implicated as blocking factors in serum of tumor-bearing animals and patients, and reports of non-specific suppression of the immune response to SE in tumor-bearing mice and mice treated with tumor cell components (16). The system described herein may be a model which could be used in the study of blocking factors in tumor immunology.

REFERENCES

1. Weigle, W.O., Adv. Immunol. 16:61 (1973).

2. Tempelis, C.H. and Rodrick, M.L., Am. J. Trop. Med. and Hyg. 21:238 (1972).

3. Eardley, D.D. and Tempelis, C.H., J. Immunol. 115:719 (1975).

4. Mancini, G., Carbonara, A.O. and Heremans, J.F., Immunochemistry 2:235 (1965).

5. Benedict, A.A., in "Methods in Immunology and Immunochemistry," ed. by Williams and Chase, Vol. I, 1969.

6. Van Meter, R., Good, R.A. and Cooper, M.D., J. Immunol. 102:370 (1969).

7. Leslie, G.A. and Martin, L.N., J. Immunol. 110:959 (1973).

8. Evans, G.H. and Ivanyi, J., Cellular Immunol. 14:402 (1974).

9. Morgan, E.L. and Tempelis, C.H., Personal Communication.

10. Hirata, A.A. and Schechtman, A.M., J. Immunol. 85:230-239 (1960).

11. Timourian, H. and Schechtman, A.M., J. Immunol. 89:886-890 (1962).

12. Perey, D.Y.E. and Bienenstock, J., J. Immunol. 111:633 (1973).

13. Nachtigal, D., Zan-Bar, I. and Feldman, M., Transplantation Rev. 26:88 (1975).

14. Basten, A., Miller, J.F.A.P. and Johnson, P., Transplantation Rev. 26:131 (1975).

15. Pross, H.G. and Eidinger, D., Adv. Immunol. 18:133 (1974).

16. Pikovski, M.A., Ziffroni-Gallon, Y. and Witz, P., Eur. J. Immunol. 5:447 (1975).

THE ROLE OF THE ADHERENT CELL IN ANTIGEN-ANTIBODY COMPLEX INDUCED IMMUNE UNRESPONSIVENESS

Edward L. Morgan, Constantine H. Tempelis

and Hans A. Abplanalp

Department of Biomedical and Environmental Health Sciences, School of Public Health, University of California Berkeley; Department of Avian Sciences, University of California, Davis

INTRODUCTION

There is growing evidence which implicates antigen-antibody (Ag-Ab) complexes in the induction and maintenance of immune unresponsiveness (1-4). Eisen and Karush (1) proposed that a critical ratio of Ag to Ab was necessary for the establishment of tolerance. They postulated that complexes formed in Ag excess would be suppressive and this has recently been confirmed (4).

The adherent cell has been found to be essential in the immune response. Mosier (5) found that the adherent cell was needed in obtaining an in vitro response to sheep erythrocytes (SE) by mouse spleen cells. More recently this requirement has been extended to the chicken (6). The adherent cell has also been implicated in immunological unresponsiveness (7-13). We report here that bovine serum albumin (BSA)-antibody (Ab) complexes act at the level of the adherent cell in suppressing a nonspecific response to SE.

MATERIALS AND METHODS

The animals used were line 3 white leghorn chickens identical for the 10 major blood loci (14). The methods used for the preparation of BSA-Ab complexes and antibody production in vitro

147

have been described previously (4). Briefly, complexes were
prepared at equivalence (Ag$_1$Ab$_8$) and in antigen excess (Ag$_1$Ab$_{2.7}$),
incubated for 10 min. with 2x10^7 spleen cells, the cells washed
extensively, and cultured with SE in modified Marbrook chambers.
Splenic adherent cells were collected by allowing 7x10^7 cells to
adhere to plastic petri plates for 24 hours (6). Adherent cells
were depleted from spleen cell populations by Sephadex G-10
passage (15). The number of adherent cells in the preparations were
determined by their ability to take up neutral red (16). Sephadex
G-10 passage depleted the adherent cell population by 90%-95%.
Suppressor serum was prepared by giving chicks less than 24 hours
old 1250 mg BSA/kilogram body weight intraperitoneally. Fourteen
days later sera from these and uninjected hatchmates were collected,
pooled, and heat inactivated (56°C. for 30 minutes) before use
(4).

RESULTS

The basic protocol for determining the role of the adherent
cell is shown in Figure 1.

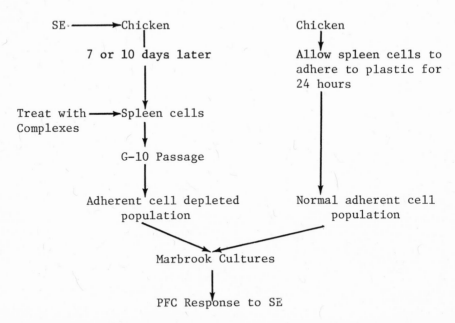

FIGURE 1   Experimental Design for Determining the Role of
the Adherent Cell in Immune Complex Mediated
Suppression.

The suppressive effects of complexes on cells from birds primed 7 days prior to culture are shown in Table 1. Only the direct (IgM) response was suppressed by antigen excess complex treatment (48%). Incubation with BSA alone was taken as 0% suppression. The direct response was adherent cell dependent because G-10 passage of the cells suppressed the response (30%), and was restored by the addition of normal adherent cells. However, G-10 passage had no effect on the indirect response. The suppressive effect of $Ag_1Ab_{2.7}$ complex treatment on the direct response was diminished by the addition of normal adherent cells indicating that Ag excess complexes were probabily acting upon the adherent cell. The above experiments were repeated with cells from birds primed 10 days previously with SE (Table 2). In addition suppressor serum was found to suppress the direct response (60%) and the indirect response (66%). Both the direct and indirect responses were adherent cell dependent, as evidenced by the effect that adherent cell depletion had on the responses and as shown for the 7-day group, the responses were restored by the addition of normal adherent cells (Table 1). The addition of normal adherent cells to G-10 passed spleen cell populations that were treated with suppressor serum restored both direct and indirect responses whereas only the indirect response was restored in those with Ag excess complexes.

Table 1

Secondary Response to SE from Birds Primed 7 Days Previously[a]

Treatment[c]	% Suppression[b]	
	Direct Response	Indirect Response
None	0	0
Ag_1Ab_8[d]	0	0
$Ag_1Ab_{2.7}$	48	0
None; adherent cell depleted	30	0
Ag_1Ab_8; adherent cell depleted	45	0
$Ag_1Ab_{2.7}$; adherent cell depleted	78	0
None; adherent cell depleted + 10^5 Adh.[e]	0	0
Ag_1Ab_8; adherent cell depleted + 10^5 Adh.	60	7
$Ag_1Ab_{2.7}$; adherent cell depleted + 10^5 Adh.	70	0
None; adherent cell depleted + $5x10^4$ Adh.	0	0
Ag_1Ab_8; adherent cell depleted + $5x10^4$ Adh.	20	10
$Ag_1Ab_{2.7}$; adherent cell depleted + $5x10^4$ Adh.	30	0

[a] Average of three experiments

[b] $\left[1 - \dfrac{\text{Plaque Forming Cells/Culture (test)}}{\text{Plaque Forming Cells/Culture (BSA)}} \right] x\ 100$

[c] $2x10^7$ spleen cells were incubated for 10 min. with these reagents

[d] BSA_1 Chicken anti-BSA_8 on a weight basis

[e] Adherent Cells

Table 2

Secondary Response to SE from Birds Primed 10 Days Previously[a]

Treatment[c]	% Suppression[b] Direct Response	Indirect Response
None	0	0
Ag_1Ab_8[d]	0	3
$Ag_1Ab_{2.7}$	49	45
Sup. Serum[e]	60	66
Normal Serum[f]	0	17
None; adherent cell depleted	75	86
Ag_1Ab_8; adherent cell depleted	76	90
$Ag_1Ab_{2.7}$; adherent cell depleted	77	91
Sup. Serum; adherent cell depleted	56	75
Normal Serum; adherent cell depleted	48	83
None; G-10 Passed+10^5 Adh.[g]	6	14
Ag_1Ab_8; adherent cell depleted+10^5 Adh.	20	23
$Ag_1Ab_{2.7}$; adherent cell depleted+10^5 Adh.	78	13
Sup. Serum; adherent cell depleted+10^5 Adh.	18	33
Normal Serum; adherent cell depleted+10^5 Adh.	0	42
None; G-10 passed + 5×10^4 Adh.	8	18
Ag_1Ab_8 G-10 passed + 5×10^4 Adh.	0	38
$Ag_1Ab_{2.7}$ G-10 Passed + 5×10^4 Adh.	75	24
Sup. Serum G-10 Passed + 5×10^4 Adh.	ND[h]	ND
Normal serum; adherent cell depleted + 5×10^4 Adh.	ND	ND

[a] Average of three experiments

[b] $\left[1 - \dfrac{\text{Plaque Forming Cells/Culture (test)}}{\text{Plaque Forming Cells/Culture (BSA)}} \right] \times 100$

[c] 2×10^7 spleen cells were incubated for 10 min. with these reagents

[d] BSA_1 Chicken anti-BSA_8 on a weight basis

[e] Serum from birds rendered unresponsive to BSA 14 days previously

[f] Serum from hatchmates of the unresponsive birds

[g] Adherent Cells

[h] Not done

DISCUSSION

We have previously shown that serum from birds unresponsive to BSA and prepared BSA-Ab complexes, formed in Ag excess, suppressed both homologous BSA and heterologous SE secondary responses (4). The results reported here implicate the adherent cell as being the cell type upon which suppressor serum and complexes prepared in antigen excess act in suppressing the heterologous response. The data showing the effect of immune complexes and the dependency of the immune response on adherent cells are summarized in Table 3. It can be seen that susceptibility to suppression by complexes in Ag excess and suppressor serum is correlated with the dependency of the response on the adherent cell population. At least one other cell type is involved because the addition of normal adherent cells did not reconstitute the 10 day direct response of cells treated with $Ag_1Ab_{2.7}$ complexes (Table 2). This response was shown to be adherent cell dependent because G-10 passage of spleen cells resulted in a suppression of the response. These data can be resolved if one postulates that another cell type is being affected by the complexes in addition to the adherent cell. Thus, when normal adherent cells were added no restoration of the response was observed because of a probable second cell defect. Others have shown the secondary response to SE to be T cell as well as adherent cell dependent at the times we have tested (6), therefore, the T cell could be the second cell type affected by the immune complexes.

Adherent cells have been shown to be necessary for the processing and presentation of antigen to lymphocytes (17). It has also been demonstrated that they release soluble products which promote lymphocyte viability and inhibit in vitro antibody production (11, 18-20). Overloading of the adherent cell surface has been suggested for other forms of unresponsiveness (7, 9). Diener et al. (12) suggested, however, that mere saturation of the surface receptors was not sufficient to induce suppression but an internal "off" signal needed to be generated.

A receptor for the constant portion of the immunoglobulin has been found on B cells (21), T cells (22-23), and adherent cells (17). Nussenzweig (24) postulated that the Fc receptor may play a role in the regulation of immunological responses by lymphocytes. The Fc portion of antibody was found to be necessary for the generation of complex mediated unresponsiveness (25), suppression of a mitogenic response to lipopolysaccharide (26), and paralysis of the adherent cell's phagocytic ability (10). Feldmann's model of suppression (8) suggested that adherent cell Fc receptors were overloaded with "IgT"-Ag complexes which allowed complexes to interact with B cells inducing the suppression. We

have previously shown that spleen cells were able to bind approximately 25 times more BSA in the form of an immune complex (4)
which could be accounted for the Fc receptor binding.

To determine whether the BSA–Ab complexes in the suppressor
serum (3-4) were responsible for the suppressive effects, they
were removed by affinity chromatography and the serum assayed in
the above system. It was found that the suppressive capacity was
removed from the serum (27), indicating that the complexes were
responsible.

The exact effect that the immune complexes have on the
spleen cell population are presently being evaluated.

Table   3

Summary of AgAb Suppression and Adherent Cell Dependency

Type Response	Adherent Dependency	Cell Susceptibility to Ag$_1$Ab$_{2.7}$[a] Tol. Serum[b]		Restoration with Adherent Cells Ag$_1$Ab$_{2.7}$ Tol.Serum	
Direct 7 Day	Yes	Yes	ND	Yes	ND[c]
Direct 10 Day	Yes	Yes	Yes	No[d]	Yes
Indirect 7 Day	No	No	ND	NA[d]	NA
Indirect 10 Day	Yes	Yes	Yes	Yes	Yes

[a]BSA$_1$Chicken anti-BSA$_{2.7}$ on a weight basis
[b]Serum from birds rendered unresponsive to BSA 14 days Previously
[c]Not Done
[d]Not Applicable

ACKNOWLEDGEMENTS

This work was supported by a Grossman Foundation Award.
E.L.M. is the recipient of H.E.W. grant Award 1A03-AH00535-02.
This work is in partial fulfillment for the degree of Doctor of
Philosophy from the University of California, Berkeley.

REFERENCES

1. Eisen H.N. and Karush, F., Nature 202:677, 1964.

2. Diener, E. and Feldmann, M., Transpl. Rev. 8:76, 1972.

3. Eardley, D.D. and Tempelis, C.H., J. Immunol., 115:719, 1975.

4. Morgan, E.L. and Tempelis, C.H., Submitted for publication.

5. Mosier, D.E., Science 158:1573, 1967.

6. Evans, G.H. and Ivanyi, J., Eur. J. Immunol., 5:747, 1975.

7. Feldmann, M. and Basten, A., Eur. J. Immunol., 2:213, 1972.

8. Feldmann, M., Nature New. Bio. 242:82, 1973.

9. Chan, P.L. and Sinclair, N.R. StC., Immunol., 24:289, 1973.

10. Rabinovitch, M., Manejias, R.E. and Nussenzweig, V., J. Exp. Med. 142:827, 1975.

11. Calderon, J. and Unanue, E.R., Nature 253:359, 1975.

12. Diener, E., Kraft, N., Lee, K.C. and Shiozawa, C., J. Exp. Med. 143:805, 1976.

13. Oppenheim, J.J., Shneyour, A. and Kook, A., J. Immunol., 116: 1446, 1976.

14. Benedict, A.A., Pollard, L.W., Morrow, P.R., Abplanalp, H.A., Maurer, P.H. and Briles, W.E., Immunogen. 2:313, 1975.

15. Ly, I.A. and Mishell, R.I., J. Immunol. Meth. 5:239, 1974.

16. McCombs, C., Hom, J., Talal, N. and Mishell, R.I., J. Immunol. 115:1695, 1975.

17. Unanue, E.R., Adv. Immunol. 15:95, 1972.

18. Pierce, C.W., Kapp, J.A., Wood, D.D. and Benacerraf, B., J. Immunol., 112:1181, 1974.

19. Rosenstreich, D.L., Farrar, J.J. and Dougherty, S., J. Immunol. 116:131, 1976.

20. Dutton, R.W., McCarthy, M.M. and Mishell, R.I., Cell. Immunol. 1:219, 1970.

21. Warner, N.L., Adv. Immunol. 19:67, 1974.

22. Stout, R.D. and Herzenberg, L.A., J. Exp. Med. 142:1041, 1975.

23. Basten, A., Miller, J.F.A.P., Warner, N.L., Abraham, R., Chia,
     E. and Gamble, J., J. Immunol. 115:1159, 1975.

24. Nussenzweig, V., Adv. Immunol. 19:217, 1974.

25. Lees, R.K. and Sinclair, N.R. StC., Immunol. 24:735, 1973.

26. Ryan, J.L., Arbeit, R.D., Dickler, H.B. and Henkart, P.A.,
     J. Exp. Med. 142:814, 1975.

27. Morgan, E.L. and Tempelis, C.H., Manuscript in preparation.

INFECTIOUS AGAMMAGLOBULINEMIA: SUPPRESSOR T CELLS WITH SPECIFICITY

FOR INDIVIDUAL IMMUNOGLOBULIN CLASSES

R. Michael Blaese, Andrew V. Muchmore, Irma Koski,
and Nancy J. Dooley

Cellular Immunology Section, Metabolism Branch
National Cancer Institute, National Institutes of
Health, Bethesda, Maryland   20014

Immunoregulatory cells with potent suppressive effects on immunoglobulin or specific antibody production have been described in many experimental systems. In the chicken, bone marrow cells from adult birds rendered agammaglobulinemic by bursectomy and irradiation at hatching will induce agammaglobulinemia in recipients when transplanted into normal adult chickens of the same strain (1). This "infectious agammaglobulinemia" is induced by donor suppressor T cells which appear in the donor birds in detectable quantities by about 10 weeks of age. Suppressor cells can be demonstrated in spleen, thymus and peripheral blood in addition to bone marrow. The immunodeficiency which develops in the recipient chickens is characterized by their failure to produce specific antibody after challenge with any of several thymic dependent or thymic independent antigens, the rapid disappearance of existing serum IgG, IgA and IgM, the persistence of an intact bursa of Fabricius, and the persistence of a normal number of B lymphocytes in the spleen of these birds at least until after serum immunoglobulin has become undetectable (2,3,4).

In this report we will describe the identification of suppressor T cells with specificity for each individual class of immunoglobulin. The result of such class specific suppression is detected as dysgammaglobulinemia appearing in the recipients of limiting dilution transfers of suppressor cells from aγ donors. The pattern of dysgammaglobulinemia developing in the recipient birds varies depending upon the cell dose given and more significantly upon the specific donor bird employed.

155

MATERIALS AND METHODS

Line 6, subline 1 chicks were obtained immediately after hatching from the RPRL, East Lansing, Michigan. Chicks were surgically bursectomized and given 550 R whole body irradiation (Bx-X) within 3 days of hatching. In this chicken strain, Bx-X results in an incidence of agammaglobulinemia at 8 weeks of age of 80-85%.

Antisera to chicken IgG, IgA and IgM were produced in rabbits or sheep by injection of purified chicken immunoglobulins obtained from chicken serum or bile. The antisera were rendered specific by absorption with insolubilized sera from agammaglobulinemic, newly hatched, or dysgammaglobulinemic chickens. Serum immunoglobulin levels were determined by radial immunodiffusion in antibody containing agarose or estimated by dilution Ouchterlony analysis. Cells with membrane bound immunoglobulin of each Ig class were determined by indirect immunofluorescence on unfixed spleen cell suspensions.

Cell suspensions for transplantation were prepared by mincing spleen or thymus with fine scissors followed by sequential aspiration of the fragments through needles of progressively smaller size to 27 G. Bone marrow cells were obtained by flushing the long bones with balanced salt solution and then passing the marrow elements through needles. Peripheral blood mononuclear leukocytes were obtained by density centrifugation on Ficoll-Hypaque. Injections of the cell suspensions were given to 2 week old recipient chicks intravenously in the wing vein or intraperitoneally.

RESULTS AND DISCUSSION

Table I shows the results obtained when varying doses of lymphoid cells from thymus, bone marrow, spleen or blood from a single donor were given to fourteen 2 week old syngeneic recipient chicks. With each source of donor lymphoid cells, recipient chicks were found with abnormal immunoglobulin patterns. With thymocyte injection for example, the recipient of 10^9 cells was agammaglobulinemic 55 days after transplant. The recipient of 3×10^7 cells had no detectable abnormalities in serum immunoglobulin at 55 days. Surprisingly, recipients of 10^8 and 3×10^8 thymocytes developed a dysgammaglobulinemia characterized by the presence of IgM in normal or elevated concentrations, but with deficiency of IgG and IgA. One recipient of 10^8 thymocytes (chicken 3) lacked only IgG with IgM and IgA present in normal concentrations.

These data suggested that suppressor cells were present in the donor bird with specificity for each individual immunoglobulin class and that the class specific suppressor cell in highest

Table I: Serum immunoglobulin levels in recipients of graded doses
           of cells from a single agammaglobulinemic donor

Recipient	Cell Source	Cell Number	Ig level at 55 days*		
			IgM	IgA	IgG
1	Thymus	3×10^7	NL	NL	NL
2		"	NL	NL	NL
3		10^8	NL	NL	< 0.1
4		"	NL	20%	< 0.1
5		3×10^8	NL	< 2.0	< 0.1
6		10^9	< 1.0	< 2.0	< 0.1
7	Bone Marrow	10^8	NL	NL	NL
8		3×10^8	NL	NL	NL
9		"	NL	NL	NL
10		10^9	NL	< 2.0	< 0.1
11	Spleen	3×10^8	NL	< 2.0	< 0.1
12		"	NL	< 2.0	< 0.1
13	Blood	3×10^8	NL	NL	NL
14		"	< 1.0	< 2.0	< 0.1

*Ig level presented as a percentage of a standard pool of normal
adult line 6,1 chicken serum. NL signifies at least 75% of
standard value.

frequency was revealed by the limiting dilution transplantation.
In this case, IgG suppressors appeared to be most prevalent, followed by IgA and then IgM. In numerous subsequent experiments
with different donor birds, a similar cell dose dependent suppression was observed, but importantly, different patterns of dysgammaglobulinemia developed. Thus, some donor birds had predominantly
IgG suppressor cells while other had IgA suppressors as the predominant cell revealed by limiting dilution. In one experiment,
chickens developed IgA normally but lacked IgM and IgG.

     The distinctly different patterns of dysgammaglobulinemia
associated with different donors argues strongly that the class
specific suppression observed is not simply due to a quantitative
effect of dilution of a "panimmunoglobulin suppressor." If IgG
were easier to suppress than IgA or IgM, then one should not see
birds with normal IgG levels in the presence of deficiency of IgA

Table II: Serial transplantation of class specific immunoglobulin
            suppression*

	Recipient Ig level	1st transplant/cell dose & source	2nd transplant/cell dose & source	3rd transplant/cell dose & source
Donor 1		10^8 thymus	60×10^8 thymus	10×10^8 thymus
	IgM[†]	89	103	85
	IgG	< 1	< 1	< 1
	IgA	80	95	70
Donor 2		3×10^8 blood	10×10^8 thymus	
	IgM	110	90	
	IgG	85	108	
	IgA	< 2	< 2	

*Cells from Bx-X agammaglobulinemic donors 1 and 2 were given to 2
week old syngeneic recipients. 12 weeks after transplant, cells
were obtained from these recipient birds and transplanted into a
2nd generation of recipients. For donor 1, a third generation
transfer was also performed.

[†]Serum levels of IgM, IgG and IgA are presented as a percentage of
that found in a standard pool of adult 6,1 chicken serum.

and/or IgM.   Another observation which tends to support the true
class specific nature of the suppression observed is the fact that
the suppression "breeds true" to class. As shown in Table II, when
cells from dysgammaglobulinemic birds were transplanted to secondary and tertiary recipients, only the class suppressed in the
original bird became suppressed in the recipient, even when as
many as 60 fold more cells were transplanted.

We have previously shown that "B" lymphocytes persist in the
birds with "infectious agammaglobulinemia." To determine the
presence of B cells bearing the specific class of Ig suppressed in
birds with "infectious dysgammaglobulinemia," spleens of these
birds were examined with reagents specific for IgG, IgA, and IgM.
B cells bearing the "suppressed" immunoglobulin class were present
in readily detectable quantities even though serum Ig of that class
was undetectable.

The mechanism of the suppression of Ig production in these
experiments is obscure. The recipient chickens with "infectious
agammaglobulinemia or dysgammaglobulinemia" continue to have B
lymphocytes and a Bursa of Fabricius. T cells obtained from

birds with suppressor activity are not cytotoxic in ^{51}Cr release
assays for bursa "B" cell targets. Antibody responses to both
thymic dependent and thymic independent antigens are suppressed
equally so that the suppressor effect would not seem to be directed at a helper T cell. Since Ig production apparently ceases
immediately when recipients are given suppressor cells, the suppressive effect may well be exerted at the level of the mature Ig
secreting plasma cell. Whatever the ultimate mechanism of suppression may be, suppressor cells clearly can have a profound effect on the production of individual classes of immunoglobulin and
therefore the potential effect of these cells must be considered
when evaluating data on the ontogeny of the humoral immune system
and the sequence of appearance of various immunoglobulin classes
during the course of an antibody response to specific antigens.

REFERENCES

1. Blaese, R.M., Weiden, P.L., Koski, I., and Dooley, N.J., J.
    Exp. Med. 140:1097, 1974.
2. Blaese, R.M., Muchmore, A.V., Koski, I., and Dooley, N.J. in
    Mechanisms of Lymphocyte Activation (D.O. Lucas, Ed.) (Academic
    Press, New York) in press.
3. Palladino, M.A., Lerman, S.P., and Thorbecke, G.J., J. Immunol.
    116:1673, 1976.
4. Grebenau, M.D., Lerman, S.P., Palladino, M.A., and Thorbecke,
    G.J., Nature 260:46, 1976.

FURTHER CHARACTERIZATION OF THE SENSITIZING BURSA CELLS AND OF THE TARGET FOR SUPPRESSION IN THE TRANSFER OF AGAMMAGLOBULINEMIA

S. P. Lerman, M. D. Grebenau, M. A. Palladino,
and G. J. Thorbecke

Department of Pathology
New York University Medical Center
550 First Avenue, New York, N. Y. 10016

In previous studies, we have investigated the phenomenon of the transfer of agammaglobulinemia in chickens (first described by Blaese et al.)(1) and have extended their findings to 2 additional chicken strains (2). We have also described a phenomenon in which the T cells of agammaglobulinemic (BX) chickens develop the capacity to suppress the adoptive antibody response of histocompatible bursa cells after "presensitization" of the agammaglobulinemic donors with bursa cells from chickens of the same strain (3). The present studies were undertaken to: 1) define the target of suppression in recipients, 2) identify the "immunizing" antigen on bursa cells, and 3) tolerize agammaglobulinemic birds against bursa cells.

<u>Ability of bursa-"immune" BX lymphoid cells to inhibit adoptive antibody response of bursa cells.</u> The general protocol followed in these experiments is shown in Figure 1. Hy-Line FP (B15/B21) strain chickens rendered agammaglobulinemic by prior treatment with testosterone and cyclophosphamide (Cy) (4) were injected intravenously (i.v.) with histocompatible bursa cells from 6 to 21 days prior to killing (day 0). On day 0, spleen cells from such chickens were admixed with histocompatible bursa cells and killed <u>Brucella abortus</u> (BA) and injected i.v. into Cy-treated and γ-irradiated FP strain neonates. Seven days later recipient sera were obtained and assayed for agglutinating antibody to BA.

Table 1 demonstrates that spleen cells obtained from an FP strain BX chicken 25 days after preinjection with FP strain bursa cells markedly suppressed the adoptive antibody response of histocompatible bursa cells to BA. Indeed, even 2.5×10^6 bursa "immune" BX spleen cells caused a significant inhibition of the antibody response produced by a 10-fold excess of bursa cells. In contrast, 25×10^6 thymus cells from the same BX donor only marginally

Day -7 to -21
~10^7 Bursa cells   ⟶   12- to 15-week old
agammaglobulinemic
BX chicken

Day 0   Take BX donor spleen
(4 X 10^7), mix with
4 X 10^7 normal bursa
cells and B. abortus

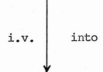

i.v.   into

XR + Cy-treated neonatal
chicken

Day 7   Take recipient sera,
titrate for Ab to
B. abortus

Fig. 1. PROTOCOL FOR DEMONSTRATION OF SUPPRESSION
BY "BURSA-IMMUNE" BX CHICKEN SPLEEN OF
ANTIBODY PRODUCTION BY BURSA CELLS

TABLE 1

COMPARATIVE ABILITY OF SPLEEN AND THYMUS CELLS FROM BURSA-"IMMUNE" BX CHICKENS
TO INHIBIT ADOPTIVE IMMUNE RESPONSE TO B. ABORTUS

NO. BX LYMPHOID CELLS ADDED*	BURSA IMMUNIZATION*	MEAN LOG$_2$ AGGLUTININ SERUM TITERS ± S.E.			
		BX SPLEEN	p	BX THYMUS	p
None	−	11.5 ± 0.76		11.5 ± 0.76	
2.5X10^6	+	7.5 ± 0.43	p<.001	10.7 ± 1.40	0.6<p<0.7
6.25X10^6	+	7.3 ± 0.67	p<.01	10.8 ± 1.10	0.6<p<0.7
25X10^6	+	5.8 ± 0.48	p<.001	9.2 ± 0.48	.02<p<.05
25X10^6	−	10.9 ± 0.50			

*Where indicated, the BX donor was injected with 2X10^7 bursa cells 25 days before killing. BX cells admixed with 25X10^6 bursa cells and B. abortus and injected into CY-XR treated neonates on day 0. Serum titers determined on day 7.

TABLE 2

INCIDENCE OF INHIBITORY ACTIVITY ON ANTIBODY PRODUCTION (SUPPRESSOR ACTIVITY) IN SPLEENS OF BX CHICKENS WITH OR WITHOUT PRIOR INJECTION OF BURSA CELLS

BURSA INJECTION*	INCIDENCE OF POSITIVE SUPPRESSOR ACTIVITY AT AGE**				
	9-11 WEEKS	11-13 WEEKS	13-15 WEEKS	15 WEEKS
+	0/3	4/7	8/12	26/26
-	0/0	0/2	1/19	2/13

*2 X 10^7 bursa cells were injected i.v. into BX chickens from 6 days to 3 weeks prior to testing.

**Suppressor activity = inhibition of adoptive antibody response to Brucella abortus by cells simultaneously injected into irradiated recipients.

TABLE 3

ROLE OF Ig IN "IMMUNIZING" BX DONORS FOR SUPPRESSOR ACTIVITY

BX SPLEEN CELLS ADDED*	BX DONOR INJECTED WITH**	MEAN LOG$_2$ AGGLUTININ SERUM TITER $\pm$ S.E.	
		EXPT. 1	EXPT. 2
-	-	10.92 ± 1.77	9.75 ± 1.35
+	-		10.40 ± 0.68
+	2X10^7 B. Cells		3.25 ± 0.57
+	5X10^6 NRS + C Treated B. Cells	8.13 ± 0.45†	
+	5X10^6 anti-Ig + C Treated B. Cells	13.25 ± 0.84†	
+	2X10^7 Chicken IgM-Coated SE	10.25 ± 1.31	
+	600 μg Chicken Ig + CFA, subc.		9.96 ± 0.48‡

*On day 0, 4X10^7 BX spleen cells, 4X10^7 bursa cells, and B. abortus were injected into neonatal recipients. Bleedings taken day 7.

**Donors all preinjected on day -7 to -6; cells all given i.v.

†Results of 2 individual donors pooled. p <.001 (n = 16).

‡Results of 2 individual donors pooled.

suppressed (.02 < p < .05) antibody production. It should be noted
that it has previously been reported that pretreatment of bursa-
"immune" BX spleen cells with anti-T cell serum and C removed suppressive capacity, indicating that the cell responsible for the suppression was a T cell (3). The relative inability of thymus cells
to inhibit the adoptive antibody response of bursa cells could have
resulted either from an absence of T cells in the thymus capable of
acquiring suppressor capacity or from an inability of a sufficient
number of injected bursa cells to reach and "immunize" the T cells
resident in the thymus. When spleen cells were obtained from a BX
chicken that had not been preinjected with bursa cells, suppression
of the adoptive immune response to BA could not be demonstrated
(Table 1). Furthermore, it has previously been reported that spleen
cells can also prime BX chickens for suppression but that preinjection of BX chickens with thymus cells does not lead to the generation
of suppressor cells (3).

The results in Table 2 indicate that there was little spontaneous development in the spleen cells of BX chickens of this ability
to inhibit the adoptive antibody response. An age-dependent maturation of the responsiveness of BX chickens to "immunization" with
bursa for the expression of suppressor capacity was also apparent.
By the time BX chickens were 15 weeks of age or older, suppressor
cells were demonstrable in all (26/26) birds after bursa "immuni-
tion." The inability of BX chickens younger than 11 weeks of age
to exhibit suppressor cells might be attributed to the stage of
maturation of their T cells although other factors cannot be ruled
out. When BX chickens were not injected with bursa cells, 31 out
of a total of 34 chickens tested failed to exhibit suppressor cells
in their spleens emphasizing that immunization with bursa was necessary.

Role of Ig in immunizing BX donors for suppressor activity.
Since both bursa and spleen cells but not thymus had been found to
"immunize" BX chickens for suppressor activity, it was decided to
investigate the role of Ig in priming for this phenomenon. As seen
in Table 3, treatment of bursa cells with rabbit anti-Ig + C prior
to injection into BX donors removed their capacity to "immunize" the
T cells of BX chickens. Despite this result, however, it was not
possible to "immunize" BX donors for suppressor activity with an
i.v. injection of IgM-coated sheep erythrocytes or with a mixture
of chicken IgM and IgG injected subcutaneously with complete Freund's
adjuvant or i.v. without adjuvant (not in Table). While these data
argue against IgM or IgG as the "antigen" on bursa cells to which
the T cells of BX chickens respond, a role for a class of Ig unique
to the cell surface cannot be excluded, and an avian analog of IgD
must still be considered. In addition, a unique "immunogenic" presentation of the surface Ig on B cells, possibly in association with
other cell surface components, also remains a possibility.

Abilities of embryonic and allogeneic bursa to immunize BX chickens. Among other B cell specific antigens which needed to be considered were those histocompatibility antigens present on B but not on T cells. Recent evidence (5) suggests the presence of Ia-like antigen on chicken B cells similar to that on B cells of other species.

It was reasoned that if allogeneic bursa cells could still "immunize" BX T cells to suppress syngeneic B cells, the likelihood of Ia antigen serving as the responsible antigen in question on the B cells would become rather remote. Indeed, it was found that bursa cells from the EL6 (B2/B2) strain chickens (from USDA, Agricultural Research Station, Regional Poultry Research Laboratory, East Lansing, Michigan) successfully primed BX FP strain chickens to inhibit the adoptive antibody response of FP strain bursa cells (Table 4). Similar results were obtained after "immunization" with SC strain (B2/B2) bursa cells. Unless significant crossreactivity exists between the B2 and the B15 or B21 haplotypes, such putative B cell specific antigens as Ia antigens do not appear to be relevant to this phenomenon.

Of possible assistance in identifying the antigen on bursa cells to which the T cells of BX chickens become "activated" would be a determination of when during ontogeny bursa cells develop the capacity to "immunize" BX chickens. As seen in Table 4, bursa cells from 17-day old embryos "immunized" BX chickens for suppressor activity. In contrast, bursa cells from 14-day old embryos "immunized" much less effectively. These data could be interpreted as indicating that cells possessing the antigen which sensitizes the T cells from BX chickens have not yet appeared in quantity in the bursas of 14-day old embryos. In data not shown, injection with 9×10^6 bursa cells from 14-day old embryos also failed to "immunize" for suppressor capacity.

Attempts to tolerize agammaglobulinemic chickens to B cells. Numerous protocols were employed in the hope of "tolerizing" BX chickens to B cells (Table 5). In Expt. 1 it was reasoned that T cells of BX chickens "activated" by prior injection of bursa cells would become susceptible to the effect of the alkylating agent, Cy. Such a protocol, however, was unsuccessful and spleen cells from BX chickens treated in this manner still were able to inhibit adoptive antibody formation by bursa cells after "immunization" with bursa. In Expt. 2, it was felt that an i.v. injection of chicken Ig might render chickens tolerant if a determinant on Ig were the antigen to which T cells of BX chickens responded. In other experiments in this laboratory it has recently been shown that the T cells of BX chickens can readily be tolerized to a protein antigen such as human γ-globulin by a single i.v. injection (6). However, in the present experiments chickens subjected to i.v. injection of chicken Ig still demonstrated suppressor capacity. In Expt. 3 large doses of the drugs Cy or 6-mercaptopurine were administered to 6 to 7 week old BX chickens followed by the injection

TABLE 4

ABILITY OF ALLOGENEIC AND EMBRYONIC BURSA CELLS
TO "IMMUNIZE" FP STRAIN BX CHICKENS FOR SUPPRESSOR ACTIVITY

GROUP	BX SPLEEN ADDED (4X10⁷)	BX DONOR INJECTED WITH BURSA			MEAN LOG$_2$ AGGLUTININ SERUM TITER $\pm$ S.E.			
		CELL NO.	STRAIN	AGE OF BURSA DONORS (DAYS)	EXPT. 1	p	EXPT. 2	p
1	-	-	-	-	13.2 ± 1.0		14.5 ± 1.4	
2	+	-	-	-	11.2 ± 1.7	$.4 > p > .3$		
3	+	20X10⁶	FP	60	1.0 ± 0.03	$p << .001$		
4	+	20X10⁶	SC	60	8.8 ± 0.5	$p < .001$		
5	+	20X10⁶	EL6	60	2.8 ± 2.8	$.01 > p > .001$		
6	+	5X10⁶	FP	17, embryo			3.8 ± 0.8	$p < .001$
7	+	5X10⁶	FP	14, embryo			9.8 ± 1.4	$.02 < p < .05$

BX spleen cell donors given single preinjection with bursa on days -12 to -6. BX spleen cells admixed with 4X10⁷ bursa cells + B. abortus and injected into neonatal FP recipients day 0. Sera assayed for antibody on day 7.

TABLE 5

ATTEMPTS TO "TOLERIZE" AGAMMAGLOBULINEMIC CHICKENS TO B-CELLS

PROCEDURES	EXPT. 1	EXPT. 2	EXPT. 3	EXPT. 4	EXPT. 5
Day of "tolerizing" injections	77	86	44-49	4-22	4
"Tolerizing" material	5×10^7 B.cells + Cytoxan 3 days later	10 mg Chicken Ig i.v.	4×10^8 B. & 2×10^7 BM cells + Cytoxan or 6 m.p. 3-5 days earlier	4 injections 2×10^7 B.cells	5×10^7 Spleen cells
Day of "bursa immunization"	90	91	70 & 146	55	84
Assay result*	Inhibition of antibody production (2/2)	Inhibition of antibody production (1/1)	Inhibition of antibody production (2/2)	Inhibition of antibody production (3/4) Partial re-constitution Ig levels (1/4)	Inhibition of antibody production (0/2) Normal Ig levels (4/4)

*Assay = Injection of spleen cells from bursa-"immunized" BX chickens along with bursa cells and Brucella abortus into neonatal chicks.

of large doses of bursa cells (4×10^8) and 2×10^7 bone marrow cells
for reconstitution. Spleen cells from such birds, however, still
could suppress adoptive antibody formation after subsequent "immunization" with bursa. The only procedures which led to an absence
of suppressor cells in BX chickens after immunization with bursa
was the injection of bursa cells (Expt. 4, in 1 of 4 animals) or
spleen cells (Expt. 5, in 4 of 4 animals) during neonatal life.
Suppressor activity could not be induced and remained absent even
after "immunization" attempts only in those cases where partial or
complete reconstitution of serum Ig levels had occurred.

Histological basis for the suppression mediated by T cells from
BX chickens. In order to determine the histological effects of the
suppressor cells from BX chickens a protocol described previously
was employed (2). Briefly, chickens were surgically bursectomized at
2 weeks of age (day -7), γ-irradiated 400 R on days -3, -2, and -1,
and injected i.v. with 1.8×10^8 spleen cells from histocompatible
BX donors on day 0. At various times after transfer, recipients
were sacrificed, their lymphoid tissues fixed in Carnoy's and sections stained with methyl green pyronin (7). Grading for plasma
cells and IgM ranged from - to 4+. It should be noted that all recipients had been primed with multiple injections of BA prior to irradiation so that numerous germinal centers and plasma cells would
be present in the irradiation-only controls.

As seen in Table 6, the most marked defect was evident in the
FP strain on day 7 with one chicken showing a total absence of plasma
cells in the spleen and intestines and a lack of detectable IgM in
its serum. In the SC strain, the defect was most pronounced on day
14 with plasma cells in the spleen and intestines virtually absent
and serum IgM also lacking. It should be noted that the data in
this table may be skewed in favor of the more positive animals in
that the presumably most deficient birds were dying during the course
of the experiment. Controls which were not injected with BX cells
had normal levels of plasma cells and IgM. Concomitant with the
destruction of plasma cells in the recipients of BX spleen cells
was a decrease and sometimes a total absence of germinal centers
in some birds (data not shown). Germinal centers occurred in
greater numbers in chickens of the SC strain and appeared also somewhat more resistant to the effects of the suppressor cells in this
strain. This difference in germinal centers between the two strains
might account for the fact that recovery from the effects of the
suppressor cells occurred more frequently in the SC than in the FP
strain (as also noted previously). More recent experiments (not
included in Table 6) have confirmed and extended these data, again
showing a complete absence of plasma cells from the mucosal lining
of the intestines in a number of recipients of BX spleen cells and
never in controls.

"Immunization" of BX donors with bursa cells was not required
in order to transfer agammaglobulinemia (2), probably because the
donor cells responded to B cells in the recipients to which they

TABLE 6

TISSUE PLASMA CELL CONTENT AND SERUM IgM LEVELS AFTER
INJECTION OF SPLEEN CELLS FROM AGAMMAGLOBULINEMIC HISTOCOMPATIBLE DONORS

CHICKEN STRAIN	BX SPLEEN CELLS INJECTED* (Day 0)	TIME AFTER BX SPLEEN (Days)	PLASMA CELL LEVEL IN:		SERUM IgM LEVEL
			SPLEEN	INTESTINES	
FP	-	7	2+, 3+	2+, 2+	2+, 2+
	-	14	3+, 4+	3+, ND	4+, 4+
	+	7	-, 1+	-, 1+	-, 2+
	+**	14	2+, 2+	2+, 2+	1+, 1+
SC	-	7	2+	2+	2+
	-	14	2+	3+	4+
	+	7	1+	1+	1+
	+≠	14	w+, vw+	vw+, vw+	-, -

*Recipients surgically BX at 2 weeks of age (day -7), γ-irradiated, 400 R on days -1, -2, -3, and
injected i.v. with 1.8 X 10⁸ spleen cells from agammaglobulinemic BX donors on day 0.

**Of 10 FP in this group, 1 died before day 14 and 4 between days 14 and 21.

≠Of 9 SC in this group, 3 died between days 14 and 21.

became exposed after transfer. Thus for the transfer of agammaglobulinemia there is no need for preimmunization of donors, but
when an immediate inhibition of B cell activity in recipients is
desired the preimmunization of donors causes sufficient accelera-
tion of the phenomenon to allow its detection.

     The suppressor system described above and that reported
Blaese et al. (these Proceedings) and Leslie and Kermani-Arab
(these Proceedings) may serve as experimental models of the suppression reported in patients suffering from common variable hypogammaglobulinemia (8). The analogies between the phenomenon described
here and those of allotype (9, 10) and idiotype (11, 12) suppression
are obvious. Allotype suppression has been reported to be mediated
by the action of T suppressor cells on allotype specific T-helper
cells (13). In contrast, in the case of the transfer of agammaglobulinemia in the chicken, suppressor cells would appear to act
directly on bursa derived cells for several reasons: 1) Spleen
cells from bursa-"immunized" BX chickens can suppress the adoptive
antibody response of bursa cells to BA, a T-cell independent immune
response (14); 2) Destruction of plasma cells and germinal centers
occurs in recipients of BX spleen cells; 3) The suppression can be
primed for by the injection of Ig positive bursa cells. The target
for T cell suppression in idiotype suppression is also likely to be
a B cell in view of the recent demonstration that the suppressor
T cells bind the idiotype containing Ig on their surface (15).

     The stage of development of B cells at which the suppressor
cells act remains to be determined. Preliminary data (not shown)
indicate that there is little decrease in numbers of surface Ig
bearing or Fc receptor bearing cells in the spleens of recipients
of BX cells, possibly implying that the suppression (or cytotoxicity?)
may act at the level of the more differentiated germinal center and
plasma cell. In our experiments we have always observed simultaneous depression of IgM and IgG production without any evidence for
isotype specific suppression such as was reported by Blaese et al.
(these Proceedings).

Summary

     Presensitization of BX donors with B cells appears obligatory
in order for their T cells to acquire suppressor capacity against
the adoptive humoral antibody response of bursa cells to B. abortus.
Although anti-Ig + C treatment of bursa cells removes their capacity
to "immunize" BX chickens for suppressor activity, BX chickens cannot
be sensitized for this effect by the injection of chicken IgM + IgG.
Both embryonic and allogeneic bursa cells can "immunize" the T cells
of BX chickens. The observation that spleen cells from BX chickens
can cause absence of plasma cells and germinal centers in the spleen
and mucosal lining of cecal tonsils of histocompatible recipients
within 1-2 weeks after transfer suggests that the suppressor cells
mediate their effect by acting directly on B cells at one or more
stages during their development.

References

1. Blaese, R. M., Weiden, P. L., Kaski, I. and Dooley, N., J. Exp. Med. 140: 1097 (1974).
2. Palladino, M. A., Lerman, S. P. and Thorbecke, G. J., J. Immunol. 116: 1673 (1976).
3. Grebenau, M. D., Lerman, S. P., Palladino, M. A., and Thorbecke, G. J., Nature 260: 46 (1976).
4. Lerman, S. P. and Weidanz, W. P., Bact. Proc. 69: 91 (1969).
5. Ziegler, A. and Pink, R., J. Biol. Chem. 215: 5391 (1976).
6. Grebenau, M. D. and Thorbecke, G. J., Fed. Proc. 36: 1226 (1977).
7. Brachet, J., Quart. J. Micr. Sci. 94: 1 (1953).
8. Waldman, T. A., Broder, S., Blaese, R. M., Durm, M., Blackwell, M. and Strober, W., Lancet 2: 609 (1973).
9. Jacobson, E. B., Herzenberg, L. A., Riblet, R. and Herzenberg, L. A., J. Exp. Med. 135: 1163 (1972).
10. Jacobson, E. B., Eur. J. Immunol. 3: 619 (1973).
11. Hart, D. A., Wang, A. L., Pawlak, L. L. and Nisonoff, A., J. Exp. Med. 135: 1293 (1972).
12. Eichmann, K., Eur. J. Immunol. 5: 511 (1975).
13. Herzenberg, L. A., Okumura, K., Cantor, H., Sato, V. L., Shen, F. W., Boyse, E. A. and Herzenberg, L. A., J. Exp. Med. 144: 330 (1976).
14. Takahashi, T., Mond, J. J., Carswell, E. A. and Thorbecke, G. J., J. Immunol. 107: 1520 (1971).
15. Owen, F. L. and Nisonoff, A., Fed. Proc. 36: 1184 (1977).

Acknowledgments

S.L. is a Special Fellow of the Leukemia Society of America. M.D.G. is a Trainee under USPHS Training Grant 5T05-GM01668. M.A.P. is a Trainee under USPHS Training Grant 5T01-GM00127. This work was supported by Grant #AI-3076 from the National Institutes of Health.

Valuable assistance was given by Melvin Bell and Pedro Sanchez. B. abortus ring test antigen was generously supplied by Dr. C. E. Watson, U.S. Dept. Agriculture, Nat'l Animal Disease Lab., Ames, Iowa.

REGULATORY LYMPHOCYTES FROM ANTI-μ BURSECTOMIZED AGAMMAGLOBULINEMIC CHICKENS

Gerrie A. Leslie and Vali Kermani-Arab

Department of Microbiology & Immunology
University of Oregon Health Sciences Center
Portland, Oregon 97201

INTRODUCTION

Due to the clear distinction between the bursa of Fabricius and thymus that serve as central organs for the generation of B lymphocytes and T cells, respectively, the avian immune system provides a unique model to study the mechanisms involved in various immunological deficiency diseases of man. In the chicken various techniques have been used to remove or ablate potential antibody-forming B cells during embryonic or early post-embryonic life (1-11). During the course of maturation, these bursectomized chickens usually exhibited a state of hypogammaglobulinemia or agamma-globulinemia without an apparent change in T cell function (12). Of recent interest is the development of a progressive humoral immunodeficiency in chickens that had received lymphoid cells from syngeneic agammaglobulinemic donors (13-15). The suppressive factor(s) responsible for induction of the agammaglobulinemic state is apparently a T cell. Consistent with this report is the observation that T cells from some individuals with common variable hypo-gammaglobulinemia exert a suppressive effect on the synthesis of immunoglobulin by normal B cells in vitro (16).

The exact mechanism whereby chicken T cells suppress immuno-globulin synthesis remains to be elucidated. In one system, pre-sensitization of bursectomized donor birds with bursa cells was required for the transfer of agammaglobulinemia, which suggested that suppression was mediated by cytotoxic T anti B cells (14). In contrast, Blaese et al. (13,17) were able to transfer agamma-globulinemia successfully without prior immunization of the donor birds.

TABLE I

Production of Agammaglobulinemia by the Injection of Anti-μ During Embryonation[a]

Injection. Day	No. of Animals	Dose of Anti-μ (mg)	Proportion Survivors Agammaglobulinemic[b]
13-14	27	2-5	17/27
16-18	10	5	8/10

[a] All chickens were bursectomized at hatch.

[b] Chickens having IgM, IgY, and IgA levels less than 3% of control values at 50 days of age.

Class specific immunoglobulin suppression has been reported in chickens that, at hatch, received suppressor T cells from surgically bursectomized irradiated donors (17). This is in contrast with the findings of Grebenau et al. (14) and Palladino et al. (15) who showed that transfer of lymphocytes from chemically bursectomized agammaglobulinemic donors consistently resulted in both IgM and IgY isotype suppression. These differing results may be reconciled by application of more selective techniques for the abrogation of B cells, which should not affect T cell or T subset maturation.

In this study we conducted experiments to determine the suppressive nature of lymphoid cells from various organs of Line 6 subline 3 donor chickens. Donor animals were made agammaglobulinemic by treatment of 14 day embryos with anti-μ and surgical bursectomy at hatch. Our results indicate that B cell, but not T cell, maturation has been blocked in these anti-μ-Bx birds.

Previous studies from my laboratory and that of Dr. Cooper have shown the effectiveness of embryonic anti-μ plus neonatal bursectomy in producing agammaglobulinemia (Table I).

We have had birds survive and remain agammaglobulinemic for more than 16 months. The evidence that these birds are truly B-cell deficient is given in Table II.

Thus, the B cell compartment apparently has been ablated in anti-μ-Bx chickens and in contrast the T cell compartment or at least certain subsets of it remained intact and functional in these birds (Table III).

TABLE II

Evidence for Ablation of B-Cell Compartment by Treatment with
Anti-μ and Neonatal Bursectomy

	Lymphocytes From:	
Parameter Measured	Adult Normal Chicken	Adult Anti-μ-Bx Chicken
1. Capacity to reconstitute CP treated agammaglobulinemic chickens	+	−
2. Expression of Ig (a) surface (b) membrane bound (c) intracytoplasmic	+ + +	− − −
3. Germinal centers in the spleen	+	−
4. Serum Ig's IgM IgY IgA	+ + +	− − −
5. In vitro stimulation by anti chicken IgM or IgY	+	−

TABLE III

Responsiveness to Phytohemagglutinin (PHA) and Concanavalin A of
Splenic Lymphocytes from 3 Month Old Chickens Treated with Anti-μ
and Bursectomized at Hatch

Chickens	Response To: (Stimulation Index)	
	PHA[a]	Con A[b]
Anti-μ plus Bx	17.2[c] (±1.2)	12.4 (±1.0)
Normal	20.0 (±1.8)	14.1 (±1.2)

a 10 μg soluble PHA was added to each culture on first day of culture.
b 5 μg Con A was added to each culture on first day of culture.
c Mean and standard error of the triplicate 3 day cultures from 4 different samples.

TABLE IV

Surface Immunoglobulin Determinants on Peripheral Blood Lymphocytes
of 42 and 90 Day Old Anti-μ Bursectomized Donors, 42 Day Old
Transplanted and Control Birds

Chickens' age in days	Anti-μ bursectomized donors			Recipients			Control		
	IgM	IgY	IgA	IgM	IgY	IgA	IgM	IgY	IgA
42	0	0	0	10[a] (±1)	8 (±1.2)	1 (±0.1)	17 (±0.7)	15 (±1.1)	1 (±0.1)
90	0	0	0	N.D.	N.D.	N.D.	N.D.	N.D.	N.D.

0 = undetected.

N.D. = not done.

[a] Mean and standard error of the mean.

We next asked the question, what is the biological status and
possible regulatory role of various lymphoid cells in anti-μ
bursectomized chickens? To determine the regulatory role of these
cells on B-cell maturation and differentiation, lymphocytes from
the blood, spleen, thymus, and bone marrow of 3 month old anti-μ-Bx
chickens were injected into newly hatched syngeneic chicks. At
various times after cell transfer, the recipients were examined for
Ig-bearing lymphocytes and their capacity to synthesize humoral
immunoglobulins (Table IV).

Thus, recipients of cells from agammaglobulinemic donors
possessed lymphocytes with surface immunoglobulins of all three
isotypes. The number of IgM and IgY-bearing cells were slightly
less than the number found in age matched control birds. In contrast to the near normal percentages of Ig-bearing lymphocytes the
concentration of serum IgM, IgY, and IgA were markedly suppressed
in comparison with the values obtained for control birds (Figures
1-3).

Experiments were next undertaken to confirm the nature and the
specificity of anti-μ-Bx T suppressor cells.

Donor cells were treated with rabbit anti chicken T-cell antiserum plus complement prior to their adoptive transfer. As shown
in Table V, anti T + C' treated lymphocytes from the spleen, bone

marrow, or thymus lost their suppressive capacity, whereas, normal
chicks that received lymphocytes from the same donor but incubated
with normal rabbit serum and guinea pig complement exhibited
severely suppressed humoral immunoglobulins.

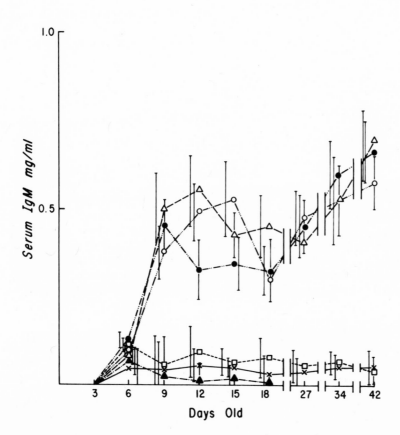

Fig. 1. Concentration of serum IgM in chickens transplanted with
7.5×10^6 splenic (x —— x), PBL (o —···——··· o), thymic
(▲ —·—·—·—▲), bone marrow (▢— — ▢) lymphocytes from 12 week
old anti-μ-Bx chickens, splenic cells from normal birds (●—··—··●)
or injected with suspending media (△————△)during the first day
after hatching. Each point represents the mean. (I) = standard
error of the mean.

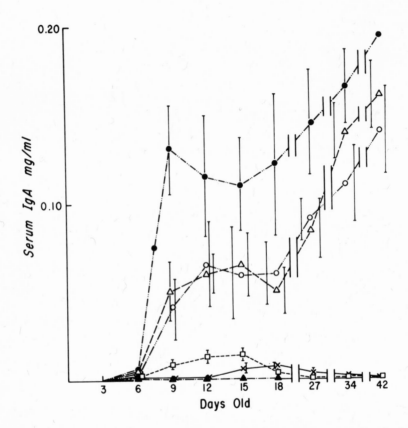

Fig. 2.   Concentration of serum IgA in chickens transplanted with
7.5 x 10⁶ splenic (x ——— x), PBL (o —••• —•••o), thymic (▲— •— • ▲),
bone marrow (□ ——— □) lymphocytes from 12 week old anti-μ-Bx
chickens, splenic cells from normal birds (●—••—••●) or injected
with suspending media (△———△) during the first day after hatching.
Each point represents the mean. (I) = standard error of the mean.

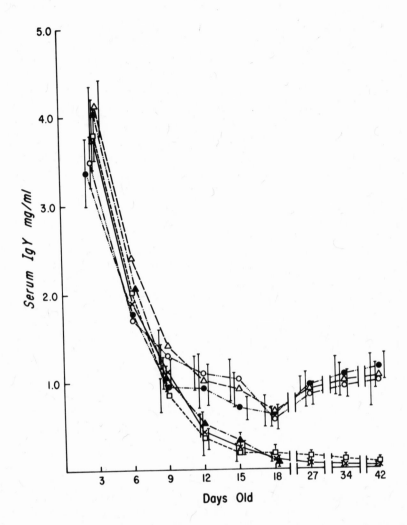

Fig. 3. Concentration of serum IgY in chickens transplanted with
7.5 x 10⁶ splenic (x —— x), PBL (o —··—···o), thymic (▲—·—· ▲),
bone marrow (□ ———□) lymphocytes from 12 week old anti-μ-Bx
chickens, splenic cells from normal birds (● —··—··●) or injected
with suspending media (△———△) during the first day after hatching.
Each point represents the mean. (I) = standard error of the mean.

TABLE V

The Effect of Anti Thymocyte Antibody Plus Complement Treatment of Splenic, Bone Marrow, and Thymic Lymphocytes from Anti-μ Bursectomized Donor Chickens on Serum Immunoglobulin Ontogeny of Recipient Birds

Pre-treatment[a]	Donor[b] cell type	Mg/ml[c] serum immunoglobulin after adoptive transfer					
		DAY 18			DAY 42		
		IgM	IgY	IgA	IgM	IgY	IgA
Rabbit anti T + C	spleen	0.28	0.78	0.10	0.63	1.1	0.15
	bone marrow	0.23	0.80	0.11	0.49	1.0	0.15
	thymus	0.20	1.0	0.07	0.58	1.3	0.13
NRS + C	spleen	0.04	0.11	–	0.07	0.05	–
	bone marrow	0.09	0.17	0.005	0.08	0.09	0.03
	thymus	0.07	0.10	0.003	0.11	0.07	0.01
None	spleen	0.06	0.10	0.007	0.05	–	–
	bone marrow	0.07	0.20	0.004	0.05	–	–
	thymus	0.02	0.08	–	N.D.	N.D.	N.D.

a,b 7.5×10^7 lymphoid cells from anti-μ bursectomized 3 month old donors were treated with rabbit anti T serum (1/50) + guinea pig complement (1/6) or equal concentrations of normal rabbit serum plus complement for 1 hr at 37 C before transplantation.

c   Mean of 7 individual samples.

–   Undetectable.

N.D. = not done.

DISCUSSION

These results clearly show that in birds rendered agamma-globulinemic by anti-μ plus bursectomy, the B cell compartment is non-functional, whereas, the T-cell compartment is intact and active. Transfer of splenic, bone marrow, or thymic but not blood lymphocytes from these birds into newly hatched recipients resulted in total suppression of serum IgM, IgY, and IgA development. The adoptive suppression was prevented by pretreatment of the cells with anti-T plus complement prior to transplantation thus indicating that the suppression was T cell mediated. Although these suppressor T-cells blocked immunoglobulin secretion, the transplanted recipients still possessed lymphocytes with all 3 classes of surface Ig determinants. Thus, it appears that the suppressor T-cells can prevent the terminal maturation and differentiation of B-cells capable of producing each of the 3 classes of immunoglobulins.

The mechanism(s) involved in the generation of T suppressor cells in anti-μ-Bx chickens and the role of these suppressor cells in maintaining agammaglobulinemia in the anti-μ plus bursectomized recipients remains to be elucidated. Anti-μ plus Bx may have rendered the donor birds agammaglobulinemic by one or a combination of the following mechanisms (Table VI).

Regarding the concept of suppressor cells with a specificity for chicken Ig, we have recently observed in anti-μ-Bx chickens a high frequency of T-cells capable of binding IgM but not IgY or IgA (Table VII).

TABLE VI

Possible Mechanisms for the Production of Agammaglobulinemia by Anti-μ Plus Bursectomy

1. Anti-μ mediated modulation of B-lymphocyte surface IgM.

2. Generation of anti heterologous antibody suppressor lymphocytes e.g. goat IgG.

3. Generation of B-cell antigen specific suppressor T cells.

4. Generation of suppressor cells with suppressive activity against helper T cells.

5. Generation of suppressor cells with chicken Ig specificity.

TABLE VII

Receptors for Chicken IgM on Peripheral Blood Lymphocytes of 2-3 Month Old Anti-μ-Bursectomized Chickens

Incubation of Cells With:	Anti-μ-Bx Chickens			Normal Chickens		
	μ	υ	α	μ	υ	α
NCS	20.3	-	-	13	15	1
AγCS	-	-	-	10	15	1
C-IgM	17.3			12	ND	ND
PBS	-	-	-	9	15	1

ND = not determined; NCS = normal chicken serum; AγCS = agammaglobulinemic chicken serum; C-IgM = purified chicken IgM; PBS = phosphate buffered saline.

It is likewise possible that suppressor T cells bear small amounts of surface IgM or that the embryo has a very low level of circulating IgM. Passive administration of anti-μ could interact with the free or bound IgM and result in proliferation of a T-cell subset with suppressor activity.

Very preliminary data using frog anti-human IgD antisera have suggested the presence of IgD on normal but not agammaglobulinemic chicken lymphocytes. Thus, it is also possible that the suppressor cells may be operating through IgD-isotypic determinants.

Suppression of Ig synthesis in the recipients of T suppressor cells has been suggested by Grebenau et al. (14) to be due to sensitized T cells with cytotoxic reactivity against B cells. This explanation cannot totally explain our results, since in our immuno-suppressed recipients, despite the lack of detectable serum immuno-globulins, lymphocytes with surface Ig are present. It is interesting that our transplanted birds are very similar to some patients with common variable hypogammaglobulinemia wherein T-cells have a suppressive influence on B cell differentiation. In this context the direct interaction of a single population of suppressor T cells, or their product(s), on potential IgM, IgY and IgA synthesizing B lymphocytes may result in suppression of Ig secretion. Alternatively, 3 subsets of suppressor T cells, or their products, may specifically block differentiation of each class of Ig-producing B cells.

REFERENCES

1. Cooper, M.D., Peterson, R.D.A., South, M.A. and Good, R.A., J. Exp. Med. 123: 75 (1966).
2. Cooper, M.D., Cain, W.A., Van Alten, P.J. and Good, R.A., Int. Arch. Allergy Appl. Immunol., 35: 242 (1969).
3. Van Meter, R., Good, R.A. and Cooper, M.D., J. Immunol. 102: 370 (1969).
4. Warner, N.L., Uhr, J.W., Thorbecke, G.J. and Ovary, Z., J. Immunol. 103: 1317 (1969).
5. Kincade, P.W., Lawton, A.R., Bockman, D.E. and Cooper, M.D., Proc. Nat. Acad. Sci. 67: 1918 (1970).
6. Linna, T.J., Frommel, D. and Good, R.A., Int. Arch. Allergy Appl. Immunol., 42: 20 (1972).
7. Leslie, G.A. and Martin, L.N., J. Immunol.,110: 959 (1973).
8. Leslie, G.A. and Martin, L.N., Int. Arch. Allergy Appl. Immunol., 45: 429 (1973).
9. Toivanan, P., Toivanen, A. and Good, R.A., J. Exp. Med., 136: 816 (1973).
10. Leslie, G.A., Am. J. Vet. Res., 36: 482 (1975).
11. Luster, M.I. and Leslie, G.A., Cell. Immunol., 20: 269 (1975).
12. Warner, N.L., Ovary, Z. and Kantor, F.S., Int. Arch. Allergy Appl. Immunol., 40: 719 (1971).
13. Blaese, R.M., Weiden, P.L., Koski, I. and Dooley, N., J. Exp. Med., 140: 1097 (1974).
14. Grebenau, M.D., Lerman, S.P., Palladino, M.A. and Thorbecke, G.J., Nature, 260: 46 (1976).
15. Palladino, M.A., Lerman, S.P. and Thorbecke, G.J., J. Immunol., 116: 1673 (1976).
16. Waldmann, T.A., Broder, S., Blaese, R.M., Durm, M., Blackman, M. and Strober, W., Lancet, 2: 609 (1974).
17. Blaese, R.M., Muchmore, A.V., Koski, I.R. and Dooley, N.J., 11th Leukocyte Culture Conference, Tucson, Arizona, September 19-23, 1976.

REGULATORY LYMPHOCYTES IN T CELL FUNCTIONS IN CHICKENS

Edward J. Moticka

The University of Texas Health Science Center at Dallas

5323 Harry Hines Boulevard; Dallas, Texas   75235

Our contemporary understanding of the immune system involves the concept of two distinct expressions of immunity as well as the division of lymphocyte types into functional subpopulations. Inherent in the development of this complexity is the discernment that some form of control mechanism must have evolved simultaneously. The study of regulatory mechanisms responsible for directing the response (normally) for the benefit of the organism has recently occupied a large number of immunologists. Their results have been frequently reviewed (1-8), and it is unnecessary to add to this literature burden. Rather, this paper will focus on the evidence which is accumulating that chicken thymocytes are capable of regulating the responsiveness of cells present in peripheral lymphoid tissue. Although these cells can regulate both T and B cell functions, emphasis will be placed on the role of these cells in the control of two phenomena which have been classically described as involving T cells.

The chicken thymus develops as a multi-lobed structure in the neck lying on either side of the trachea. While the epithelial elements of the organ develop locally, the lymphoid constituents are derived from blood-borne mesenchymal precursors which begin populating the organ at about the tenth day of embryonic development (9, 10). These cells undergo some, as yet ill-defined, maturational steps and emerge as functional T cells which subsequently populate peripheral lymphoid tissue (spleen, cecal tonsil, peripheral blood). Unlike the mammal, the avian thymus does not remain inviolate, and shortly after hatching it becomes a mixed organ consisting of immature and mature forms of both T and B cells (11). The ontogeny of this mixing and its possible role in the development of functional T cell subclasses

187

is unknown. Several observations, however, indirectly suggest
that this relationship may be important in the normal development
of the organ. Thus, there are factors extractable from the
chicken bursa which allow the development of mature T cells from
precursor cells (12). Similarly, cells derived from embryonic
bursa but not from thymus can restore cellularity and weight to
thymuses depleted of lymphocytes by cyclophosphamide treatment
(13).

The investigations reported here were aimed at determining
the presence of a population of thymocytes which can interact and
control the activity of peripheral T cells. Such a population
has previously been reported to exist in mice (1-8), and there is
one report of an analogous subset of cells in chickens (14).
Characterization of these cells on ontogenetic and functional
criteria has been carried out. In addition, their possible
relationship to other known populations of thymocytes in the
chicken and in mammals is discussed.

MATERIALS AND METHODS

Fertile eggs of the FP and SC lines were obtained from
Hyline and incubated under usual conditions. Hatched chicks were
kept in brooders for 4 weeks and then placed in open cages. The
animals had free access to food and water at all times.

Bursectomy was performed on 18-day-old embryos using techniques previously described (15). These animals were used as
cell donors 4 to 6 weeks later.

Lymphoid cells were prepared from spleen or thymus and
washed three times in Hanks' balanced salt solution. They were
subsequently resuspended, diluted to the desired concentration,
and used in the assay system. Peripheral blood was collected
aseptically in heparinized syringes, washed three times, and used
without further purification.

Two systems were employed to test T cell function and possible immunoregulatory mechanisms. In the first, chicken lymphoid
cells (primarily from the spleen) were incubated with phytohemagglutinin (PHA) to test for the blastogenic capabilities of these
cells. These cultures were performed in 0.2 ml total volume
(semi-micro) in flat bottom welled tissue culture plates (Falcon).
Various concentrations of the cells were mixed with a 1:15 dilution of the stock solution of PHA (Wellcome). The cultures were
run at 37°C in a 5% CO_2 - air mixture. After 58 hours, 1 μCi of
[3]H-thymidine was added to each well, and the cells were harvested
14-16 hours later.

The second system involved the establishment of a graft-versus-host (GvH) reaction in allogeneic fertile eggs by the injection of 50 μl unfractionated peripheral blood. The cells were inoculated intravenously into 11-12 day-old embryos. GvH reactivity was determined by the extent of splenomegaly measured 7 days later.

Thymocytes were fractionated on the basis of their adherence to a 5 ml glass wool column. Cells were loaded on the column and then allowed to incubate for 30 min at 37°C. Non-adherent cells were washed off the column by extensive washing with pre-heated medium. Adherent cells were removed by repeated mechanical compression of the glass wool. About 50% of the cells placed on the column were recovered, and of these 70-75% were in the nonadherent fraction.

RESULTS

PHA causes uptake of ^{3}H-thymidine by splenic lymphocytes (Table I). Although the critical experiments have not been performed, one might assume from investigations with mammalian systems that this phenomenon can be equated with proliferation of T cells. As can be seen, there is an optimal concentration of cells which can respond to the mitogen; this optimal concentration is not always the same between birds but usually is in the range of 5×10^5 to 2×10^6 cells per culture. As a result of this observation, each experiment was performed at several cell concentrations, and the results reported are those where the optimal response was observed.

Thymus cells by themselves rarely were stimulated by PHA. When spleen cells were mixed with varying numbers of autologous or syngeneic thymocytes and stimulated with PHA (Table II), two interesting observations were made. First, the addition of relatively small numbers of thymocytes to cultures of suboptimal numbers of spleen cells results in an enhanced response to PHA (Group C). This response is not simply an additive effect of the two cell populations and suggests cell collaboration ("help") or synergism. Alternatively, the addition of 10^5 thymocytes to cultures of optimal concentrations of splenic lymphocytes led to a severe depression of the response (Groups E and G). That this suppression is not merely the result of crowding in the culture can be seen in the comparison of Groups E and F.

TABLE I

Response of Chicken Spleen Cells to PHA

	Stimulation Index of		
Experiment	5×10^5 Cells	10^6 Cells	2×10^6 Cells
1	18.3	19.8	14
2	2.9	19.6	14.8
3	39.8	51.2	1.1
4	1.2	7.7	13.5
5	45.2	20.1	12.0
6	2	12.2	11.5

TABLE II

Response of Spleen Cells to PHA as Affected
by Autologous or Syngeneic Thymocytes

Group	Number of Spleen Cells	Number of Thymocytes	Stimulation Index
A	10^5	——	2.0
B	——	10^5	1.3
C	10^5	10^5	10.9
D	5×10^5	——	39.8
E	5×10^5	10^5	12.2
F	10^6	——	51.2
G	10^6	10^5	13.5

Previous workers (14, 16) had reported that in the chicken, cells responsible for suppression of an antibody response are dependent during development on the presence of an intact bursa. To test if the same held true of the suppressor cells active in controlling PHA responsiveness, thymocytes were removed from 4-6 week-old chicks which had been surgically bursectomized 3 days prior to hatching. These were then mixed with syngeneic spleen cells and cultured with PHA. Table III describes typical results obtained in a series of five similar experiments. In no case has there been an indication that bursectomized thymus could result in a suppression of the normal spleen response. In fact, there has been some indication that thymocytes from bursectomized birds may synergize with normal spleen and produce more stimulation. In addition, thymuses from some of the bursectomized birds responded quite well to the mitogen (data not presented).

TABLE III

Effect of Embryonic Bursectomy on the
Presence of Suppressor Cells in the Thymus

Spleen Cells	Thymus Cells	Stimulation Index
5×10^5	----	36.3
----	10^6	1.8
5×10^5	10^6	20.4
----	10^6 Bx	8.1
5×10^5	10^6 Bx	46.0

To further characterize the suppressor cell population, chicken thymus was fractionated into adherent and non-adherent populations by passage through a glass wool column. The individual fractions were mixed with syngeneic spleen cells and stimulated with PHA. Table IV shows that the addition of non-adherent thymocytes to spleen cells resulted in virtually no depression of the response. By contrast, the adherent cell population suppressed the response to a level comparable to that observed when whole thymus is used. Neither fraction obtained from regular thymus responded to PHA any better than did whole, unseparated thymus.

TABLE IV

Effect of Adherent and Non-Adherent Fractions of Thymus on the PHA Responsiveness of Spleen

Cells Cultured (10^6)	Stimulation Index
Spleen	19.8
Thymus	4.3
Spleen + Thymus	3.9
Nonadherent Thymus	2.6
Spleen + Nonadherent Thymus	18.7
Adherent Thymus	3.4
Spleen + Adherent Thymus	4.2

The presence of suppressor cells for T cell functions has been confirmed in vivo using a graft-versus-host assay (GvH) involving the injection of allogeneic lymphoid cells into embryos and measuring the resultant splenomegaly. The injection of 50 μl of peripheral blood (containing approximately 1.5×10^5 leuko-cytes) regularly led to spleen weights five to six times as great as saline injected controls (Group A; saline control weights average 12.4 mg). Thymus cells never resulted in splenomegaly. When 50 μl of peripheral blood is mixed with 5×10^4 or more thymocytes, the increase in spleen weight is significantly reduced (Table V; Group D). This same reduction is not observed when the GvH-inducing blood is mixed with thymocytes syngeneic with the recipient embryo (control for dilutional effect; Group E). This suppression is seen to better advantage when thymuses from very young chicks (1 week of age) are used (Group F). Old thymuses (2-5 months) will not readily reproduce this phenomenon (Group G).

TABLE V

Effect of Syngeneic or Allogeneic Thymocytes on
the GvH-Inducing Capabilities of Whole Chicken Blood

Group	Cells Injected	N	Spleen Weight ± SEM*
A	50 µl B2 Peripheral Blood	(57)	91.6 ± 4.6
B	5 x 10^4 B2 Thymus	(25)	25.6 ± 3.7
C	5 x 10^5 B2 Thymus	(5)	17.6 ± 4.6
D	B2 Blood + 5 x 10^4 B2 Thymus	(20)	62.9 ± 5.2
E	B2 Blood + 5 x 10^4 B15 Thymus	(7)	103.7 ± 13.0
F	B2 Blood + B2 Young Thymus	(19)	59.2 ± 3.4
G	B2 Blood + B2 Old Thymus	(18)	85.5 ± 5.7
H	Saline	(12)	14.1 ± 1.6

*Groups D and F are significantly different (p<0.05) from
Group A.   Groups E and G are not statistically different
from Group A.

DISCUSSION

The results presented in this paper indicate that there are
present in the chicken thymus subsets of cells which can regulate
peripheral T cell functions. Such cells can either help or
suppress these immunological activities, depending on the experimental system used to detect them. This can be taken as an
indication that there are probably at least two separate subpopulations of cells responsible for the two phenomena. Other data
which support this postulate include the apparent greater sensitivity of suppressor cells to embryonic bursectomy, the ability
to remove suppressor cells by passage of thymocytes through a
glass wool column, and the different ontogenetic histories of the
cells.

Previous investigations on suppressor cells in birds have focused primarily on their activity during antibody or immuno-globulin formation. Droege and his collaborators (16, 17) have characterized a cell population in the thymus which is capable of depressing the response of immunologically mature birds to several antigens. These cells, although found in the thymus, are absent in bursectomized animals and may, therefore, be B cells. That there are T cells which can act as suppressors has been indicated in the study of several phenomena exemplified by the infectious agammaglobulinemia of Blaese and co-workers (18). In this system, lymphoid cells from birds hormonally bursectomized can transfer the lesion to normal, sublethally irradiated recipients. The cells responsible for this transfer are sensitive to anti- T cell antisera.

Suppressor cells for T cell mediated immune mechanisms have previously been demonstrated in only one system: the rejection of skin allografts (14). The present study extends this observa-tion to two other phenomena--graft-versus-host reactivity and blastogenic response to the T cell mitogen PHA. In addition, some evidence is presented which indicates that there may be synergistic interactions between two types of thymus-derived lymphocytes at least during PHA stimulation. It will be of interest to determine if a similar mechanism might be operative in other immunological responses.

Speculation on the nature of the cell type responsible for the suppressive activity reported here might be somewhat prema-ture. The cell or cells are most plentiful in the thymus, al-though there is a definite requirement for the presence of the bursa at some stage of their development. This latter fact as well as the nylon wool column data suggest that these cells are B cells which have taken up residence in the thymus. Alternatively, the cells could be of the macrophage-monocyte series; however, this appears less likely since this cell line has never previously been shown to be bursal dependent. The definitive identification of the cells must wait for the development of more clearly defined antisera.

REFERENCES

1. Allison, A. C., Contemp. Top. Immunobiol., 3: 171 (1974).

2. Basten, A., Miller, J. F. A. P. and Johnson, P., Transplant. Rev., 26: 130 (1975).

3. Dutton, R. W., Transplant. Rev., 26: 39 (1975).

4.   Singhal, S. K. and Sinclair, N. R. (eds.), Suppressor Cells
     in Immunity (University of Western Ontario Press, London,
     Ontario, Canada, 1975).

5.   Gershon, R. K., Contemp. Top. Immunobiol., 3: 1 (1974).

6.   Katz, D. H., Prog. Immunol., 2(3): 77 (1974).

7.   Tada, T., Taniguchi, M. and Takemori, T., Transplant. Rev.,
     26: 106 (1975).

8.   Pierce, C. W. and Kapp, J. A., Contemp. Top. Immunobiol., 5:
     91 (1976).

9.   Moore, M. A. S. and Owens, J. J. T., J. Exp. Med., 126: 715
     (1967).

10. Le Dourain, N. M. and Jotereau, F. V., J. Exp. Med., 142: 17
     (1975).

11. Hemmingson, E. J. and Linna, T. J., Int. Arch. Allergy Appl.
     Immunol., 42: 693 (1972).

12. Baba, T. and Kita, M., Immunology, 32: 271 (1977).

13. Eskola, T. and Toivanen, A., Cell. Immunol., 26: 68 (1976).

14. Droege, W., Proc. Natl. Acad. Sci. U.S.A., 72: 2371 (1975).

15. Van Alten, P. J., Cain, W. A., Good R. A. and Cooper, M. D.,
     Nature, 217: 358 (1968).

16. Droege, W., Nature, 234: 549 (1971).

17. Droege, W., Eur. J. Immunol., 3: 804 (1973).

18. Blaese, R. M., Weiden, P. L., Koski, I. and Dooley, N., J.
     Exp. Med., 140: 1097 (1974).

INHERITED IMMUNODEFICIENCY IN CHICKENS: A MODEL FOR COMMON VARIABLE HYPOGAMMAGLOBULINEMIA IN MAN?

A.A. Benedict, H.A. Abplanalp* L.W. Pollard and L.Q. Tam

Dept. of Microbiology, University of Hawaii, Honolulu,

Hawaii 96822, and Dept. of Avian Sciences* University of

California, Davis, California 95616

INTRODUCTION

In 1974 we observed several sera from chickens from two particular families of hybrids which by immunoelectrophoresis (IE) had greatly reduced 7S Ig (low molecular weight immunoglobulin). Some of these sera also had elevated amounts of 17S Ig (high molecular weight immunoglobulin) and will be referred to as dysgammaglobulinemic. Examples of abnormal IE patterns observed are shown in Fig. 1.

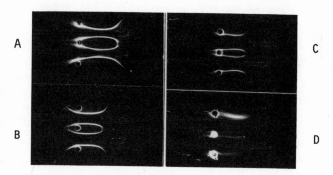

Figure 1. Immunoelectrophoretic patterns of serum from a (a) normal bird; (b) dysgammaglobulinemic bird (high 17S and no 7S Ig); (c) dysgammaglobulinemic bird; (d) hypogammaglobulinemic bird (greatly reduced 7S and 17S Ig).

Soon after we began our studies on characterization of the immunodeficiency we realized that we were dealing with an inherited dysgammaglobulinemia similar to that described by Brüggemann, et al. (1-3)
and Lösch et al. (4-7).

In this report we describe an inherited immunodeficiency characterized by a 7S Ig deficiency which occurs after several weeks
of normal 7S Ig synthesis, and is often accompanied by increased 17S
Ig. Some of the characteristics of this disease in chickens resemble those of inherited, common variable ("acquired" or "late onset") immunodeficiency in humans (8-10).

                              INHERITANCE

        Three experimental highly inbred lines, UCD 2, UCD 3, and UCD
7, which had been propagated exclusively by full-sib matings over
16 generations, were crossed in 1973 to produce F_1 progenies designated as follows:

      1972   1973   1974   1975   1976

UCD 2 x UCD 3 $\longrightarrow$ F_1-140 $\longrightarrow$ F_2-140 $\longrightarrow$ F_3-140 $\longrightarrow$

UCD 7 x UCD 3 $\longrightarrow$ F_1-142 $\longrightarrow$ F_2-142 $\longrightarrow$ F_3-142 $\longrightarrow$ F_4

The F_2 and F_3 generations, as well as crosses among the F_3 progeny
(140 x 142), served as the basis of the partial genetic analysis of
the immunodeficiency in 1976.

        The first abnormal birds, as demonstrated by IE, were observed
in a male (5266) in line 142 (3 x 7 origin) F_2 generation and in a
hen (6561) in line 140 (3 x 2 origin). If a single gene was involved, it most likely originated in line 3 in 1971 where a single
male (7047) appears to be the ancestor for all subsequent matings.
The fact that an abnormal male appeared in the F_2 generation of line
142 rules out sex linkage of a possible single gene.

        A mating between two abnormal birds was performed in 1974, but
egg production of the hen was very sporadic, and all three chicks
hatched from her died before 8 weeks of age. In 1975, line 140 was
propagated by full-sib matings of normal birds, and an abnormal male
(4275) was produced. In line 142 three affected females appeared
among offspring of a cousin mating, and one female (line 140) appeared from a brother x sister mating in a previously affected
family.

        In order to test the hypothesis of a single gene control of
the defect by a recessive gene, the abnormal male (4275) was mated
in 1975 with available abnormal hens (102, 105, 1408), as well as

several normal sisters of affected birds. Matings of normal brothers
and sisters of abnormal birds also were made. In addition, male
4275 was backcrossed to three normal UCD 3 females.

Among the families produced in 1976 from abnormal male 4275
with abnormal hens, abnormal offspring were frequent, as judged by
IE analysis and by quantitative determination of 7S and 17S Ig by
radial immunodiffusion (11). Matings of the same cock with normal
sisters of abnormal birds also produced abnormal offspring without
exception, but at a lower overall incidence than matings involving
only abnormal parents. A relatively high incidence of immunodeficient offspring also was obtained from matings of "normal" sibs
from abnormal parents. Surprisingly, two of the backcrosses in
line 3 produced abnormal offspring even though none were previously
diagnosed abnormal among tested individuals of line 3 itself.

These findings show the immunodeficiency to be highly heritable but do not allow definite conclusions about the exact mode of
inheritance. The occurrence of affected birds in backcrosses to
line 3 suggests genetic control by one or more genes with additive
action but variable penetrance. Incomplete penetrance of a possible major additive gene is also indicated by the lack of families
without normals among matings of abnormal parents. However, hetero-
zygosity of the latter for an additive gene could also be a cause
of this finding. Taken together, the breeding data must be judged
inadequate for a final conclusion about the mode of gene action and
the possible level of penetrance for the observed abnormality.

IMMUNOGLOBULIN CONCENTRATIONS

Sera from 217 offspring from the 1976 generation were examined
by IE, and 89 were judged abnormal. The 7S and 17S Ig concentrations of 28 of these birds were determined for about one year. For
about the first 40 days after hatching it has not been possible to
diagnose the deficiency by IE or radial immunodiffusion. As shown
in Fig. 2, the levels of both 7S and 17S Ig during this period were
about the same as the Ig levels for normal control birds. However,
after this time the 7S Ig concentrations of some birds decreased and
were then followed at about 50-60 days of age by a distinctive dysgammaglobulinemia (Fig. 2). Based on the mean values (Fig. 2), the
7S Ig concentrations increased between 100-150 days and continued
to increase to reach normal values (5-6 mg/ml) by 250 days. The
17S Ig concentrations also increased and reached levels about 10
times above normal.

The mean values of the Ig concentrations presented in Fig. 2
are somewhat misleading because the patterns of temporal Ig synthesis differed among individual birds, examples of which are shown

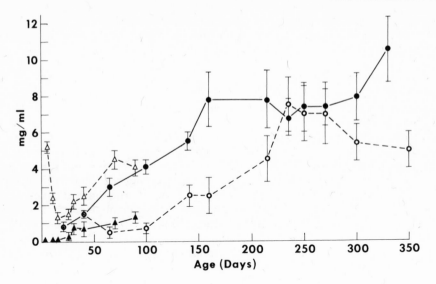

Figure 2. The synthesis of 7S Ig (----) and 17S Ig
(———) in normal outbreds (Δ) and immunodeficient (O)
birds. Values represent the means± S. E. for 10 normal
and 28 immunodeficient birds.

in Fig. 3. In Fig. 3a is a pattern essentially the same as given
by the mean values in Fig. 2; that is, early 7S Ig synthesis is
followed by a shutdown and then a gradual synthesis of 7S Ig over
a period of 200 days. The dysgammaglobulinemia also is similar to
that shown in Fig. 2. Characteristic of a few birds was a hypogammaglobulinemia (greatly reduced concentrations of both 7S and
17S Ig) for the first two months of age (Fig. 3b). Vigorous 7S Ig
synthesis in this bird (Fig. 3b) began between 100-150 days of age,
and reached a level of 33 mg/ml at 267 days of age; the bird died
at 275 days of age. In a few birds no 7S Ig synthesis occurred
except for the early initial burst (Fig. 3c). Fig. 3d shows a
bird which had only 0.6 mg/ml of 7S Ig and almost normal 17S Ig
when the serum was first examined at 100 days of age. After 200
days, 7S Ig synthesis increased sharply reaching a level of 15
mg/ml; whereas, the 17S Ig remained at a constant level throughout
this time.

Although the patterns of Ig synthesis varied, dysgammaglobulinemia was a prominent finding, similar to that described by
Lösch's group (1-7). In another group of birds hatched in late
1976 from abnormal sires and dams, 45 of 80 birds examined were

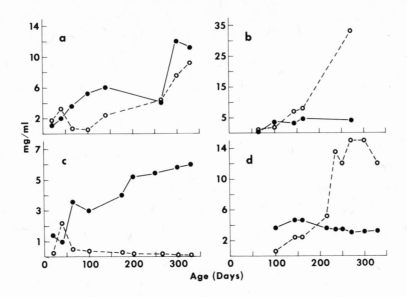

Figure 3.   The synthesis of 7S Ig (O---O) and 17S
Ig (●——●) in individual immunodeficient birds.

dysgammaglobulinemic between 70–100 days of age.

To confirm the finding that the 7S Ig deficiency represents
"late onset", the Ig concentrations of 12 birds from the late 1976
generation were followed at close intervals for two months after
hatching. Some of these birds were capable of synthesizing 7S Ig
for several weeks; however, by 68 days of age the 7S Ig concentrations in most birds were greatly reduced (Fig. 4). Since these
birds were offspring of 7S Ig deficient females, little or no 7S
Ig was of maternal origin; therefore, the presence of 7S Ig during
the first 3 weeks of age represented synthesis by the chicks. Thus,
birds destined to become dysgammaglobulinemic at 70 days of age
(Fig. 4) were capable of early 7S Ig synthesis.

                          AUTOIMMUNITY?

     After several months of age, some birds had greatly increased
7S Ig concentrations (as high as 40 mg/ml) and/or greatly increased
levels of 17S Ig suggesting autoimmune disease, a syndrome seen in
human common variable immunodeficiency (8). To test this possibility, sera from several birds with hypergammaglobulinemia at about
one year of age were examined for "autoimmune" antibodies. In none

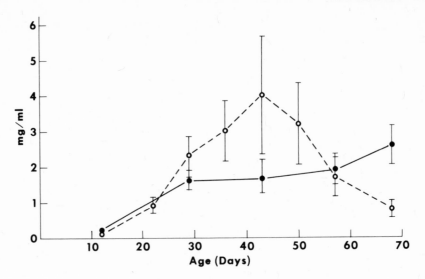

Figure 4. The synthesis of 7S Ig (O---O) and
17S Ig (●——●) in immunodeficient birds. Values
represent the means ± S. E. for 12 birds.

of these sera were anti-thyroglobulin or anti-DNA antibodies found.
No LE cells were observed. Also, their red blood cells were Coombs
reaction negative indicating the absence of acquired hemolytic
anemia at this time. Monitoring for autoimmune disease is being
continued.

    In regards to general health of dysgammaglobulinemic birds,
many were healthy appearing with no apparent illness for an observation period of about one year. However, a few birds with extremely high 17S Ig (20-40 mg/ml) and no or low 7S Ig died or were ill
during this period of time. The chief finding in these birds was
acute infections, particularly of the eyes, caused by staphylococci
and pseudomonas.

                    NATURE OF THE GENETIC DEFECT

    There was no association of the abnormality with sex, 7S Ig
allotypes, or B blood group genotypes (histocompatibility).

    In regards to T lymphocyte function, delayed-type hypersen-
sitivity (wattle reaction) to tuberculin in sensitized dysgammaglobulinemic birds was as intense as in normal birds. Also,

transformation of peripheral lymphocytes by PHA-P yielded stimulation indices no less than those obtained with cells from normal controls (Table 1).

Peripheral lymphocytes responded to the B cell mitogens pokeweed (12) and PPD (13), and to rabbit anti-Fc antibody to the same extents as normal cells. Birds with all variations of Ig concentrations—agammaglobulinemic, dysgammaglobulinemic, and hypergammaglobulinemic—were capable of antibody responses to the synthetic polypeptide polymer, $glu^{60}ala^{30}tyr^{10}$ (GAT), to bovine serum albumin, and to the DNP group. The specific antibody concentrations tended to reflect the total Ig concentrations. Where both 7S and 17S Ig concentrations were low, the amounts of antibody produced were low.

Thus, we have developed an immunodeficient line of chickens similar to that described earlier (1-6), with particular reference to inheritability of the abnormality, variable Ig patterns with dysgammaglobulinemia as a prominent feature, and possibly lowered fertility and hatchability. In addition, we noted that an early normal 7S Ig synthesis often preceded reduced 7S Ig output. Does the defect reside in the stem cells, T cells, B cells, or both the T and B cells? Our preliminary studies seem to rule out defective stem cells and T cells with certain functions. Development of DHS, stimulation of peripheral lymphocytes with T cell mitogens, and antibody responses to GAT—which behaves as a T-dependent antigen (14)—suggest either an intrinsic B cell defect and/or a suppression of Ig synthesis by extrinsic factors. B cell defects could occur at various steps in the maturation pathway. Although peripheral lymphocytes were stimulable with B cell mitogens and rabbit anti-Fc, we do not know whether such stimulated cells were capable of normal 7S Ig synthesis if obtained during the period of reduced 7S Ig synthesis. The fact that normal 7S Ig synthesis occurred early after hatching, followed by reduced synthesis, and then greatly elevated Ig synthesis after several months in some birds, suggests a disturbed regulatory mechanism as a factor in the defect. Despite

Table 1. Stimulation of peripheral lymphocytes from immunodeficient and normal chickens as measured by uptake of ^{3}H-thymidine in vitro.

	Stimulation index (means ± S.E.)			
	PHA-P	PWM	PPD	aFc
Normals	119 ± 6.5	41 ± 3.8	23 ± 2.9	3 ± 0.3
Abnormals	104 ± 16.1	37 ± 5.3	24 ± 6.2	4 ± 0.5

the extreme variability of 7S Ig levels shown by individual birds, the transformation of peripheral 7S Ig bearing cells from some birds by anti-chicken Fc antibody was the same. Furthermore, stimulation of B cells from such animals by PPD and PWM was not different. These findings also suggest an impaired regulatory system.

Suppressor cells, presumably T cells, are generated in chickens rendered agammaglobulinemic by bursectomy (BX) as revealed by immunodeficiency in birds which had been adoptively transferred with BX donor cells (15-17). However, the immunodeficiency in BX birds probably is due to the removal of the B cell generating organ and not to suppression by regulatory cells. In the dysgamma-globulinemic birds of Lösch and Hoffman-Fezer (6), there were no histological signs of either bursal or thymus defects. If the inherited defect proves to be an abnormality of regulatory cells (T?) rather than solely an intrinsic B cell defect, it may be that we are dealing with an immunodeficiency disease(s) similar to human common variable hypogammaglobulinemia in which suppressor cells have been implicated (18,19). Work is in progress to determine this possibility.

ACKNOWLEDGEMENTS

This work was supported by United States Public Health Service Grant AI05660. We are grateful for the capable technical assistance of Philip Morrow and Ms. Jean Reid, University of California, Davis, and for the splendid cooperation of Dr. Noel Rose, Wayne State School of Medicine, for anti-thyroglobulin antibody determinations; of Sam Perry, Dept. of Comparative Medicine, University of Hawaii, for LE cell examinations; and of Leslie Chock for the Coombs reactions.

REFERENCES

1. Brüggemann, J., Merkenschlager, M., Kircher, B. and Lösch, U., Naturwissenschaften, 54: 97 (1967).

2. Brüggemann, J., Friedrich, B. and Lösch, U., Heuhner. Z. Tierphysiol., 24: 317 (1969).

3. Brüggemann, J., Friedrich, B., Lösch, U. and Schmid, D. O., Z. Immun.-Forsch., 141: 280 (1971).

4. Lösch, U., Friedrich, B. and Hoffmann-Fezer, G., Tierärztl. Umschau, 26: 338 (1971).

5. Lösch, U., Hartmann, W. and Riedel, G., Z. Immun. Forsch, 113: 16, (1972).

6. Lösch, U. and Hoffmann-Fezer, G., Huehner. Zbl. Vet. Med. A.,
    20: 596 (1973).

7. Hoffmann-Fezer, G. and Lösch, U. Zbl. Vet. Med. A., 20: 586
    (1973).

8. Park, B. H. and Good, R. A., Principles of Modern Immunobiolo-
    gy (Lea and Febiger, publishers, Philadelphia, 1974).

9. Choi, Y. S., Biggar, W. D. and Good, R. A., Lancet, 1: 1149
    (1972).

10. Gajl-Peczalska, K. J., Park, B. H., Biggar, D. W. and Good,
    R. A., J. Clin. Invest., 52: 919 (1973).

11. Mancini, G., Carbonara, A. O. and Heremans, J. F., Immuno-
    chemistry, 2: 235 (1965).

12. Weber, W. T., Cell. Immunol., 9: 482 (1973).

13. Tufveson, G. and Alm, G. V., Immunology, 29: 697 (1975).

14. Benedict, A. A., Pollard, L. W. and Maurer, P. H., Immuno-
    genetics, 4: 199 (1977).

15. Blaese, R. M., Weiden, P. L., Koski, I. and Dooley, N. J.,
    Exp. Med., 140: 1097 (1974).

16. Grebenau, M. D., Lerman, S. P., Alladino, M. A. and Thorbecke,
    G. J., Nature, 260: 46 (1976).

17. Palladino, M. A., Lerman, S. P. and Thorbecke, G. J., J.
    Immunol., 116: 1673 (1976).

18. Waldmann, T. A., Broder, S., Blaese, R. M., Durm, M., Blackman,
    M. and Strober, W., Lancet, 2: 609 (1974).

19. Waldmann, T. A., Broder, S., Krakauer, R., MacDermott, R. P.,
    Durm, M., Goldman, C. and Meade, B. Fed. Proc., 35: 2067 (1976).

Major Histocompatibility Complex

ISOLATION AND PARTIAL CHARACTERIZATION OF THE MAJOR HISTOCOMPATI-

BILITY ANTIGEN IN THE CHICKEN

R. T. Kubo, K. Yamaga and H. A. Abplanalp*

National Jewish Hospital & Research Center, Denver, Co.
80206 and the *Department of Avian Sciences, University
of California, Davis, California 95616

INTRODUCTION

In a number of mammalian species it is well documented that
the immune responses to a variety of antigens are controlled by the
major histocompatibility gene complex (1-4). Several laboratories
have recently shown that in the chicken as in mammals, the major
histocompatibility complex controls various immune responses (5-10).
These observations have resulted in increasing efforts in the study
of the structure and in the elucidation of the function of the major
histocompatibility complex and its various gene products.

This laboratory has been involved with the characterization of
a variety of lymphocyte membrane macromolecules, among these membrane immunoglobulins β_2-microglobulin (β_2m), and the major histocompatibility antigens in man and mouse. Recently we have undertaken a phylogenetic approach to the study of β_2m and the major
histocompatibility antigens to evaluate the generality of the
structure of major histocompatibility antigens in evolution. In
this report we present some of our studies on the characterization
of the B locus antigen of the chicken.

MATERIALS AND METHODS

Erythrocytes and lymphocytes were isolated from peripheral
blood of inbred line-2 chickens (genotype B/6/B/6) (University of
California at Davis). Lymphocytes were purified by the method described by Noble et al (11). Antisera against the B6 antigens were
raised by cross-immunization with whole blood as previously
described (12). Normal chicken serum or alloantisera to B antigens

209

of different genotypes (e.g., B2) were used as control reagents.
A rabbit anti-chicken red blood cell reagent was included in some
experiments.

To characterize the B locus antigen, the technique of the
lactoperoxidase-catalyzed radioiodination of membrane proteins of
viable cells was employed (13,14). In brief, radiolabeled cells
were lysed with a nonionic detergent, NP-40. Following centrifugation to remove nuclei and other debris, aliquots of the lysate were
treated with specific and control alloantiserum. Immunoprecipitation was accomplished by the indirect technique using a goat anti-
chicken immunoglobulin reagent. Lysates from radiolabeled leucocytes were first treated with rabbit anti-chicken immunoglobulin
and goat anti-rabbit IgG. Following the removal of this immune
precipitate to deplete any radioiodinated membrane-bound-immuno-
globulin, the supernatants were then treated with alloantisera.
Washed immune precipitates were analyzed by sodium dodecyl sulfate-
polyacrylamide gel electrophoresis (SDS-PAGE) (15).

Leucocytes were also metabolically labeled with ^{3}H-leucine in
short-term cultures (6 to 8 hrs) essentially as described for human
lymphocytes (16). Labeled cells were washed three times and lysed
with NP-40. Labeled lysates were treated as for surface labeled
lysates described above.

RESULTS AND DISCUSSION

The SDS-PAGE pattern of a whole radiolabeled lysate of surface
labeled line-2 erythrocyte is shown in Figure 1. The major peak of
radioactivity of the lysate corresponds to a molecular weight of
about 150,000 daltons. Several minor peaks of radioactivity with
molecular weights in the range of 10,000 to 60,000 daltons are also
discernible. The low molecular weight region between 10,000 and
20,000 daltons appears to contain several polypeptides. In contrast, the pattern of a specific immune precipitate obtained with
an alloanti-line-2 antiserum shows three peaks which are not seen
in the pattern of the control anti-line-3 immune precipitates
(Fig. 2). The peaks correspond to molecular weights of approximately 45,000, 35,000 and 11,000 daltons, respectively. Similar
patterns are seen whether the immune precipitates are analyzed in
the reduced or unreduced state. The 45,000 and 11,000 dalton polypeptides correspond to the sizes of the subunits of mammalian major
histocompatibility antigens (13,17). The peak in the 35,000 dalton
region may represent a minor red cell histocompatibility antigen
specificity, since as shown below, this peak is not readily seen in
the anti-line-2 immune precipitates of leucocytes. Absorptions of
the alloantiserum with white cells have not yet been performed to
verify this.

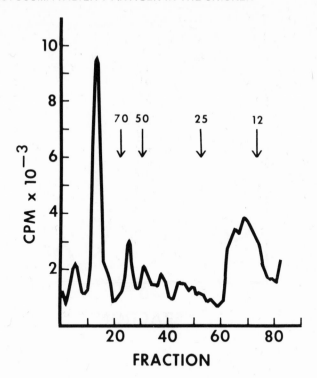

Fig. 1. SDS-polyacrylamide (7.5%) gel electrophoresis of $[^{125}I]$ surface labeled chicken red blood cell lysate. Positions of molecular weight marker proteins are indicated by arrows. Numbers above the arrows represent molecular weight x 10^{-3}.

If the 45,000 dalton and 11,000 dalton peaks truly represented the subunit structure of the chicken B locus antigen, the chicken major histocompatibility antigen would indeed be structurally similar to the mammalian major histocompatibility antigens. Furthermore, if the specific activity of labeling of the two polypeptide chains were equal, there would be approximately three to four times more radioactivity in the 45,000 dalton material compared to the 11,000 dalton component. The heavy to light chain ratios calculated from the gel patterns range from 5-6:1. In man, the comparable ratio of HL-A to β_2m is about 1.7-2:1 (Kubo, unpublished

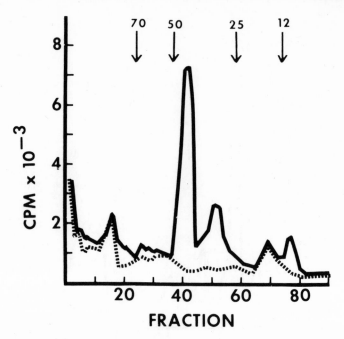

Fig. 2. SDS-polyacrylamide (7.5%) gel electrophoresis of reduced immune precipitates of $[^{125}I]$ cell lysate of line-2 erythrocytes. Solid line: specific anti-line-2 immune precipitate. Broken line: control anti-line-3 immune precipitate. Positions of molecular weight marker proteins are indicated by arrows. Numbers above the arrows represent molecular weight x 10^{-3}.

observations). The high 45,000 dalton to 11,000 dalton ratio may reflect differences in iodination of the two polypeptide chains or it may be due to the fact that the alloantiserum upon combination with the B locus antigen results in the dissociation of some of the 11,000 dalton polypeptide as had been observed in some cases with the reactivity of anti-HL-A reagents with the HL-A-β_2m complex.

We do not have a reagent directed toward chicken β_2m, but this reagent should be useful in determining which of the possibilities is most probable. Of some interest in this regard, the reactivity of a rabbit antiserum to chicken red blood cells has been evaluated.

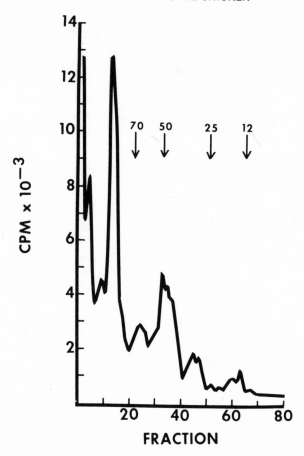

Fig. 3.   SDS-polyacrylamide (7.5%) gel electrophoresis of a reduced rabbit anti-chicken red blood cell immune precipitate of [125I] cell lysate of line-2 erythrocytes.   Positions of molecular weight are indicated by arrows.   Numbers above the arrows represent molecular weight x 10-3.

The rabbit anti-red cell reagent immune precipitate shows a pattern very similar to that of the whole red cell lysate (Fig. 3 compared to Fig. 1).   The major reactivity is in the 150,000 dalton region

and several minor peaks which differ quantitatively from the whole
lysate pattern are also observed. The peaks in the 10,000 to
20,000 dalton region seen in the whole lysate (Fig. 1) apparently
are not reactive with the anti-red cell reagent. There appear
to be at least 2 to 3 components detected in the 40,000 to 50,000
dalton region. One of these, as will be shown below, corresponds
to the B antigen. In the 11,000 dalton region, there is very little
if any, discernible reactivity.

The reactivity of various reagents directed toward the
mammalian major histocompatibility structures was tested on radiolabeled chicken erythrocyte lysates. These included a rabbit anti-
human β_2m, rabbit anti-HL-A, rabbit anti-H2, goat and anti-rabbit
β_2m, and goat anti-human β_2m. All of these reagents do not show
any greater reactivity by immunoprecipitation over normal serum controls, nor by SDS-PAGE analysis. Thus, the extent of crossreactivity, if any, that may exist between the avian and mammalian
major histocompatibility antigens must be low, perhaps in keeping
with the lack of crossreactivity with other evolutionarily-related
proteins; e.g., immunoglobulins.

The reactivity of the alloanti-line-2 antiserum with surface
proteins of peripheral blood leucocytes of line-2 chickens is shown
in Figure 4(top). In this SDS-PAGE pattern, only 2 peaks of radioactivity with molecular weights of 45,000 daltons and 11,000 daltons
are obtained with the anti-line-2 antiserum whereas the anti-line 3
antiserum (a control) shows no discernible peaks. Furthermore, no
radioactive peak is seen in the 35,000 dalton region as had been
seen in the specific immune precipitates of labeled erythrocyte
lysates. The pattern obtained for the chicken B locus antigen on
the surface of lymphocytes is strikingly similar to the patterns we
have obtained for the HL-A and H2 antigens in man and mouse, respectively (13,17). The ratio of radioactivity of the 45,000 dalton
peak to the 11,000 dalton peak is again in the range of 5:1. A
similar profile is obtained from peripheral leucocytes which were
biosynthetically labeled with ^{3}H-leucine(Fig.4 (bottom)). The similarity in profiles and ratios of 45,000 and 11,000 dalton material
suggests that there is not a preferential labeling of the 45,000
dalton component to the 11,000 dalton component in the surface
labeling technique. Biochemical comparisons of the polypeptide subunits of the chicken and mammalian major histocompatibility antigens
may yield answers to this question.

Finally, some preliminary data on the further comparison of
the avian and mammalian histocompatibility antigens using a two-
dimensional polyacrylamide gel electrophoretic technique are presented. Briefly, the method involves the separation of polypeptides
based on molecular size using the SDS-PAGE techniques of Laemmli (18)
or Maizel (15) in the first dimension. The separation in the second

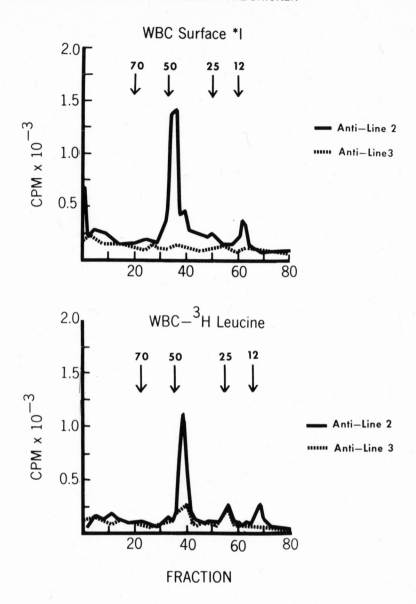

Fig. 4.   SDS-polyacrylamide (7.5%) gel electrophoresis of reduced immune precipitates of labeled cell lysate of line-2 peripheral blood leucocytes. Immune precipitates of specific anti-line-2 allo-antiserum (solid line) and control anti-line-3 alloantiserum (broken line) from [125I] surface labeled leucocyte lysate (top) or biosynthetically labeled (3H-leucine) leucocyte lysate (bottom).

dimension is based primarily on the charge of molecules. For this
purpose, a modified alkaline urea gel system (19) which incorporates
a nonionic detergent, Triton CF-10, to facilitate the dissociation
of SDS from the protein, allowing for the separation based on charge
differences is employed. Specific details of this method are
presented elsewhere (20).

When normal human IgG is analyzed by this technique, the pattern shown in Figure 5 is seen. Similar to the analysis of this
protein by the alkaline urea gel technique of Reisfeld and Small
(19), there is a heterogeneity observed in the immunoglobulin light
chains. The immunoglobulin heavy chains do not, however, display
the same extent of charge heterogeneity. In Figure 6A is shown the
pattern of the HL-A antigens of human tonsil lymphocytes. The β_2m
subunit is not readily discernible in this pattern. The HL-A polypeptides are resolved into two spots. It is not known at present
whether these components may represent the **HL-A A and B locus**
products or an indication of genetic polymorphism in both.

Analysis of the chicken erythrocyte B locus antigen immune
precipitate by the two-dimensional gel technique is shown in Figure
6B. A major spot is seen in the 45,000 dalton region. The minor
spots with the same molecular size range are seen in control precipitates and are presumably non-B locus specificities. The anti-
red cell pattern, shown in Figure 6C, shows a greater number of
spots including a spot in the same position of the B6 antigen.
Several other spots with a molecular weight of 45,000 daltons are
also discernible. Thus among the specificities recognized by the
heterologous anti-red cell antiserum is the chicken major histocompatibility antigen. Figure 6D shows the two-dimensional pattern
of the leucocyte membrane B6 antigen. Only a single spot is seen
suggesting a more restricted heterogeneity in the chicken major
histocompatibility antigen as compared to the human HL-A antigens.

In summary, the B locus antigen from the surface of chicken
erythrocytes and leucocytes have been characterized. The data show
that the major histocompatibility antigen in the chicken is structurally similar to the major histocompatibility antigens in the
mammals. Both are comprised of two polypeptide chains with molecular weights of 45,000 and 11,000 daltons held together by noncovalent bonds. Ziegler and Pink have reached a similar conclusion in
their studies on the characterization of the B locus antigen from
biosynthetically labeled leucocytes (21). The B antigens on the
surface of red cells and of leucocytes appear to be identical. If
the major histocompatibility antigens are expressed on the red blood
cells in lower vertebrate species, methodologies developed to isolate the B locus products from chicken red blood cells may allow for
the further phylogenetic evaluation of the structure of major
histocompatibility antigens in the lower vertebrates.

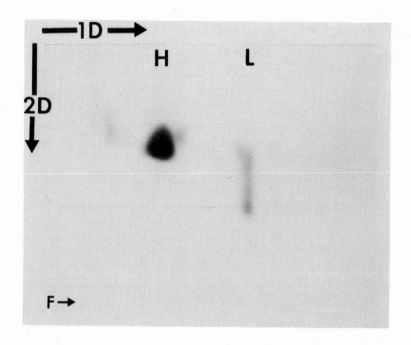

Fig. 5.   Autoradiograph of a two-dimensional separation of normal
human IgG.   Radioiodinated human IgG was separated into heavy and
light chains in an SDS-containing 10% polyacrylamide gel in the
first dimension.   The directions of the electrophoretic migration
are shown by arrows and "1D" and "2D", for the first and second
dimensional directions, respectively.   H and L represent the
positions of the IgG heavy and light chains, respectively.   The
marker dye (bromophenol blue) front indicating the extent of
migration in the second dimension electrophoresis is shown on the
left of the figure by an arrow and "F".

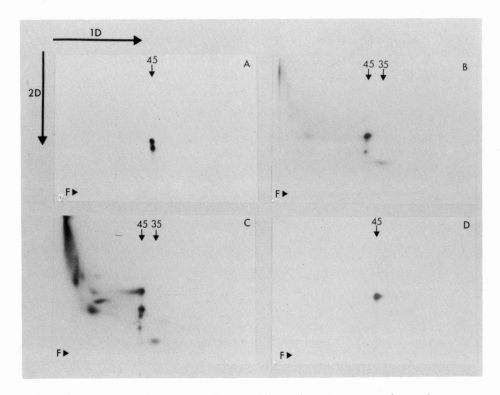

Fig. 6.   Autoradiographs of two-dimensional separation of:
A. anti-HL-A immune precipitate of surface labeled human tonsil
lymphocyte lysate; B.   anti-line-2 immune precipitate of surface
labeled line-2 erythrocytes; C. rabbit anti-chicken red blood
cell immune precipitate of surface labeled line-2 erythrocytes;
and D.   anti-line-2 immune precipitate of surface labeled line-2
peripheral blood leucocytes. The directions of the electrophoretic
migration are shown by arrows and "1D" and "2D", for the first and
second dimensional directions, respectively. The extent of migration in the second dimension is indicated by an arrow and "F". The
numbers and arrows at the top of each figure indicate the position
of various molecular weight regions (x 10^{-3}).

ACKNOWLEDGEMENTS

The authors thank Dr. H.M. Grey for his critical review of this manuscript. The patience and secretarial assistance of Charlene Griffiths are gratefully acknowledged. We thank Shelley M. Gordon for the goat anti-rabbit β_2m reagents.

This study was supported by NIH Grant AI-12136, American Heart Association Grant 74856 and NIH Research Fellowship AI-05334.

REFERENCES

1. Benacerraf, B. and McDevitt, H. O., Science, 175: 273 (1972).

2. Munro, A. J. and Taussig, M. J., Nature, 256: 103 (1975).

3. Shreffler, D. C. and David, C. S., Adv.Immunol., 20: 125 (1975).

4. Green, I., Immunogenetics, 1: 4 (1974).

5. Günther, E., Balcarova, J., Hála, K., Rüde, E. and Hraba, T., Eur. J. Immunol., 4: 548 (1974).

6. Longenecker, B. M., Pazderka, F., Law, G. R. J., and Ruth, R. F., Transplantation, 14: 424 (1972).

7. Miggiano, V. C., Birgen, I., Pink, J. R. L., Eur. J. Immunol., 4: 397 (1974).

8. Simonsen, M., Acta Pathol. Microbiol. Scand. C , 83: 1 (1975).

9. Benedict, A. A., Pollard, L. W., Morrow, P. R., Abplanalp, H. A., Maurer, P. H. and Briles, W. E., Immunogenetics, 2: 313 (1975).

10. Benedict, A. A. and Pollard, L. W., In Immunologic Phylogeny, Advances in Experimental Medicine and Biology (W. H. Hildemann and A. A. Benedict, Eds.), Plenum Publishing Corporation, New York and London), 64: 421 (1975).

11. Noble, P. B., Cutts, J. H. and Carroll, K. K., Blood, 31: 66 (1968).

12. Morrow, P. R., M.S. Thesis, University of California, Davis (1974).

13. Grey, H. M., Kubo, R. T., Colon, S. M., Poulik, M. D.,
     Cresswell, P., Springer, T., Turner, M. and Strominger, J. L.,
     J. Exp. Med., 138: 1608, (1973).

14. Vitetta, E. S., Bauer, S. and Uhr, J. W., J. Exp. Med.,
     134: 242 (1971).

15. Maizel, J. V., Jr., In Methods in Virology, 5: 179
     (K. Maramorsch and H. Kaprowski, Eds.), (Academic Press,
     New York, 1971).

16. Maino, V. C., Kurnick, J. T., Kubo, R. T. and Grey, H. M.,
     J. Immunol., (In press) (1977).

17. Kubo, R. T., Colon, S. M., McCalmon, R. T. and Grey, H. M.,
     Fed. Proc., 35: 1183 (1976).

18. Laemmli, U. K., Nature, 227: 680 (1970).

19. Reisfeld, R. A. and Small, P. A., Jr., Science, 152: 1253
     (1966).

20. Imada, M., Hsieh, P. and Sueoka, N., (Manuscript in
     preparation).

21. Ziegler, A. and Pink, J.R.L., Transplantation, 20: 523 (1975).

SOME RECENT RECOMBINANTS AT THE B LOCUS

W. Elwood Briles and Ruth W. Briles

Dept. of Biological Sciences, Northern Ill. University

DeKalb, Illinois 60115

INTRODUCTION

The multi-locus nature of the major histocompatibility complex in the mouse and in man has been well established (1,2). The association of the major histocompatibility complex of the chicken with immune response to specific antigens (3), complement activity (4), and susceptibility to Marek's Disease (5,6), has heightened interest in the genetic nature of the B chromosomal region of this species. From functional and evolutionary standpoints, it would be informative to learn to what extent such multi-locus complexity also characterizes the major histocompatibility system in this phylogenetically more primitive species.

The B system of alloantigens in chickens has generally been presumed to correspond to the H-2 of the mouse and, as such, offers a convenient avian model for study. From the time of first discovery, the B locus has been characterized by extensive multiple allelism, with broad cross-reactivity between antigens produced by the different alleles. Presently, several laboratories are cooperating in an attempt to establish an internationally acceptable terminology for distinguishing the several alleles existing in populations of chickens being utilized experimentally. For this presentation allele designations will be those employed in the original publications and for this report allele designations will be those currently used in our laboratory.

Probable genetic recombinations involving the B system have already been reported in the literature from two other laboratories. In 1969 Schierman and McBride (7) noted the occurrence of unusually rapid

221

skin rejection among a group of recipient-donor pairs matched for compatibility on the basis of B hemagglutination reactions. The exceptional recipient, a female, was originally typed as B^2/B^3, but after investigation she was redesignated B^2/B^4 to indicate the uniqueness of the "new" allele, classified earlier as B^3. Appropriate tests utilizing the cells of the exceptional individual and her progeny showed that the B_4 antigen was reactive with both anti-B_2 and anti-B_3 reagents but would absorb in each case only for the B_4 antigen, leaving reactivity for the respective homologous antigens. Finally, when normal B^2/B^3 heterozygotes received skin from the B^2/B^4 female, the graft was tolerated in a manner characteristic of non-B histocompatibility antigens. Thus, all data presented in this first report were compatible with the aberrant type B^4, having resulted from a recombination between chromosomal segments coding for the B^2 and B^3 alleles.

The second report of a probable recombinant in the B system was in 1975 by Hála, Vilhelmová and Hartmonová (8,9). Three inbred lines CB (B^1/B^1), CC (B^2/B^2), and WB (B^{10}/B^{10}), homozygous for transplantation and erythrocyte antigens were used in a special cross (CC x CB) F_1 x WB to produce B^1/B^{10} and B^2/B^{10} chicks to be grafted with skin from congenic grandparent lines CC and CB. Typical segregation of B^1 and B^2 occurred in all but two of 1,206 chicks resulting from the mating. The erythrocytes of both of these exceptional chicks (males) were agglutinated by both reagents B1 and B2, in addition to B10. One of the males is an exception in several respects and has not been satisfactorily accounted for. The other male, 744, appears to have resulted from crossing over within the region coding for serological determinants, but outside the region coding also for histocompatibility determinants. The latter is evidenced by the ability of the 744 cock to accept a skin graft from line CB (B^1/B^1) but repeatedly reject grafts from CC (B^2/B^2). That the cells of cock 744 possess only a portion of the antigenic determinants characterizing each of the antigens B_1 and B_2 is shown by the ability of B^1/B^{10} and B^2/B^{10} recipients to produce anti-B antibodies against cells from cock 744 or his B^{10}/B^{R1} (recombinant) progeny. Hála, et al. (9) designated the postulated locus determining the SD and H antigens B-F and the other locus determining the other SD antigens B-G.

This paper presents recent observations in our laboratory on recombination of serologically identified determinants of antigens of the B system; these were given earlier in a preliminary report (10).

RECOMBINANTS IN NEW HAMPSHIRE-LEGHORN CROSSES

A male of a strain of new Hampshire chickens was mated to females of White Leghorn inbred line 7_2 from the Regional Poultry Research Laboratory at East Lansing, Michigan. This cross was made

Table 1.   Reactivity of B alloantigens in sire family 532

$\underline{B}$ Genotype		Number of chicks		Reagents		
		(1974)	(1975)	B2	B23	B24
Sire	$\underline{B}^{23}/\underline{B}^{24}$			0	+	+
Dam	$\underline{B}^2/B^2$			+	0	0
Progeny:	$\underline{B}^{23}/\underline{B}^2$	10	54	+	+	0
	$\underline{B}^{24}/\underline{B}^2$	4	66	+	0	+
	$\underline{B}^{23-24}/\underline{B}^{\underline{2}}$	1[a]	1[b]	+	+	+

[a]Recombinant male, (B64883) became sire of 722 family (Table 2).
[b]Female, died when six weeks of age.

to establish a population segregating at the three major loci controlling host-range susceptibility for the respective three major subgroups of leukosis-sarcoma viruses. In the routine typing of the progeny for the eleven systems of erythrocyte alloantigens, it was found that one of the make chicks possessed an aberrant B phenotype (Table 1). The genotype of the New Hampshire sire was known from previous typing and family data to be $\underline{B}^{23}/\underline{B}^{24}$ and several years of continuous typing had established that line 7_2 was uniformly homozygous at the $\underline{B}$ locus and the allele present has been recently determined to be synonomous with $\underline{B}^2$ of the Hy-Line stocks (11,12); direct typing of all dams showed them to be $\underline{B}^2/\underline{B}^2$. Of 15 progeny resulting from this cross in the 1974 breeding season, ten were $\underline{B}^{23}/\underline{B}^2$, four were $\underline{B}^{24}/\underline{B}^2$, while one chick reacted with all three of the typing reagents--B2, B23 and B24--and was presumed to have received from the sire the ability to produce all or part of the antigenic determinants coded for by both $\underline{B}^{23}$ and $\underline{B}^{24}$. This mating was repeated again the next year (1975) using the same sire with a new generation of line 7_2 females; of 121 progeny, 54 were $\underline{B}^{23}/\underline{B}^2$, 66 were $\underline{B}^{24}/\underline{B}^2$ as expected, and again one chick (a female) possessed an aberrant B type apparently identical to that observed previously (Table 1). Unfortunately this chick died at six weeks of age; thus, the genotype of this chick can only be presumed.

That the aberrant chick hatched in 1974 was truly a recombinant is shown by data presented in Table 2. This chick developed into a vigorous male and was mated to line 7_2 females, all confirmed to be $\underline{B}^2/\underline{B}^2$. The two major classes of progeny consisted of 54 whose cells were reactive only with the B2 reagent and 49 whose cells were re-

Table 2. Reactivity of B alloantigens in recombinant sire family 722

B Genotype		Number of chicks	Reagents		
			B2	B23	B24
Sire[a]	$\underline{B}^{23-24}/\underline{B}^2$		+	+	+
Dams	$\underline{B}^2/\underline{B}^2$		+	0	0
Progeny	$\underline{B}^2/B^2$	54	+	0	0
	$\underline{B}^{23-24}/\underline{B}^2$	49	+	+	+
	$\underline{B}^{2-23}/\underline{B}^{2b}$	2	+	+	0

[a]Recombinant male chick, B64883, from sire family 532, Table 1.
[b]Genotype presumed, awaiting definitive genetic data.

active with both B23 and B24 reagents, showing that the sire, B64883, was transmitting an "allele" consisting of specificity-determining elements from both $\underline{B}^{23}$ and $\underline{B}^{24}$, for which his sire had been heterozygous. In addition, two aberrant chicks resulted from this sire, B64883. Both chicks were reactive with the B2 and B23 reagents only, suggesting that the $\underline{B}^{24}$ portion of the recombinant chromosome $\underline{B}^{23-24}$ in the sire had been lost, probably through crossing over with the $\underline{B}^2$ segment. These two chicks presumed to be $\underline{B}^{2-23}/\underline{B}^2$ were found in later tests with a battery of anti-B_{23} antisera to be non-reactive with certain antisera. Parallel non-reactivity was also exhibited by cells from birds of the $\underline{B}^{23-24}/\underline{B}^2$ genotype, as would be expected from their origin. These two chicks are females and are under further immunogenetic analysis.

Whether the recombinant $\underline{B}^{23-24}$ received all or part of $\underline{B}^{23}$ or $\underline{B}^{24}$ was not apparent from the data presented in Tables 1 and 2; two separately produced anti-B_{23} and two separately produced anti-B_{24} antisera were used as reagents in typing all progeny, with parallel results. To obtain data bearing on the complete or partial presence of the $\underline{B}^{23}$ and $\underline{B}^{24}$ specificities, chickens of the $\underline{B}^{23-24}/\underline{B}^2$ genotype were immunized with $\underline{B}^{23}/\underline{B}^2$ or $\underline{B}^{24}/\underline{B}^2$ blood. Several such recipients produced anti-B antibodies against their respective B-donor antigens, showing that the recipient genotype, $\underline{B}^{23-24}/\underline{B}^2$ failed to code for at least a portion of the specificity determinants characterizing $\underline{B}^{23}$ and those characterizing $\underline{B}^{24}$.

Currently, graft-versus-host reaction is being employed in an

effort to determine the histocompatibility interrelationships between
the recombinant $\underline{B}^{23-24}$ and the original alleles $\underline{B}^{23}$ and $\underline{B}^{24}$. In
spite of the wide array of histocompatibility antigens besides B
likely to be segregating in these stocks, we anticipate being able
to utilize at least the $\underline{B}^{23-24}$ recombinant in studies relating to
the B-F and B-G subregions of Hála, Vilhelmová, and Hartmanová (9)
and the $\underline{B}$ sublocus $\underline{AA}$ of Simonsen (13) controlling **allo-aggression.**

REFERENCES

1. Klein, Jan. Biology of the Mouse Histocompatibility-2 Complex.
    620 pp. (Springer-Verlag, New York, 1975).

2. Thorsby, E. Transplant. Rev. 8: 51 (1974).

3. Benedict, A. A., Pollard, L. W., Morrow, P. R., Abplanalp, H. A.,
    Maurer, P. H. and Briles, W. E. Immunogenetics 2: 313 (1975).

4. Chanh, T. C., Benedict, A. A. and Abplanalp, H. A. J. Exptl.
    Med. 144: 555 (1976).

5. Longenecker, B. M., Pazderka, F., Gavora, J. S., Spencer, L.,
    Stevens, E. A., Witter, R. L. and Ruth, R. F. in this conference.

6. Stone, H. A., Briles, W. E. and McGibbon, W. H. in this
    conference.

7. Schierman, L. W. and McBride, R. A. Transplantation 8: 515
    (1969).

8. Hála, K., Vilehlmová, M. and Hartmanová, J. In Proceedings of
    XIIIth International Symposium on Laboratory Animals, Hruba
    Skala (1975).

9. Hála, K., Vilhelmová, M. and Hartmanová, J. Immunogenetics
    3: 97 (1976).

10. Briles, W. E. and Briles, R. W. Proceedings of XVth Interna-
    tional Conference on Animal Blood Groups and Biochemical
    Polymorphisms, Dublin, July, 1976.

11. Briles, W. E., Allen, C. P. and Millen, T. W. Genetics 42: 631
    (1957).

12. Pazderka, F., Longenecker, B. M., Law, R. J., Stone, H. A. and
    Ruth, R. F. Immunogenetics 2: 93 (1975).

13. Simonsen, M. Acta Path. Microbiol. Scand. Sec. C, 83: 1 (1975).

THE STRUCTURE OF THE MAJOR HISTOCOMPATIBILITY COMPLEX OF THE CHICKEN

K. Hála, M. Vilhelmová, J. Hartmanová

Institute of Molecular Genetics, Czechoslovak
Academy of Sciences
166 10 Prague 6, Flemingovo nám.2, Czechoslovakia

The major histocompatibility complex (MHC) of the chicken, which had been described as a blood group system (Briles et al. 1950), shortly after its discovery attracted attention of the investigators that the genotype of this genetic system may influence viability, hatchability and a number of economically important traits (Gilmour 1960, Briles 1964). When its importance for skin graft survival (Schierman and Nordskog 1961), graft-versus-host reaction (GVHR, Jaffe and McDermid 1962) and mixed lymphocyte reaction (MLR, Miggiano et al. 1974)was found, studies on the structure of the respective region of the chromosome were initiated (Schierman and McBride 1969, Hála et al. 1975).

The availability of inbred lines of chickens homozygous for transplantation antigens and blood group systems appeared of decisive importance for the study of the structure of the MHC, because the products of the recombinant allele could be analyzed by different methods. Because three different B alleles on the same genetic background were not available, we used F_1 hybrids of two congenic lines, CB and CC, differing only at the B antigen (Hašek et al. 1966). These F_1 hybrids were crossed with another homogeneous line WB. Among progeny of this cross one bird contained the B allele derived from an F_1 hybrid which arose by recombination between the B^1 and B^2 allele. We designated it the B^{RI} allele. Transplantation analysis (Table 1) revealed that antigens responsible for skin graft survival are determined by that part of the chromosome which is derived from the CB line (Hála et al. 1976). The same holds for antigens responsible for GVHR and MLR. On the basis of the results some of which are shown in Table 1, we assume that the respective region of the chromosome was divided into two parts (Figure 1). One part determines the

Table 1. Analysis of the product of recombinant allele B^{Rl}

Genotype in the B system	Serology Reaction with serum against			Skin grafts from^x		to^xx		GVH reaction embryos	
	B1	B2	B10	CB	CC	(CBxWB)F₁	(CCxWB)F₁	(CBxWB)F₁	(CCxWB)F₁
Rl/10	+	+	+	+	–	+	–	–	+
1/10	+	–	+	+	–	+	–	–	+
2/10	–	+	+	–	+	–	+	+	–
Rl/1	+	+	–	+	–	+	NT	NT	NT
Rl/2	+	+	–	+	+	NT	–	NT	NT

+, RBC agglutination
–, no agglutination

x Skin grafts from donors CB and CC onto recipients Rl/10,1/10 etc
xx Skin grafts from donors Rl/10, etc. onto F₁ hybrids
+, grafts surviving for at least 98 days after transplantation.
–, grafts rejected within 10-40 days.
5 – 10 birds in group
NT, not tested

Splenomegaly assessed 5 days after cell injection.
+, spleens enlarged 10 times than controls.
–, spleen weight same as in controls.
NT, not tested

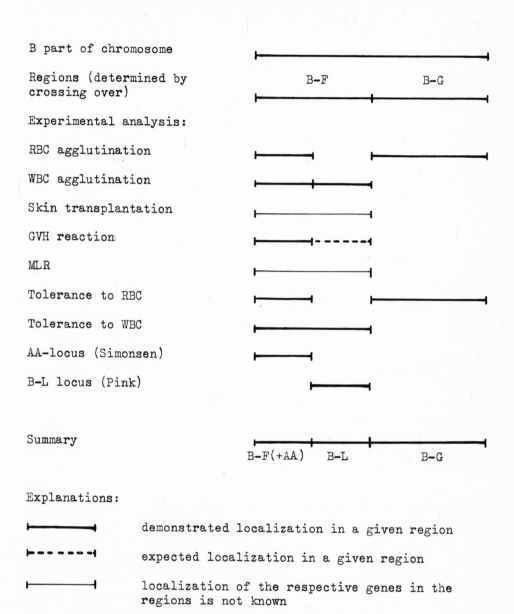

Figure 1. Structure of the MHC of the chicken

antigens capable of eliciting an immune elimination of ^{51}Cr-label-
led red blood cells (RBC) and haemagglutinating antibody formation.
The other part determines, in addition, the antigens capable of
inducing skin graft rejection and a number of other reactions.

The new allele was further studied by genetic analysis. In
the first generation we mated cock 744 with the recombinant allele
to WB, CB and CC hens and examined altogether 142 offspring. The
recombinant allele was present in 78 birds, i.e., in approximately
54% of the total number of birds. In the next generation, these
offspring were mated to CC and CB hens, 126 offspring were examined,
and 54 (approx. 43%) of them contained the B^{R1} allele. In these
two generations no other irregularities were observed. The new
allele B^{R1} is transmitted to the progeny with the genotypic ratio
1:1.

Another antigen within the MHC with a molecular weight of about
30,000 was demonstrated by biochemical analysis (Ziegler and Pink
1976). This antigen, designated B-L, is not present on erythrocytes.
In our experiments with tolerance induction, we demonstrated an
antigen with a similar distribution, i.e., it was present on lymphocytes and absent in erythrocytes. In the system in which the recipient differed from the donor only in the B system (Table 2) we
found that peripheral white blood cells (WBC) were not capable of
inducing tolerance to RBC but they induced tolerance to skin grafts.
Similarly, RBC induce tolerance to RBC only, and this tolerance does
not affect the survival time of skin grafts. Only whole blood
elicits tolerance to both RBC and skin grafts. On the basis of the
work of Ziegler and Pink (1976) and Pink et al. (1977) and our own
results (Table 2), the existence of minimally three loci and three
corresponding antigens can be assumed:

1. Antigens common to WBC and RBC, i.e., antigens determined by the
   B-F region of the chromosome. AA locus antigens belong to this
   group (Simonsen 1973).

2. Antigens present on WBC and absent in RBC, i.e., antigens determined by the B-L region.

3. Antigens present on RBC, which have not yet been demonstrated on
   WBC. These antigens were proved not to have any influence on
   skin graft survival, GVHR and MLR. They are controlled by the
   B-G region.

On the basis of the same molecular weight (Ziegler and Pink
1976) and on the basis of the distribution (Ziegler and Pink 1976,
and Table 2), it can be supposed that B-L antigens and Ia antigens
of the mouse are identical. Yet, the function of these antigens in
chickens is still unclear. If B-L antigens should be responsible
for the GVHR in chickens, as are Ia antigens in mice (Shreffler and
David 1975), then at least two loci within the MHC of the chicken

Table 2. Test of tolerance by means of elimination of allogeneic ^{51}Cr-labelled RBC and skin grafts[a]

Pretreatment	Test by	
	^{51}Cr-labelled RBC of CB	Skin grafts of CB
Whole allogeneic blood (CB)	nonimmune elimination	accepted
Allogeneic RBC (CB)	nonimmune elimination	rejected
Allogeneic WBC (CB)	immune elimination	accepted
Whole syngeneic blood (CCxIC)F$_1$	immune elimination	rejected

[a]The recipients (7-12 birds/group) were (CCxIC)F$_1$ hybrid chickens of the genotype B^2/B^{13}. Tolerance was induced by injecting whole blood or corresponding amounts of RBC or WBC on the day of hatching, and 6 and 12 days after hatching. At 18 days of age tolerance was tested by elimination of ^{51}Cr-labelled RBC and by skin grafts. Tolerance was induced to CB cells, i.e., only to the difference in the MHC (B antigen).

are responsible for GVHR: AA locus antigens (they belong rather to B-F antigens because of their presence on WBC and RBC) and B-L antigens.

It seems that the frequency of recombination in the MHC of chickens is lower than that of the H-2 of mice. In mice the frequency of crossing over between the K and D regions was found to be 0.5%, in chickens one recombinant was found among 1,206 birds typed (Hála et al. 1976). Another difference between the mouse and the chicken MHC is an obvious asymmetry in the arrangement of this complex in chickens. It was found that the B-F region controls antigens responsible for RBC agglutination and skin graft survival, while the B-G region controls only erythrocyte antigens (Hála et al. 1976, Pink et al. 1977). There may be several reasons behind this asymmetry in the arrangement of MHC and at least 5 times lesser frequency of crossing over in chickens compared to the frequency in mice. For example, the MHC of chickens may represent the original state of an ancestor common to mammals and birds before subsequent duplication in mammals occurred (Ziegler and Pink 1976). Further, only serologically defined determinants present on erythrocytes are typed. If the arrangement of the chicken MHC would not correspond to the mouse model, but rather to the human model, then merely serological analysis would not be sufficient to detect all possible recombinants. Another reason may be the similarity (identity) of one chromosome region between the B1 and B2 haplotypes. Both B haplotypes originate from the C line, which was established in 1933. It was since maintained by brother x sister matings. These 2 haplotypes segregated within this line up to 1964. With some 3,000 offspring obtained during this period the chromosome region determining some transplantation antigens might have been exchanged, for example, by crossing over. In this way, identity of that region of the chromosome which lies, for example, opposite to the B-F region, might have been obtained.

Chickens are suitable experimental models for various experiments. The study of the structure of the MHC provides a possibility of investigating the differentiation antigens determined by this complex and the role thereof in immunity.

REFERENCES

Briles, W. E., Tierzüchtung Züchtungsbiol., 79: 371 (1964).

Briles, W. E., McGibbon, W. H. and Irwin, M. R., Genetics, 35: 633 (1950).

Gilmour, D. G., Brit. Poultry Sci., 1: 75 (1960).

Hála, K., Vilhelmová, M. and Hartmanová, J., Folia Biol. (Praha), 21: 363 (1975).

Hála, K., Vilhelmová, M. and Hartmanová, J., J. Immunogenet., 3: 91 (1976).

Hašek, M., Knížetová, F. and Mervartová, H., Folia Biol. (Praha), 12: 335 (1966).

Jaffe, W. P. and McDermid, E. M., Science, 137: 984 (1962).

Miggiano, V. C., Birgen, I. and Pink, J. R. L., Eur. J. Immunol., 4: 397 (1974).

Schierman, L. W. and McBride, R. A., Transplantation, 8: 515 (1969).

Schierman, L. W. and Nordskog, A. W., Science, 134: 1008 (1961).

Shreffler, D. C. and David, C. S. in Adv. Immunol., 20: 125 (1975).

Simonsen, M., J. Immunol., 111: 1607 (1973).

Pink, J. R. L., Droege, W., Hála, K., Miggiano, V. C. and Ziegler, A., Immunogenetics (1977, submitted to publication).

Ziegler, A. and Pink, J. R. L., J. Biol. Chem., 251: 5391 (1976).

IMMUNE RESPONSE GENES IN CHICKENS: THE MULTIFARIOUS RESPONSIVENESS TO (T,G)-A--L

Claus Koch[1], Karel Hála[2] and Per Sørup[1]

[1]Institute for Experimental Immunology
University of Copenhagen
Nørre Alle 71
DK 2loo Ø, Denmark and

[2]Institute of Molecular Genetics
Czechoslovak Academy of Sciences
Flamingovo Nam. 2
Prague

ABSTRACT.   Immune response in chickens to the multi-chain copolymer (T,G)-A--L 2o3o is analysed. Previous work has shown that responsiveness is not linked to the B-complex. Three different antibody specificities could be distinguished. From the data it is proposed that the response to the backbone of (T,G)-A--L (poly-DL-alanine) influences the responses to the side chain determinants (primarily the (T,G)-determinant). Thus the anti-(T,G) response in chickens is determined by at least two different loci, the B-complex, and another, as yet unidentified locus which determines the response to the poly-DL-alanine determinant. A third antibody specificity is directed against G-A--L and is only detectable in chickens which are high responders to poly-DL-alanine.

INTRODUCTION

During the last few years several data on antibody production in chickens have stressed the importance of genes, located within the major histocompatibility complex (MHC) of the chicken for the immunogenecity of certain antigens. Thus the antibody responses to (T,G)-A--L (4),

233

PPD (5), and DNP-CGG (1) are all influenced by the MHC,
The so-called B-complex.

In a previous paper (8) we have described a B-
complex linked immune response to the (T,G) part of a
certain (T,G)-A--L preparation, whereas responsiveness
to the back-bone part of (T,G)-A--L was not influenced
by the MHC.

Furthermore we found that the antibody response in
chickens to the random copolymer GT was solely governed
by the B-complex, a point which makes the response to GT
a potential genetic marker within the chicken MHC. Benedict et al. (2) have previously described responsiveness
to GA and GAT as useful markers.

In this presentation we shall elaborate some of the
problems which were raised in our previous paper (8). It
involves a further analysis of the specificity of the
antibody response to a particular (T,G)-A--L preparation
(no. 2o3o), the immunogenecity of which was found unlinked to the B-complex. Our results indicate, that the
response to the poly-DL-alanine determinant of (T,G)-A--L
may have a marked influence on the concomitant response
to the (T,G) determinant.

                    MATERIALS AND METHODS

     Our methods for immunization (8), titration (7) and
inhibition tests (11) have been fully described in the
references.

     Animals.   Chickens of the CB, CC, WA and M lines
are kept at the Institute of Molecular Genetics in Prague.
Outbred White Leghorns (W. L.) were obtained from a
local hatchery.

     Antigens.   The preparation of (T,G)-A--L 2o3o is
described in detail in (11). It has a molecular weight
of about 2oo.ooo and the amino acid ratios are:
T: G: A: L 1.2: 2.o: 14.7: 1. GT was obtained from Miles-
Yeda, molecular weight 3o.8oo and G: T ratio 1: 1.
Poly-DL-alanine was prepared as described in (11).

     Immunoadsorbents.   GT and poly-DL-alanine was
coupled to CNBr-activated Sepharose 4B (Pharmacia Fine
Chemicals) as described by Porath et al. (1o).

Fig. 1.   Titration of inbred chicken strains, immunized
            with (T,G)-A--L 2o3o.

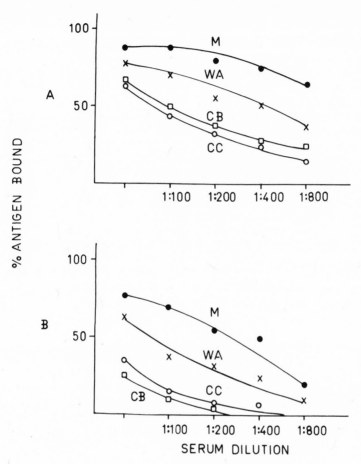

A: Titrated with [125]I-(T,G)-A--L 1383.
B: Titrated with ^{125}I-poly-DL-alanine-BSA.

25 µl serum dilution was incubated with 2.5 ng. radioiodinated antigen in 5o µl. After ½ hr. at 37°C and 1 hr.
at 4°C the incubation procedure was repeated with an ap-
propiate amount of rabbit anti-chicken Ig in 5o µl. After
centrifugation 5o µl of the supernatant was counted and
antibody titer was expressed as % antigen bound. All
points represent the mean of 6 individual chickens.

RESULTS

I.   Antibody response in inbred chicken strains to (T,G)-A--L 2o3o

Four inbred strains (CB, CC, WA and M) were immunized with 25o µg (T,G)-A--L 2o3o in Freunds complete
adjuvant (FCA). A primary response could not be detected
in any of the strains, but 7 days after boosting with the
same amount of antigen they all developed a significant
secondary response. Fig. 1 A shows a titration of antisera from the four strains performed at different serum
dilutions. The radioiodinated antigen used for titration
was (T,G)-A--L 1383. From the figure it appears that the
M and WA chickens are high responders whereas the response in CB and CC chickens is significantly lower.

However, when the same sera are titrated with iodinated poly-DL-alanine, coupled to BSA since poly-DL-alanine as such cannot be iodinated by the chloramin T
method, titration curves appear as shown in fig. 1 B.
Again M and WA are high responders, while CB and CC are
low.

With the purpose of further distinguishing between
various antibody specificities which might be present in
the antisera from the four chicken strains we pooled the
individual sera from each strain and examined them in
inhibition studies and after specific immunosorptions.
The inhibition experiments were performed by preincubation
of sera with an excess of cold inhibitor (GT, GA, GAL,
TGAL and poly-DL-alanine), and the immunosorption experiments were carried out by passing the sera through Sepharose columns coupled with either GT or poly-DL-alanine.
The final titrations were made with ^{125}I-(T,G)-A--L 1383.

Specific immunosorption on Sepharose-GT

loo µl of pooled antiserum from each strain was
passed through a 1 x 3 cm column of Sepharose coupled
with GT. The effluent was diluted 1 : 25 as compared to
the original serum. A proportion of the effluent was further preincubated with poly-DL-alanine, after which three
samples from each strain was titrated: a) serum before
immunosorption, b) effluent from specific immunosorption
and c) effluent from specific immunosorption preincubated
with poly-DL-alanine. Fig. 2 shows the titration curves.
Both the sera from the M and WA strains contain considerable amounts of antibodies which are retained on the GT
columns whereas the sera from CB and CC chickens have an
almost identical antibody titer before and after passage
through the columns. Further preincubation with poly-DL-

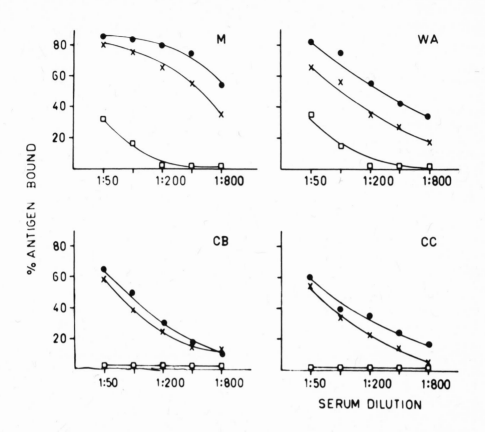

Pooled sera from each strain were passed through
Sepharose-columns coupled with GT.

●————● Serum before passage

x————x Serum after passage

□————□ Serum after passage but further preincu-
        bated with an excess of poly-DL-alanine

The x————x curves represent mainly the anti-poly-
DL-alanine response.

Fig. 2.   SPECIFIC IMMUNOSORPTION ON SEPHAROSE-GT.

alanine completely inhibits the antibodies from CB and CC
sera, while there still remain a significant antibody
titer in the M and WA sera. Later experiments (not shown)
have shown that this particular response is totally inhibited with (T,G)-A--L and G-A--L, whereas no inhibition
was seen after preincubation with GA or A--L. We therefore
designate this specificity G-A--L.

Specific immunosorption on Sepharose-poly-DL-alanine
        The procedure was essentially the same as described
in the previous section except that the column-passed
sera were now preincubated with GT. Fig. 3 shows the titration curves. The titrations of sera after passage
through Spharose-poly-DL-alanine represents mainly the
anti (T,G) response and thus emphasizes the point mentioned above that CB and CC are nearly non-responders to
(T,G). Again the G-A--L specificity in M and WA sera is
significant.
        The results shown in fig. 2 and 3 are thus in com-
plete accordance and illustrates that we are dealing
with three non-crossreacting specificities; a poly-DL-
alanine specificity, a GT specificity, and a G-A--L
specificity. It is noteworthy that these responses are
correlated such that the M and WA strains are high responders, whereas the CB and CC strains are low responders
to all three specificities. Immunization of outbred
chickens further emphasized this correlation.

II.   Antibody response in outbred White Leghorns to
(T,G)-A--L 2o3o
        14 White Leghorns were immunized twice with 25o µg
(T,G)-A--L 2o3o. The secondary antibody response to:
a) (T,G)-A--L (titrated with (T,G)-A--L 1383), b) poly-
DL-Alanine (titrated with poly-DL-alanine-BSA) and
c) (T,G) (titrated with (T,G)-A--L 1383 after preincubation with poly-DL-alanine) were measured. The results
are seen in table 1. Using a non-parametric statistical
analysis (Spearman's ranking coefficient) we found a
significant positive correlation between the antibody
responses to poly-DL-alanine and to (T,G).

DISCUSSION

        Immunization of chickens with the commonly used
synthetic multichain copolymer (T,G)-A--L has not led to
the same neat situation as in mice where (T,G)-A--L
evokes a clear anti (T,G) response, linked to the H2
complex (for review see 6).

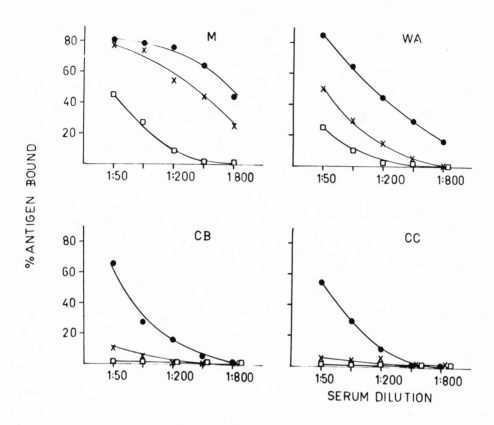

Pooled sera from each strain were passed through
Sepharose-columns coupled with poly-DL-alanine.

●————● Serum before passage

x————x Serum after passage

□————□ Serum after passage but further preincubated with an excess of GT

The x————x curves represent mainly the anti-(T,G)
response.

Fig. 3.

SPECIFIC IMMUNOSORPTION ON SEPHAROSE-POLY-DL-ALANINE.

The main reason for this discrepancy seems to be that chickens show an additional and very significant antibody response to the back bone of (T,G)-A--L. Further analysis of this particular antibody specificity has revealed that it is directed against poly-D-alanine, as judged from inhibition studies with poly-L-alanine, poly-D-alanine and poly-DL-alanine (11).

The complexity of the response to (T,G)-A--L is further emphasized by the different immunogenecity of different (T,G)-A--L preparations. Thus the antibody response to (T,G)-A--L JC 42o is mainly directed against the (T,G) determinant, and the response is clearly linked to the B-complex (8). The anti-DL-alanine response to this particular preparation is rather small and is not linked to the B-complex (8). In contrast, (T,G)-A--L 2o3o gives rise to a brisk anti-DL-alanine response, which is also unlinked to the B-complex (unpublished).

The main surprise in the present work was the finding that even the (T,G) response may, with some (T,G)-A--L preparations, be unlinked to the B-complex. The formal proof of this point is not at hand. Nevertheless, it is a conclusion which is difficult to avoid on the following grounds: a) The poly-DL-alanine response has so far been found to be unlinked to the B-complex, b) The (T,G) response to (T,G)-A--L 2o3o has been found to be strongly positively correlated to the former response in both the inbred Prague strains and in outbred White Leghorns.

Poly-D-amino acids are known to be T-cell independent antigens, and T-cell independent antigens (including poly-D-amino acids) seem to be polyclonal B-cell activators (PBA) (3). Granted that the poly-DL-alanine response is in fact due to poly-D-alanine (11), many of the apparant inconsistencies in the response of chickens to various (T,G)-A--L preparations may be explained as follows. Different (T,G)-A--L preparations are quantitatively different in their poly-D-alanine constitution. Different chicken strains react differently to the mitogenic stimulus of the D-alanine moieties. The net result may be great differences in anti-poly-DL-alanine responses to different (T,G)-A--L preparations. The (T,G)-specific B-cells binding (T,G)-A--L are triggered by a mitogenic stimulus (poly-D-alanine) and the degree of mitogenecity could therefore greatly influence also the anti-(T,G) response.

The anti-(T,G) responses are probably thus determined by at least three factors, i.e. 1) a B-complex linked Ir gene, 2) the mitogenic properties of the particular (T,G)-A--L preparation, and 3) unmapped genes controlling the mitogenic response to poly-D-alanine.

TABLE 1.

   Correlation between antibody response to poly-DL-
alanine and antibody response to (T,G) after immunization with (T,G)-A--L 2o3o.

W. L. No.	Response to		
	(T,G)-A--L[a]	(T,G)[b]	poly-DL-alanine[c]
37o1	66	53	21
3624	65	43	57
32o9	64	59	39
3739	61	34	46
3598	6o	32	47
1482	44	13	29
343o	44	5	21
2735	37	23	31
3348	32	17	1o
3634	28	9	8
3644	25	o	13
364o	24	1	11
3699	21	7	3o
3725	12	o	6

a) Titrated with ^{125}I-(T,G)-A--L 1383 at a serum dilution
   1:4oo.

b) Sera preincubated with poly-DL-alanine 2 mg/ml, titrated with ^{125}I-(T,G)-A--L 1383, final serum dilution
   1:4oo.

c) Titrated with ^{125}I-poly-DL-alanine-BSA at a serum
   dilution 1:2oo.

All titers are expressed as % antigen bound.

Antibody titers to poly-DL-alanine were compared with
antibody titers to (T,G). Using Spearman's rank correlation analysis we found the rank correlation coefficient
R=o.78o2 which means a significant correlation (p<o.o1).

Particular (T,G)-A--L preparations such as (T,G)-A--L JC 42o, which show a low poly-DL-alanine response, are probably little mitogenic and display therefore neatly the effect of the Ir gene. So does of course the poly-GT preparation (8). Our present experiments do not give grounds for distinguishing between the B-complex linked anti-(T,G)-A--L response and the anti-GT response.

Further elucidation of these problems will involve a direct test of the mitogenicity of poly-DL-alanine in chicken lymfocytes, and a further analysis of the GT response in the inbred chicken strains in Prague together with a genetic analysis of the antibody response to (T,G)-A--L 2o3o in these strains.

In mice Watson and Riblet (12) have demonstrated what may be a similar effect of another PBA, lipopoly-saccharide (LPS). They found that two inbred mouse strains differed considerably in their in vitro mitogenic respon-ses to LPS, and coupled with these were marked differences in the amounts of antibody formed in vivo against LPS. Such genetically determined differences in mitogenic in vitro responses have already been described in chickens with respect to a T-cell mitogen (Con A) (9).

ACKNOWLEDGEMENTS

Birgitte Christensen, Dorthe Kolding and Hanne Braae are thanked for excellent technical assistance. The work was supported by grants from the Danish medical research Council (512-5686) and F.L.Schmidt and Co's Jubilæumsfond.

REFERENCES

1. Balcarova, J., Derka, J., Hala, K. and Hraba, T., Folia Biol. (Praha), 2o: 346 (1974).

2. Benedict, A.A., Pollard, L.W., Morrow, P.R., Abplanalp, H.A., Maurer, P.H. and Briles, W.E., Immunogenetics, 2: 313 (1975).

3. Coutinho, A. and Møller, G., Nature (New Biology), 245: 12 (1973).

4. Günther, E., Balcarova, J., Hala, K., Rüde, E. and Hraba, T., Eur. J. Immunol., 4: 548 (1974).

5. Karakoz, I., Krejci, J., Hala, K., Blaszczyk, B., Hraba, T. and Pekarek, J., Eur. J. Immunol. 4: 545 (1974).

6.   Klein, J., Biology of the mouse histocompatibility
      2 complex, Springer Verlag, Berlin, N.Y. (1975).

7.   Koch, C., Immunogenetics, 1: 118 (1974).

8.   Koch, C. and Simonsen, M., Immunogenetics,
      In press (1977).

9.   Miggiano, V., North, M., Buder, A. and Pink, J.R.L.
      Nature, 263: 61 (1976).

lo.   Porath, J., Axen, R. and Ernback, S., Nature,
      215: 1491 (1967).

11.   Sørup, P. and Koch, C., Scand. J. Immunol., 6:
      31 (1977).

12.   Watson, J. and Riblet, R., J. exp. Med., 14o:
      1147 (1974).

IMMUNE RESPONSE AND ADULT MORTALITY ASSOCIATED WITH THE B LOCUS IN CHICKENS[1]

A. W. Nordskog, I. Y. Pevzner, C. L. Trowbridge
and A. A. Benedict

Dept. of Animal Science, Iowa State University, Ames,
Iowa, and University of Hawaii, Honolulu

OVERVIEW

We are studying immune response to natural and synthetic
antigens as related to viability and disease and are attempting to
determine the extent to which the major histocompatibility complex
(the B blood group system) is involved. We are using a noninbred
line, S1, segregating for 3 B alleles and 7 inbred lines with
inbreeding coefficients ranging from 60-97%. This gives us the
opportunity to compare the experimental efficiency of inbreds and
noninbreds for studies of immune response. A unique feature of
our approach concerns the B^1B^1 genotype. In particular, B^1B^1
chickens show consistently high adult mortality, 4- or 5-fold
higher than controls, and they are highly susceptible to Marek's
disease virus. Also, they have proved to be low responders to
Salmonella pullorum bacterin, human serum albumin, GAT^{10}, and
(T,G)-A--L. We think that there is some broad immunodeficiency
associated with B^1B^1 but as yet we have not discovered it.

The B^1 allele has been transferred to each of 6 inbred lines.
We are now in the 4th backcross generation. The purpose is to
expedite the study of B alleles unique to each inbred line and
also to make possible a study of the overall behavior of the B^1B^1
genotype in different genetic backgrounds.

[1] Journal Paper No. J-8833 of the Iowa Agriculture and Home Economics
Experiment Station, Ames, Iowa; Project 1980. In cooperation with
the Northeastern States Regional Poultry Breeding Project, NE-60.
Supported in part by USPHS NIH Grant AI 12746, and AI 05660.

INTRODUCTION

Our interest is in immune response as it relates to disease resistance and to the B locus--the major histocompatibility locus in chickens. A principal objective is to identify and characterize immune response genes (Ir) with special reference to linkage with the B complex.

To characterize the B blood group region or complex, we employ routine hemagglutination tests supplemented with skin-grafting and the graft vs. host reaction (GVHR) using immune competent lymphocytes on the 12-day chorioallantoic membrane (CAM).

Evidence that the B blood group locus is involved in the allograft reaction was first reported by Schierman and Nordskog (1). The C locus is a second, but minor, blood group histocompatibility system in chickens (2). However, for both B and C, the histocompatibility (H) antigens are found on both erythrocytes and lymphocytes, but the C allograft reaction is weaker than the B.

By using the CAM test for GVHR, we demonstrated a dosage effect of the B antigens: more CAM foci were produced when the host embryo differed from the lymphocytes donor by 2 B antigens compared with one antigen (3).

In a study involving 712 inbred chickens, incompatibility at the B locus accounted for 3/4 of the total variance in graft rejection within lines (4).

The B complex has been shown to influence adult mortality in a synthetic line of Leghorns derived from a 2-way inbred-line cross segregating for 4 B alleles (5). The B^1 homozygotes were consistently lowest in adult viability. However, viability seemed to improve somewhat in each successive generation. This suggested to us that a major fitness gene is linked to B. We now think that such a "fitness" gene may be an Ir gene. So far, we have been unable to demonstrate a single specific cause of death, although the immune response of B^1B^1 to S. pullorum has proved to be markedly lower than control genotypes (6).

MATERIAL AND METHODS

Genetic Stocks

Leghorn S1. This noninbred line originated from a cross of 2 Hy-line[1] inbred lines in 1964. It currently segregates for B^1,

---

[1]Hy-Line International, Des Moines, Iowa.

B^2 and B^{19} blood group alleles (5).

Leghorn inbreds. Lines 8, 9, 19, GH and HN. The range in inbreeding coefficients is between 60 and 97%. Lines 8 and 9 have colored plumage. The others are white.

Spanish SP. About 75% inbred. A black-plumaged breed with the sex-linked barring gene segregating. Segregation has been deliberately maintained.

Fayoumi (Egyptian) Line M. About 60% inbred, resistant to Marke's disease, and we think it carries the B^{21} allele.

Currently, we are attempting to identify all segregating B alleles in our inbred lines. To aid this purpose, we have introduced a known allele (B^1) into each line followed by backcrossing. At the same time, we plan to make a special study of the immune response and mortality associated with the B^1 allele, having introduced it into several inbred lines each with different genetic background. Because we maintain both noninbred and inbred stocks, we have the opportunity to gain some knowledge of their comparative experimental efficiencies for immune response studies.

Laboratory Procedures

Antigens – _Salmonella pullorum_ bacterin, human serum albumin (HAS) GAT^{10} and (T,G)-A--L. Assays – passive hemagglutination, ordinary agglutination, modified Farr technique, radioelectro-complexing (REC) and radioimmunoelectrophoresis (RIE).

Routinely, birds were bled at 7 or 14 days after the first injection of antigen and then one week after the second injection on the 21st day. In general, birds were 20 to 30 weeks of age at the start of an experiment. Both males and females were used as test birds.

Immune response to _S. pullorum_ was assayed by agglutination. Immune response to HSA and (T,G)-A--L was assayed by the modified Farr technique and passive hemagglutination at Iowa State; GAT^{10} was assayed by REC and RIE at the University of Hawaii (7). Samples were shipped from Ames to Honolulu.

Challenge – chicks from the S1 population were challenged with Marek's disease virus in collaboration with the U.S. Regional Poultry Laboratory at East Lansing, Michigan. Also, mortality of growing birds and adults from the Poultry Research Center at Ames was considered important observation data.

RESULTS

B locus and skin graft rejection. Fig. 1 demonstrates the
role of the B locus on histocompatibility in inbred Leghorn GH.
Similar experiments performed with noninbreds have shown that
about 3/4 of the variance in skin graft rejection is controlled
by the B locus. From this we deduce that minor histocompatibility
loci (as the C blood group locus) control up to 25% of the variance.

B locus and mortality. Fig. 2 shows overall adult mortality
by years from 1965 to 1977 for the B^1B^1 genotype and controls.
Although considerable variation occurred from year to year, the
B^1B^1's had consistently higher mortality. The unusually high
mortality in 1974 of both groups was attributed to an outbreak of
Marek's, even though the chicks were vaccinated, possibly due to
faulty vaccination technique.

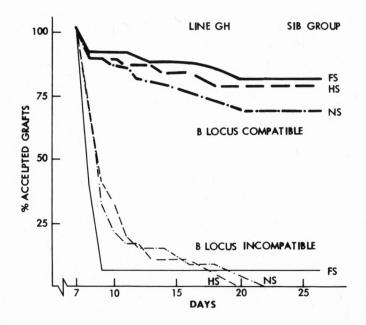

Fig. 1.   Percentage of accepted skin grafts of Line GH chicks
          grafted at 17 days to 25 days post-grafting. Heavy lines
          are B locus compatible transplants; light lines are
          incompatible. Sib groups are: FS - full sibs, HS - half
          sibs and NS - nonsibs (from reference 4).

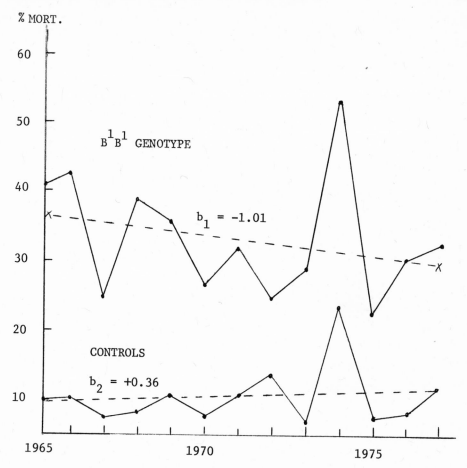

Fig. 2.   Adult mortality from all causes of B1B1 females
          of the S1 Leghorn line.

Gene model.   If we assume that an Ir gene is linked to B^1
and that, in the case of the B^1B^1 genotype, high mortality is
associated with Ir^1, then the hypothetical possible genotypes

would be:

$$P_1 \quad \dfrac{B^1 \quad Ir^1}{B^1 \quad Ir^1} \qquad \text{- High mortality [observed]}$$

$$P_2 \quad \dfrac{B^2 \quad Ir^2}{B^2 \quad Ir^2} \qquad \text{- Normal} \qquad \text{[observed]}$$

$$F_1 \quad \dfrac{B^1 \quad Ir^1}{B^2 \quad Ir^2} \qquad \text{- Normal} \qquad \text{[observed]}$$

$$F_2 \quad \dfrac{B^1 \quad Ir^1}{B^1 \quad Ir^2} \qquad \text{- Normal (?)}$$

$$\dfrac{B^1 \quad Ir^2}{B^1 \quad Ir^2} \qquad \text{- Normal (?)}$$

$$\dfrac{B^2 \quad Ir^1}{B^2 \quad Ir^1} \qquad \text{- High mortality (?)}$$

With this genetic model, we expect some crossovers giving the recombinant genotypes indicated in F_2 above. If linkage is close, as for Ir and H-2K in the murine model, then only a low frequency of the crossover genotypes, $B^1B^1Ir^1Ir^2$ and $B^1B^1Ir^2Ir^2$ with normal viability, would be expected. Natural selection, however, would favor such genotypes over $B^1B^1Ir^1Ir^1$ and, year by year, viability of the B^1B^1 genotype would improve. The negative regression ($b = -1.01$) of percent mortality by years for the B^1B^1 genotypes (Fig. 2) is evidence for this model. The difference between the 2 regressions $(b_1-b_2) = (-1.01-0.36) = -1.37$ is statistically significant at the $P = 0.05$ level of probability. If the regressions are taken at face value, it can be deduced that B and Ir are between 1 and 2 crossover units apart. In other words, this much crossing over would allow the B^1B^1 serotyped individuals to increase in viability an average 1.37% per year because of recombination.

Immune Response

S. pullorum bacterin. Confirming earlier studies (6), we find that the B^1B^1 genotype is a low responder to S. pullorum antigen. Table 1 presents a summary of three separate experiments showing observed adult mortality over a 9-month period, plus mortality from inoculation with JM Marek's disease virus, and anti-pullorum titers of 3 genotypes in our S1 line.

Table 1. Adult mortality, resistance to Marek's virus and immune response to S. pullorum bacterin of 3 B locus genotypes.

Genotype	% Overall mortality (9 months)	% Chick mortality[1] following inoculation with JM Marek's disease virus at 1 day of age	Anti-pullorum Titer (log 2) at 20 weeks of age	
			1°	2°
B^1B^1	36 (206)	43 (154)	5.4	9.7
B^2B^2	30 (52)	10 (40)	5.9	10.0
$B^{19}B^{19}$	20 (45)	45 (38)	6.7	11.4

Figures in parentheses are number of birds

The results show that overall mortality was highest for the B^1B^1 genotype, as observed in previous years. After inoculation with the JM Marek's virus, both the B^1B^1 and $B^{19}B^{19}$ genotypes proved to be highly susceptible but the B^2B^2 genotype was resistant with only 10% of 40 birds dying in the test. Anti-pullorum titers demonstrate that B^1B^1 is consistently lower than both B^2B^2 and $B^{19}B^{19}$ and also for both the primary and secondary responses.

GAT^{10}. The injection schedule was 100 µg in Freund's Complete Adjuvant (FCA) as the primary dose and 100 µg in saline as the secondary dose. Fig. 3 presents a comparison of B^1B^1 with the two heterozygotes, B^1B^2 and B^1B^{19}. B^1B^1 proved to be a low responder, B^1B^2 was intermediate, and B^1B^{19} was a high responder.

Fig. 4 gives the results of an experiment comparing the homozygous genotypes B^1B^1, B^2B^2, and $B^{19}B^{19}$ and the two heterozygotes, B^1B^2 and B^1B^{19}. B^1B^1 gave essentially no response in either the primary or secondary period. B^2B^2 and $B^{19}B^{19}$ were high responders. B^1B^2 was a low primary responder but a high secondary period responder. B^1B^{19} was intermediate in both periods.

Table 2 presents some preliminary results of immune response of inbred lines to GAT^{10} using the RIE assay. The birds tested from the various lines were those available as surviving breeders of

[1] These tests were kindly made with the cooperation of Howard Stone at the U.S. Regional Poultry Laboratory, East Lansing, Michigan.

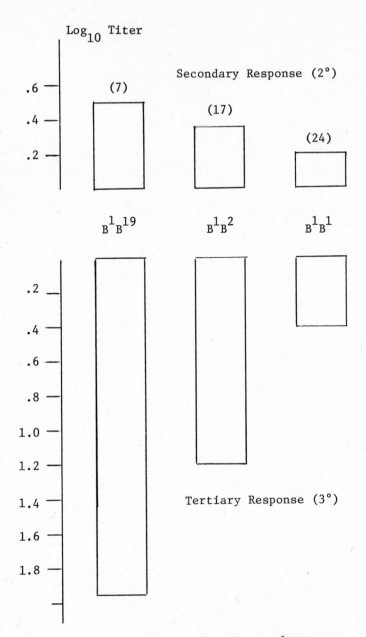

Fig. 3.   Immune response of B^1B^1, B^1B^2 and B^1B^{19} genotypes to
          GAT^{10} assayed by REC. Primary dose was 100 μg in FCA.
          The secondary dose (2°) was 100 μg in saline with the
          same dose given as a booster (3°) about 12 weeks later.
          Only responses to 2° and 3° are shown.

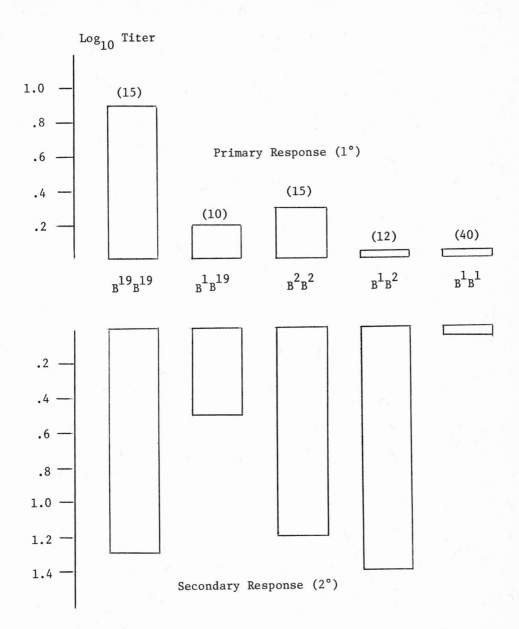

Fig. 4.   Immune response to 5 B genotypes to 100 µg of GAT^{10} given in FCA as a primary dose (1°) and 100 µg in saline as a secondary (2°) dose.

the 1976 generation. Numbers are sufficient to draw only tentative conclusions. In the primary response period, lines 8, 9 and GH were nonresponders and lines HN, 19, SP and M were responders. In the secondary response period, only line GH was a nonresponder but unfortunately, only 4 birds were available for the test.

Table 2.   Immune response to GAT^{10} in 7 inbred lines injected with 100 µg/ml (FCA) followed by 100 µg/ml in saline assayed by RIE

Inbred Line	No. of Birds	% of birds testing positive	
		1°	2°
8	9	0	29.
9	5	0	50.
GH	4	0	0.
HN	10	50.	75.
19	3	33.	40.
SP	12	58.	83.
M	12	75.	75.

Experiments with (T,G)-A--L and human serum albumin (detailed results to be published elsewhere) show that the B^1B^1 of our S1 line is again a low responder, the $B^{19}B^{19}$ is a high responder and B^2B^2 gives a low to intermediate response under both the Modified Farr and Passive hemagglutination techniques. Response to both antigens was, in general, completely dominant to nonresponsiveness.

Similar tests in the inbred lines showed that the Fayoumi line was a strong immune responder while the GH line was a low responder to either antigen. The other 5 lines showed different degrees of intermediate response.

DISCUSSION

Most of the immune response work we have under way is in the beginning stage, especially with the inbreds. The unique feature of our approach is to develop congenic inbreds by incorporating the B^1 allele as a genetic marker into each line. We are now in our fourth generation of backcrossing so that each line is now 93.75% of the original inbred line genome. The B^1 allele will aid in the production of individual inbred line test antisera, and at the same time we shall be able to test the effects of the B^1 on mortality in different genetic backgrounds.

We are aware of the importance of perfecting a system of monitoring the genetic integrity of our inbreds. We have this essentially under control in lines 8, 9, SP and M because these are easily identified by their different plumage colors. On the other hand, lines GH, HN and 19 being white-plumaged Leghorns, require a more sophisticated system of monitoring such as blood typing or other genetic markings.

The S1 population, although not inbred, was derived originally from a commercial 2-way inbred line cross. The population has been maintained for more than 10 years by controlled matings as to pedigree and the B locus. With the 3 genes of B^1, B^2 and B^{19}, we have each year produced all combinations of homozygotes and heterozygotes. Thus, if each genotype (or haplotype of the B complex) has a unique Ir gene, our breeding system makes possible the formation of B-Ir recombinants. We, therefore, believe that much can be learned about immune response, disease and the major histocompatibility complex without the necessity of first developing inbred lines. For this reason we plan to continue with the non-inbred S1 line population. That we have generally good reproduction in S1 compared with inbreds means that many more birds are available for testing. Also one can argue that the results obtained from an outbred population are more relevant to the real world of birds and people than are results from inbreds.

From an experimental design point of view, it is of interest to ask the question as to how much more efficient inbreds are than noninbreds in the production of experimental information on some heritable response. For example, assume that the heritability of a response under genetic control is of the order of 90%. Further, assume that 70% of the individual variation in response is associated with the B complex, and 20% is associated with other genetic loci. Let the remaining 10% be due to random environmental effects. For this hypothetical case,it is possible to compare the relative efficiency of an experiment using inbreds, say, derived from this population compared with an experiment using the base population of noninbred birds. Suppose that two congenic lines, differing only at the B locus, are formed from the base population. The individual or experimental error variation within congenic lines would then be only the 10% associated with random environment. For the noninbred base population, the experimental error variation would be 30% (i.e., 20% genetic plus 10% random experiment). In this case the experimental error variation of the noninbreds would be 3 times greater than that within the congenic inbreds. In practice, this would mean that more birds of the noninbreds would be required for testing to equal the accuracy of a experiment using congenic lines. It is easy to show that to reduce the experimental error of the noninbreds to equal that in the inbreds in this hypothetical example would require three times as many test birds as for the congenic inbreds, i.e., 30/10 = 3. On the other hand, if

all the genetic variance is associated with the b locus, say 90%
with 10% random environmental effects, then inbred lines, with
segregation at the B locus (congenic lines), would be no more
efficient for testing immune response effects than would a non-
inbred population.

Benedict et al. (7) found the responses to GAT^{10} in chickens
to be associated with certain B alleles; however, in the present
study with GAT^{10}, we found considerable variation in differences
between genotypes. This could well represent genetic differences
between individuals not linked to the B complex. However, a significant part of the variation probably results also from random
environmental-variable factors, not subject to experimental control,
which influence both test birds and serum samples differently. We
believe that it will be useful to further explore this question
experimentally to more clearly assess the relative values of
outbreds and inbreds as subjects for studies of the B complex
and as related to immune response and disease.

REFERENCES

1.   Schierman, L. W. and Nordskog, A. W. Science 134:1008 (1961).

2.   Schierman, L. W. and Nordskog, A. W. Transplantation 3:44 (1965).

3.   Schierman, L. W. World's Poul. Sci. J. 21:6 (1965).

4.   Marangu, J. P. and Nordskog, A. W. Theor. Appl. Genet. 45:
     215 (1974).

5.   Nordskog, A. W., Rishell, W. A., and Briggs, D. M. Genetics
     75:181 (1973).

6.   Pevzner, I. Y., Nordskog, A. W., and Kaeberle, M. L.
     Genetics 80:753 (1975).

7.   Benedict, A. A., Pollard, L. W., Morrow, P. R., Abplanalp,
     H. A., Maurer, P. H., and Briles, W. E. Immunogenetics
     2:313 (1975).

HISTOCOMPATIBILITY REQUIREMENTS FOR CELLULAR COOPERATION IN THE CHICKEN[1]

Auli Toivanen, Matti Viljanen and Pekka Tamminen

Departments of Medicine and Medical Microbiology

Turku University, SF-20520 Turku 52, Finland

In the studies regarding the B cell differentiation we have been using the chemical bursectomy model in the chicken. Newly-hatched chickens are treated with cyclophosphamide on four consecutive days starting on the day of hatching. The treatment results in virtually complete and life-long humoral immune deficiency, including atrophy of the bursa of Fabricius and absence of germinal center formation. On the fourth day of life such birds are transplanted with different lymphoid cells to be studied, and the effects of the transplantation are assessed at the age of 4-6 weeks using morphological and functional criteria. On the basis of these studies we have found that during late embryonic development and around the time of hatching the bursa contains a special cell population which we have chosen to call *bursal stem cells* (1-4). These cells are still unable to produce antibodies by themselves. When transplanted into cyclophosphamide-treated recipients they induce a full functional and morphological restoration, including normalization of the bursal morphology and germinal center formation in the spleen. In order to differentiate further these cells need a close contact to the bursal reticulum.

Bursa cells lack the capacity to induce graft-versus-host reaction, and thus it is possible to study whether bursal stem cells can undergo differentiation in the bursal environment of an allogeneic host. Table 1 shows the most important findings of one series of experiments where bursal stem cells were transplanted into cyclophosphamide-treated allogeneic recipients.

---

[1]Supported by a grant from the Sigrid Jusélius Foundation, and by NIH Contract NO1-CB-43971.

Table 1

Transplantation of histocompatible, allogeneic or semiallogeneic
bursal stem cells in cyclophosphamide-treated newly-hatched recipients. The parameters indicated were measured at 7 wks after the
transplantation. Mean values are given.

Transplanted bursal stem cells	Bursal weight[1]	Ig+ cells[2]	Antibody formation[3]		Germinal centers[4]
			Brucella	SRBC	
None	69	2.3	0.0	0.0	0.1
Histocompatible	335	27.2	8.6	5.8	15.7
Allogeneic	273	40.0	6.4	0.8	1.0
Semiallogeneic	341	ND[5]	6.4	3.9	21.1

[1] Mg/100 g of body weight
[2] Per cent in spleen
[3] Log_2 secondary titers
[4] Per cross section of spleen
[5] Not done

We have at our use two White Leghorn chicken lines, derived
originally from the Hy-Line lines; one is type B^2B^2 (line P) and
the other is $B^{15}B^{15}$ (line V). Cyclophosphamide-treated control
birds had an atrophic bursa and very few if any surface immunoglobulin positive cells in the spleen (Table 1). They failed to
produce antibodies both to *Brucella* and sheep red blood cells
(SRBC), and they had no germinal center formation in the spleen.
If these birds had been transplanted with histocompatible or semiallogeneic bursal stem cells, all of these functions became restored to a normal level. If the donors of the bursal stem cells
had been allogeneic to the recipient, the results differed in two
interesting respects. The bursal weight became restored, immunoglobulin positive cells appeared in the periphery, and antibody
production to *Brucella* occurred. However, no antibody production
to T-dependent SRBC and no germinal center formation occurred in
these birds (5, 6).
    The absence of antibody production against T-dependent anti-
gens was confirmed in carrier-priming experiments with a subsequent
immunization with a hapten coupled to a homologous or heterologous
carrier. Figure 1 shows the results regarding immunization with
dinitrophenyl (DNP). Again 4-day-old cyclophosphamide-treated
birds had been transplanted with bursa cells taken from 4-day-old
donors that were histocompatible, semiallogeneic or allogeneic to
the host. Four weeks after the transplantation the birds were
primed with methylated bovine serum albumin (MBSA) and boostered
seven days later with DNP coupled to bovine serum albumin (DNP-BSA).

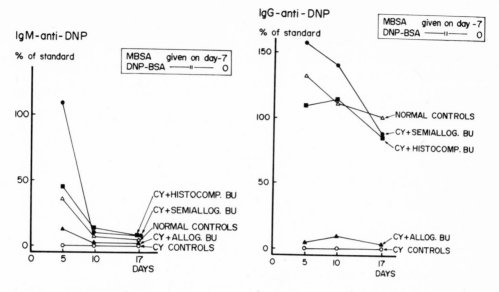

Fig. 1. Development of anti-DNP antibodies in birds primed with MBSA and challenged with DNP-BSA. Cyclophosphamide (CY) was given in the newly-hatched period, and histocompatible, allogeneic or semiallogeneic bursal stem cells (BU) immediately thereafter. Day 0 refers to the age of 5 weeks. IgM and IgG antibodies were measured by a solid-phase radioimmunoassay (7). Mean values are given.

Blood samples were drawn 5, 10 and 17 days after the booster. The results are very clear-cut. Cyclophosphamide-treated birds and those that had received allogeneic bursa cells failed completely to produce any anti-DNP antibodies. Birds that had received bursa cells from semiallogeneic or histocompatible donors produced normal levels of antibodies, and the immune response in these cases was a typically secondary one.

Figure 2 demonstrates a similar type of experiment where the priming had been carried out by using human gamma globulin instead of BSA. Otherwise, the experimental groups were the same as in Fig. 1. On day 0 the birds had been given DNP-BSA and blood samples were drawn as described above. Cyclophosphamide-treated control birds and those that had received allogeneic bursa cells failed again to produce any antibodies. Those that had received semiallogeneic bursa cells or bursa cells from histocompatible donors produced good primary response.

It could be suspected that the transplanted cells had not survived in the allogeneic host, but rather had been rejected. This

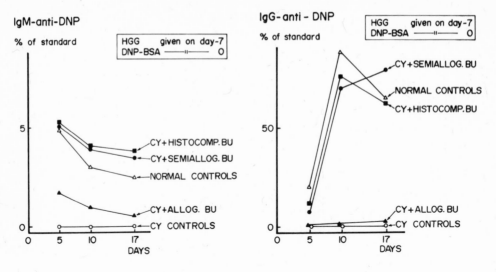

Fig. 2. Development of anti-DNP antibodies in birds primed with HGG and challenged with DNP-BSA. Otherwise, the experimental conditions were the same as described in Figure 1.

was not the case. The transplanted cells induced full tolerance to the donor line as indicated by survival of the donor line skin grafted at the age of 4-6 weeks, whereas third party skin grafts were rejected in a normal time. Furthermore, it was demonstrated that the cells had remained functionally active even in the allogeneic environment. Table 2 shows antibody response by the same birds as in Figures 1-2 to a thymus-independent antigen, *Brucella*. It is clearly evident that all these birds produced good quantities of IgM class anti-*Brucella* antibodies. Furthermore, using a serial transplantation experiment (5), we could show that the cells had retained their ability to form antibodies and also germinal centers (Table 3). In these experiments, we first transplanted bursa cells from 3-day-old donors into cyclophosphamide-treated recipients of the same age and let these birds mature for 4 weeks. Thereafter we took out the bursa and put the cells now into new 3-day-old cyclophosphamide-treated recipients of either the same line as the cells were originally derived from, or again in an allogeneic environment. We let the birds mature for 4 weeks and tested their antibody production to SRBC and *Brucella* and the germinal center formation in the spleen. If the cells in the second transfer ended into their own original environment, good antibody production both to SRBC and *Brucella* occurred, as well as good

Table 2

Antibody response to *Brucella* in the same birds as described in Figures 1 and 2. IgM and IgG antibodies were measured by a solid-phase radioimmunoassay (7). Mean values are given.

Treatment	Anti-*Brucella*[1]	
	IgG	IgM
CY + histocomp. BU	3.8	18.6
CY + semiallog. BU	0.4	7.6
CY + allog. BU	1.5	18.8
CY	0.0	0.0
None	16.2	63.5

[1] Per cent of standard

Table 3

Antibody response and germinal center formation in the secondary hosts after a serial transfer of bursa cells. Mean values are given.

1st transfer		2nd transfer	Antibody response[2]		Germinal centers[3]
Line of		Line of	SRBC	*Brucella*	
Donors	Recipients[1]	Recipients			
V	P	V	4.4	4.8	20.6
V	P	P	0.0	0.0	1.2
P	P	V	0.0	0.0	0.5
P	P	P	3.0	7.0	13.7

[1] At 4 wks after the cell transfer, these birds served as bursa cell donors for the 2nd transfer
[2] Log_2 titer
[3] Per cross section of spleen

Table 4

Number of germinal centers in the spleen of cyclophosphamide-
treated line V birds five weeks after transplantation of B and T
cells (bursa and thymus cells from 3-day-old donors). Different
combinations of line P and line V cells were used.

Line of cell donors		Line of recipients	Germinal centers[1]	P
B cells	T cells			
P	P	V	9.0)	
P	V	V	3.0)	< 0.05
P	-	V	2.3	
-	P	V	0.1	
-	V	V	0.8	
-	-	V	0.1	

[1] Per a cross section of spleen; mean values are given

germinal center formation. But if they now again came into an allogeneic host, all these functions failed.

The results of all these experiments have been interpreted to
indicate that the descendants of the transplanted bursal stem cells
and the T cells provided by the allogeneic host have failed to cooperate in order to produce anti-SRBC antibodies and germinal centers. These two functions seem to go hand in hand in all experimental set-ups described above.

In order to study whether, indeed, both B and T cells are required for germinal center formation and also to study the histocompatibility requirements in these functions we transplanted 3-
day-old cyclophosphamide-treated birds with both B cells and T
cells (8). The B cells were bursa cells and the T cells were thymus cells, both from 3-day-old normal donors. The cyclophosphamide-
treated recipients received allogeneic bursa cells that were combined with T cells of either their own type or allogeneic. At the
age of 6 weeks, after immunization, we studied the germinal center
formation in the recipients' spleens. The results are summarized
in Table 4. If the recipients have been of line V (genotype $B^{15}B^{15}$)
and the transplanted B cells have been of type P (genotype B^2B^2),
germinal center formation occurs only when the B cells have been
complemented with T cells of their own type. In the experiments
where the recipients were of line P and the B cells transplanted
of line V, the significance of this difference was even greater
(Table 5). However, the number of germinal centers in the spleen
of a host that had received B and T cells that were histocompatible

Table 5

Number of germinal centers in the spleen of cyclophosphamide-treated line P birds five weeks after transplantation of B and T cells (bursa and thymus cells from 3-day-old donors). Different combinations of line V and line P cells were used.

Line of cell donors		Line of recipients	Germinal centers[1]	P
B cells	T cells			
V	V	P	10.2)	< 0.001
V	P	P	3.0)	
V	–	P	2.4	
–	V	P	1.5	
–	P	P	1.4	
–	–	P	0.4	

[1] Per a cross section of spleen; mean values are given

with each other but not with the host was only half of that observed when all these three - the host, the B cells and the T cells - were histocompatible with each other. Thus it appeared that there would be a third, augmenting factor involved in the germinal center generation. The most obvious possibility would have been the splenic stroma.

To study this, we carried out still another type of experiments. "Empty" splenic stromas of different types were transplanted under the thoracic skin of cyclophosphamide-treated 4-day-old chickens (8). These stromas were obtained from 3-day-old cyclophosphamide-treated donors. Each recipient had three spleens: one of its own, one of line P, and one line V. The transplanted spleens were well accepted, they became revascularized and filled with lymphoid cells. At the age of 4 days the recipients were transplanted with B and T cells that were histocompatible with each other but either allogeneic or histocompatible to the recipient. Table 6 shows the main results of this type of experiments. Both line P and line V recipients were used; each of them had been cyclophosphamide-treated and had three spleens. When such line P recipients received B and T cells that both were of type P, germinal center formation occurred in all three spleens. The same was the case when line V recipients received B cells and T cells of line V. Germinal center formation occurred in all three spleens, and expectedly the best production was in the host's own spleen. In the cases where the transplanted cells were allogeneic to the host, even if histocompatible with each other, some germinal center formation occurred in the host's own spleen but only very poorly in both transplanted spleens,

Table 6

Capacity of transplanted B and T cells to form germinal centers in different splenic environments in cyclophosphamide(CY)-treated chicks.

Recipients		Line of cell donors		Germinal centers[1]		
CY	Line	B cells	T cells	P spleen	V spleen	Own spleen
+	P	P	P	4.3	5.8	12.8
+	P	V	V	0.9	2.7	7.6
+	V	P	P	1.3	1.0	9.0
+	V	V	V	8.0	5.1	28.1
+	P	-	-	0.0	0.0	0.0
-	P	-	-	14.1	7.6	17.5
+	V	-	-	0.0	0.2	1.4
-	V	-	-	11.9	11.2	25.0

[1] Per a cross section of spleen; mean values are given

no matter whether they were of type P or type V. Thus it appears that, indeed, in addition to B and T cells, there is a third factor augmenting germinal center formation, but this factor does not seem related to the splenic stroma.

We would like to draw three conclusions on the basis of the results. First, when an immune response requires cooperation between B and T cells, a histocompatibility or at least identity of one haplotype between these cells seems to be necessary. Results have been presented where a cooperation across this barrier has been obtained (cf. 8-11), and an explanation has been offered that when the B cells have undergone differentiation or have been primed in the allogeneic environment, they might be able to cooperate even with allogeneic T cells. Now, in our experimental set-up the B cells both were primed and had undergone a differentiation in the allogeneic host and yet no cooperation occurred. Therefore this explanation of adaptive differentiation has to be excluded. Thirdly, also the germinal center formation requires cooperation between the B and T cells. Here a third augmenting factor may be needed, although not absolutely necessarily. This third factor seems not to be related to the splenic stroma.

REFERENCES

1. Toivanen, P. and Toivanen, A., Eur. J. Immunol., 3: 585 (1973).

2. Toivanen, P., Toivanen, A. and Tamminen, P., Eur. J. Immunol., 4: 220 (1974).

3. Sorvari, T., Toivanen, A. and Toivanen, P., Transplantation, 17: 584 (1974).

4. Sorvari, T. E. and Toivanen, A., Scand. J. Immunol., 5: 317 (1976).

5. Toivanen, P., Toivanen, A. and Sorvari, T., Proc. Nat. Acad. Sci. USA, 71: 957 (1974).

6. Toivanen, P., Toivanen, A. and Vainio, O., J. Exp. Med., 139: 1344 (1974).

7. Viljanen, M. K., Granfors, K. and Toivanen, P., J. Immunol. Meth., 14: 111 (1977).

8. Toivanen, A. and Toivanen, P., J. Immunol., 118: 431 (1977).

9. von Boehmer, H., Hudson, L. and Sprent, J., J. Exp. Med., 142: 989 (1975).

10. Heber-Katz, E. and Wilson, D. B., J. Exp. Med., 142: 928 (1975).

11. Katz, D. H. and Benacerraf, B., in The Role of Products of the Histocompatibility Gene Complex in Immune Responses (D. H. Katz and B. Benacerraf, Eds.) (Academic Press, New York, 1976).

ALLO-AGGRESSION IN CHICKENS: ANALYSIS OF THE B-COMPLEX

BY MEANS OF GVH SPLENOMEGALY AND BY INHIBITORY ANTIBODIES

M.Simonsen, K.Hála, and M.Vilhelmová

Institute of Experimental Immunology
University of Copenhagen
71, Nørre Alle, 2100 Ø., Denmark and
Institute of Molecular Genetics
Czechoslovak Academy of Sciences
Prague 6 Czechoslovakia

We will present in this paper some new data which
contribute to the analysis of the recombinant B-haplotype in Prague, RI, which was mentioned already in the
preceding section of this meeting. In addition, there
will be new data concerning the extent of the similarity
in B-haplotypes of the inbred CC strain in Prague and
the B-complex-homozygous American strain, G-Bl, which is
maintained in Europe both in Copenhagen and in Basel.

The analytical methods employed represent three
different forms of the GVH splenomegaly test, namely (1)
the direct compatibility test, (2) the GVH-inhibition
test, and (3) the GVH-inhibition-removal test. These 3
tests are in principle measuring different things. They
will be discussed successively in connection with the
use they have been put to in the present work.

THE GVH TEST OF DIRECT COMPATIBILITY

It has been known for some 15 years (1, 2) that the
B-complex determines the histocompatibility differences
which cause the severe splenomegaly of a typical GVH
reaction at 4-6 days after i-v injection of the donor
lymphocytes. Hence the absence of a grossly enlarged
spleen with necrotic nodules (pocks) after injection of
a cell dose which would normally result in such changes
is a sign of compatibility. It indicates that the
recipient did not contain stimulatory B-antigens which

were lacking in the donor. The word stimulatory has to
be stressed because it is known that it is only some of
the antigens coded for by a given B-haplotype which are
stimulatory in the sense of provoking splenomegaly (3, 4).
Clearly, the absence of splenomegaly is only an indication
of a one-way compatibility; the donor may in principle
contain any number of antigens lacking in the host and
yet cause no reaction because of the immunological
immaturity of the host.

The first experiment to prove that the Rl-haplotype
had derived its GVH-stimulatory antigen(s) from CB, and
none from CC, was performed as a direct compatibility test
by injecting peripheral blood cells from the recombinant
cock # 744 into CB and CC embryos. It was found that only
the latter responded with splenomegaly. Later experiments
with blood lymphocytes from the Rl-containing offspring
has fully confirmed the original conclusion (Vilhelmova
et al., to be published). Thus, as far as the direct
compatibility test can tell, there are no GVH-stimulatory
antigens encoded in the B-G region of the B-complex. They
are all in the B-F region. However, exactly because the
direct compatibility test is only a measure of gross
compatibility which by no means excludes the presence of
minor histocompatibility differences, other tests are
required for further elucidating the possible role of
the B-G region in histocompatibility.

THE GVH-INHIBITION TEST

The GVH-reactive donor cells can be suppressed
completely in the spleen test by allo-antibodies against
B-complex antigens, (5, 6), and by heterologous antibodies
against chicken thymus (6, 7, 8), but not by anti chicken
Ig. Complement does not appear to be required for the
inhibition. Lydyard and Ivanyi have provided evidence of
the fact that the inhibitory effect of both allo- and
heteroantibodies is due to an Fc-requiring process,
probably opsonization. Crone et al. (6) found on the
contrary that also F(ab) preparations of the alloantibodies were inhibitory, even when the injection was
delayed by several hours after injection of the donor
cells. This finding clearly argued against opsonization,
and it was seen instead as evidence of inhibition of a
receptor system involving MHC products.

However, recent experiments with improved techniques
(Koch and Simonsen, to be published) have not yielded F
(ab) preparations of inhibitory capacity unless when
rabbit-anti-chicken-Ig is added to the system. Furthermore it is now known that also alloantibodies to non-B

loci can inhibit the GVH reactivity of donor cells
injected into B-incompatible embryos. This is for example
what we have recently found with several antisera raised
by hyperimmunization with WBC in chickens which were B-
locus identical though differed by an unknown number of
non-B loci. Table 1 shows the data from an inhibition
experiment with two such antisera.

The interpretation of a positive GVH-inhibition
experiment which now seems the more tenable is that it
simply proves the presence of a molecule in the T-cell
membrane which can react with one or more antibody
specificities in the antiserum used. We are not aware
so far of a case where antibodies are sure to react
with a T-cell without inhibiting its GVH reactivity.

Table 1. GVH-inhibition in a G-Bl panel with 2 alloanti-
         sera, # 2971 & # 2991, directed against non-B
         antigens.

| G-Bl # | 2×10^6 Leukocytes preincubated with | | |
	Diluent	Serum 2971	Serum 2991
877	2.09 + 0.14	1.33 + 0.09	1.16 + 0.11
888	2.05 + 0.04	1.83 + 0.09	1.30 + 0.08
890	1.91 + 0.07	1.72 + 0.05	1.31 + 0.03
946	1.92 + 0.09	1.43 + 0.04	1.37 + 0.03
970	2.04 + 0.15	1.37 + 0.04	1.32 + 0.04
984	1.66 + 0.10	1.44 + 0.05	1.25 + 0.04
1007	1.96 + 0.10	1.42 + 0.04	1.27 + 0.07
1054	2.02 + 0.09	1.98 + 0.07	1.38 + 0.06
1100	2.13 + 0.05	1.92 + 0.03	1.44 + 0.01

The antisera were raised by hyperimmunization with WBC
in B-complex identical birds differing at unknown "minor"
loci. Both sera were employed here in dilutions 1:10.

The data represent mean log spleen weight + S.E. at
day 5 after the i-v. injection of 13 day embryos of
outbred stock. The underscored entries differ from
diluent controls with a p-value < 0.001 (t-test).

Returning now to the further analysis of the B-G
and B-F regions by means of GVH-inhibition, the following
4 antisera were produced by 6-8 weekly i-v injections
of 1-2 ml of whole blood in the following combinations:

CC/WB anti Rl/WB = anti B-F $\frac{CB}{CB}$ = anti CB "Head" (9)
Rl/CC anti CB/CB = anti B-G $\frac{CB}{CC}$ = anti CB "Tail"   "
Rl/CB anti CC/CC = anti B-F $\frac{CC}{CC}$ = anti CC "Head"   "
CB/WB anti Rl/WB = anti B-G = anti CC "Tail"   "

The effect of 4 hemagglutinating specimens of such sera
were now tested in GVH-inhibition of CC and CB cells
with the results shown in Fig. 1. It is clear that none
of the 2 sera against the B-G region antigens had any
inhibitory effect, whereas both the sera directed against
B-F antigens gave very solid inhibition. Apparently the
B-G antigens, which are well expressed in erythrocytes,
are lacking in T-cells, just as they have earlier
appeared to be missing in skin cells (4). Also recent
biochemical analysis (10, 11) suggests that the B-G
antigens are pure blood group antigens. However, in view
of the fact that the antibodies were raised by injection
of whole blood, i.e. in a vast erythrocyte excess,
renewed attempts should be made by injections of WBC
alone.

THE GVH-INHIBITION-REMOVAL TEST

The inhibitory antibodies can naturally be removed
by absorption with cells from the original donor which
provoked them. If a third-party has a phenotype sharing
some T cell-expressed antigens with the original donor,
then the same inhibitory antibodies can also inhibit the
GVH-reacting T-cells from the third-party. Assuming
this being the case, it does not follow, however, that
the third-party's cells can also absorb away all the
inhibitory activity for the original donor's T-cells.
In order to do that it must share all the T-cell antigens,
which are defined by the antiserum employed. Therefore,
the GVH-inhibition-removal test is a more demanding test
than is the simple inhibition test. It was earlier
established (3) that only the former correlated well
with the direct compatibility test in the screening of
outbred birds.

Tables 2 and 3 summarize two experiments which aimed
at testing the degree of similarity between the CC
strain in Prague and the G-Bl strain in Copenhagen by
means of the GVH-inhibition-removal test.

Table 2 shows that an antiserum CB-anti-CC, which
inhibited CC cells, had its inhibitory antibodies
removed equally well by prior absorption with CC and
G-Bl cells, but not of course by CB cells.

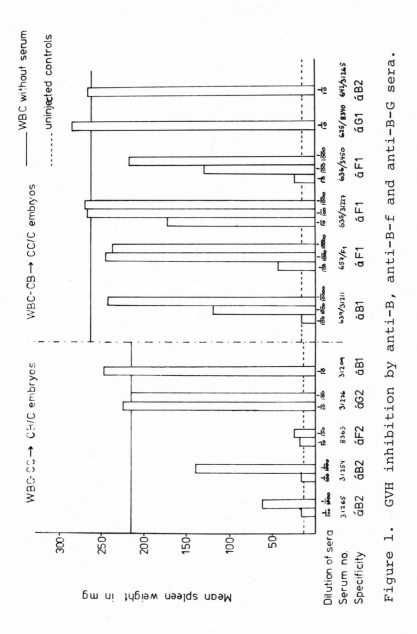

Figure 1. — GVH inhibition by anti-B, anti-B-f and anti-B-G sera.

Table 2. GVH-inhibition-removal test showing absorption
of inhibitory CB-anti-CC antibodies by CC and G-Bl cells.

Antiserum and absorption[x) Dilution 1:50	0.6×10^6 CC leukocytes[xx) injected into outbred embryos log spleen weight ± S.E.
Diluent (PBS)	1.56 ± 0.08
CB-anti-CC, abs CC	1.63 ± 0.07
- - - - G-Bl	1.61 ± 0.11
- - - - CB	1.05 ± 0.02
- - - non-absorbed	1.07 ± 0.06

[x) Absorptions performed at room temperature with 3 times
washed whole blood cells. Half vol. of washed cells
per vol. of antiserum dilution.

[xx) Equal vol. of leukocyte suspension and antibody
dilution preincubated for 1 h. at 37°C.
Embryos injected at day 13 and killed 6 days later.

Table 3. GVH-inhibition-removal test showing absorption
of inhibitory G-B2-anti-G-Bl antibodies by G-Bl and CC,
but not by CB or RI/CB.

Antiserum and absorption	1.5×10^6 G-Bl leukocytes injected. Outbred embryos. 2 independent experiments.	
	I[x) log spleen weight + S.E.	II[xx) log spleen weight + S.E.
Diluent (TCM-199)	1.67 ± 0.10	1.30 ± 0.04
G-B2-anti-G-Bl, abs G-Bl RBC	1.39 ± 0.07	1.45 ± 0.07
- - - - CC -	1.52 ± 0.08	1.51 ± 0.12
- - - - RI/CC -	1.41 ± 0.08	1.57 ± 0.11
- - - - CB -	1.18 ± 0.07	1.24 ± 0.06
- - - - RI/CB -	1.12 ± 0.11	1.14 ± 0.06
- - - - G-B2 -	n.d.	1.09 ± 0.07
- non-absorbed	1.03 ± 0.05	0.98 ± 0.12

[x) Antiserum (1:200 dilution) used was raised against
purified leukocytes.
[xx) Antiserum (1:10 dilution) used was raised against
purified erythrocytes. Other footnotes are the same
as in Table 2.

Table 3 shows the complementary situation where the antiserum was directed against G-B1 and was absorbed equally well by G-B1 and by CC, but not demonstrably so by either CB or by R1/CB. The failure of removal by the latter cells is in keeping with the results from the GVH-inhibition experiments of Fig. 1. R1 contains only the B-G region of the CC-haplotype and, since the B-G region antigens are not apparently expressed in T-cells, absorption with R1/CB could not be expected to remove the inhibitory antibodies either. On the basis of these GVH-inhibition-removal experiments it was expected that the G-B1 and CC strains would also prove compatible in the direct compatibility test. In actual fact they did so only one-way, as shown by the data of Table 4.

In experiment I, CC blood was flown from Prague to Copenhagen and injected on the same day into embryos homozygous for either the G-B1 or G-B2 haplotype. Controls received either G-B1 blood or PBS. It is seen that the spleen weights recorded after injection of the 2 kinds of blood into G-B1 embryos are indistinguishable, in either case only slightly above the PBS controls. In G-B2 embryos they both gave the expected gross splenomegaly.

Table 4.   Direct compatibility test of the B-haplotypes of strains CC and G-B1.

Donor blood	Log spleen weight ± S.E. in recipient embryos	
	G-B1	G-B2
Exp.		
I CC, 0.1 ml, dil. 1:10	1.31 ± 0.04	1.85 ± 0.09
– – , undil.	1.41 ± 0.06	1.95 ± 0.18
G-B1, – , dil. 1:10	1.34 ± 0.04	1.73 ± 0.09
– – , undil.	1.36 ± 0.10	2.01 ± 0.08
PBS	1.15 ± 0.04	1.15 ± 0.08
Exp.		
II G-B1	CC	CB
#891, 0.2 ml, undil.	1.77 ± 0.05	2.19 ± 0.02
#971, – –	1.82 ± 0.05	2.22 ± 0.03
#984, – –	1.86 ± 0.03	2.15 ± 0.02
#1055, – –	1.86 ± 0.05	2.16 ± 0.02

Embryos injected at 13-14 days of incubation and killed 5 days later.

In experiment II, where G-Bl blood from 4 donors was flown from Copenhagen to Prague and injected the same day into CC and CB embryos, the result was markedly different. Although all 4 donors gave a significantly stronger reaction in CB than in CC embryos, the spleen weights recorded in the latter were certainly also grossly enlarged. Simultaneous controls with CC blood were not performed, but numerous earlier control injections of this kind performed by one of us (M.V.) have regularly yielded small spleens of 10-20 mg.

It is noteworthy that Pink et al (10) found the CC and G-Bl strains compatible in 2-way MLC tests, which is clearly in contrast with the result of the direct compatibility test just mentioned. The reason for this discrepancy is not yet understood but will be further investigated.

REFERENCES

1. Jaffe, W.P. and McDermid, E.M., Science, 134: 984 (1962).

2. Schierman, L.W. and Nordskog, A.W., Nature, 197: 511 (1963).

3. Simonsen, M., Acta path. microbiol. scand., Sect. C., 83: 1 (1975).

4. Hálá, K., Vilhelmová, M., and Hartmanová, J. Immuno-genetics 3: 97 (1976).

5. McBride, R.A., Coppleson, L.W., Nisbet, N.W., Simonsen, M., Skowron-Cendrzak, A. and Wigzell, H.L.R., Immunology, 10: 63 (1966).

6. Crone, M., Koch, C. and Simonsen, M., Transplant. Rev. 10: 36 (1972).

7. Lydyard, P. and Ivanyi, J., Transplantation, 12: 493 (1971).

8. Lydyard, P. and Ivanyi, J., Transplantation, 17: 400 (1974).

9. Simonsen, M., Transplant. Proc. 8(3): 329 (1976).

10. Pink, J.R.L., Droege, W., Hálá, K., Miggiano, V.C. and Ziegler, A., In press (1977).

11. Ziegler, A. and Pink, R., J. Biol. Chem. 251: 5391 (1976).

CELL TRANSFER STUDIES WITH THE DK/OR INBRED CHICKEN LINES

Frank Seto

Zoology Department, The University of Oklahoma

Norman, Oklahoma 73019, U. S. A.

INTRODUCTION

Early cell transfer studies with chickens were hampered by histoincompatibility interactions between allogeneic immunocompetent cells of donors and the hosts. To avoid the host allograft rejection response, immunologically immature embryos and baby chick hosts were employed (1,2,3,4,5,6) and the growth and function of the allogeneic cells were often improved (7,8,9) when the hosts were pre-treated with x-irradiation or cylophosphamide to suppress the host's responsiveness. However, the immunologic immaturity of the host fostered the graft-versus-host reaction (GVHR) and allogeneic enhancement effects (7,10). Since the major histoincompatibility factors in chickens are associated with the B and C blood cell antigen systems (11,12,13), such complications are avoidable with the judicial use of genetically histocompatible donors and hosts. The adverse effects of the GVHR were less when certain inbred lines were used (14,15) and successful cell transfer and reconstitution experiments have been reported with inbred adult chickens (16) and with genetically uniform chicks and juvenile birds (17,18,19,20,21,22). With the availability of many inbred lines, several approaching syngeneic level of uniformity according to reports at this conference, cell transfer experiments will be utilized more in avian immunology.

Early Studies with the DK/OR Inbred Lines

Although our allogeneic cell transfer system has been useful for some adoptive cell transfer experiments in the past (8,9,23), its application to reconstitution and cell interaction studies has

been restricted by histoincompatibility interactions between the
participating donor and host cell populations. With the availability of the DK/OR inbred lines, we have initiated such studies.
The White Leghorn chicken lines were initiated at the Biology Division of the Oak Ridge National Laboratory, Oak Ridge, Tennessee,
U.S.A., with eggs obtained from Dr. W. E. Briles. The eggs were
from crosses of established commercial inbred lines with B and C
red cell antigen markers. Before the Oak Ridge colony was phased
out, Dr. J. F. Albright and Dr. T. Makinodan generously provided
eggs to establish a new colony at the University of Oklahoma,
Norman, Oklahoma, U.S.A. Since 1970 we have continued the inbreeding program initiated by Dr. Albright and have extracted four lines
homozygous for the B^{13}, B^{19}, C^2 and C^4 blood group markers. These
have been maintained by brother-sister matings. The original B
allele designations in these lines were B^1 and B^2 and were so reported in earlier papers (10,26,27,28). In accordance with a proposed International Nomenclature System, the numbering of the alleles in the DK/OR lines have been changed to B^{13} and B^{19}, respectively. The histoincompatibility within each line was analyzed
with the embryonic spleen assay, a direct test for the GVHR. Splenomegaly is one of the more constant and measurable features of
histoincompatibility interaction (24,25). When whole blood from
immunocompetent donors were injected into 13 to 14 day assay hosts
of the same or different lines, only those combinations where the
host differed from the donor in a B antigen was significant splenomegaly observed. All other combinations were negative. Representative data from this study (26) are shown in Table 1.

TABLE 1

Spleen weights of embryonic hosts inoculated with blood from immunocompetent donors. Donor cells were administered into 14-day embryos and spleen weights measured six days later.

Donor	Hosts		
Line	Line	Number	Mean Spleen Weights
DK/OR-1	DK-OR-1	43	12.5 ± 3.1[a]
DK/OR-3	DK-OR-3	23	13.4 ± 3.6
DK/OR-1/3	DK-OR-1/3	13	8.8 ± 1.1
DK/OR-1	DK/OR-3	25	23.4 ± 7.6[b]
DK/OR-3	DK/OR-1	25	35.6 ± 10.1[b]

[a] Weights in mg with s.d.

[b] P of 0.01

The in vivo culture antibody assay was used in reverse to measure indirectly the allograft-rejecting capacity of hosts in incompatible donor-host combinations (8). Immunocytes from immunized donors when mixed in vitro with MRBC and administered to embryonic hosts will produce moderate to high hemagglutinin titers within a week of in vivo culture. Various combinations of donors and hosts with respect to B^{13} and B^{19} antigens were tested and the hemagglutinin output measured. For comparable amounts of donor immunocytes, the antibody output with 14-day hosts was high in both B antigen-matched and mismatched donor-host combinations. With 17-day embryo and baby chick hosts, however, the in vivo titers were significantly reduced in many mismatched hosts. The decrease was directly correlated with B antigen disparity between donor and host. Moreover, when older hosts pretreated with cyclophosphamide prior to cell grafting were similarly tested, significantly greater improvement in antibody production was observed in the mismatched hosts than in B antigen-matched hosts. Representative data from this study (10) are shown in Table 2.

Observations from these earlier studies (10,26) and those reported in this paper indicate that the DK/OR lines are sufficiently histocompatible for use in cell transfer studies.

MATERIALS AND METHODS

Most of the experiments described here have been performed with eggs and chickens of the DK/OR-1($B^{13}B^{13}$ C^2C^2) and DK/OR-3

TABLE 2

In vivo culture hemagglutinin titers of baby chicks inoculated with immunocyte-MRBC mixtures at hatching. Different combinations of donors and hosts were tested.

Donor	Hosts		
Line	Line	Number	Mean Antibody Titers
DK/OR-1	DK/OR-1	11	8.0 ± 0.8[a]
DK/OR-1	DK/OR-3	13	3.6 ± 1.2[b]
DK/OR-3	DK/OR-3	7	6.5 ± 1.6
DK/OR-3	DK/OR-1/3	6	7.0 ± 1.3
DK/OR-3	DK/OR-1	5	3.0 ± 0.7[b]

[a] Hemagglutinin titers in $\log_2$ units and s.d.

[b] P of 0.01

($B^{19}B^{19}C^2C^2$) inbred lines of White Leghorn chickens. Unless indicated otherwise, embryos and chicks used for the in vivo antibody
assay and cell transfer experiments were of the same line as the
donors.

Mortality Counts

Blood and cell suspensions of bone marrow cells or thymocytes
were prepared from juvenile donors, 5 to 9 weeks of age. One-tenth
ml of whole blood in Alsever's solution, 10^7 bone marrow cells in
Alsever's solution or 10^7 thymus cells in Medium 199 was administered intravenously to each 14-day embryo host. Survival counts
were made at hatching, 1 week and 5 weeks of age depending on the
experimental group.

The In Vivo Antibody Assay

This assay method was used to estimate the relative content of
antigen responsive cells (ARC) in bone marrow. Femurs were dissect-
ed from the donors, cleaned of adherent tissues, rinsed in sterile
saline and the marrow flushed out with sterile Alsever's solution.
The marrow was dispersed by lightly aspirating the fragments through
a 20 gauge needle attached to a plastic syringe. The resulting cell
suspension was lightly centrifuged to remove cell clumps and washed
in fresh sterile Alsever's solution. Alsever's solution was used
to avoid clot formation in the cell suspension which often occurred
with tissue culture media. All tissue preparations were made at
room temperature in siliconized glassware. One-tenth ml of the
suspension containing 10^7 "lymphoid" cells, with or without sterile
MRBC suspension depending on the experiment, was intravenously administered to 14-day embryo hosts. Six days later, serum samples
were collected and stored in a freezer. The anti-MRBC hemagglutinin
titers were quantitated with the limiting dilution method in U-type
Microtiter plates (Cooke Engineering, Alexandria, Va.) and recorded
in $\log_2$ units.

Baby Chick Immune Enhancement Assay

Bone marrow cells, with or without MRBC depending on the experiment, were administered into 14 or 18 day embryo recipients.
Upon hatching, the chicks were challenged with MRBC and bled six
days later for antibody titration. Since the untreated newly
hatched chicks respond poorly to MRBC immunization, elevated hemagglutinin production in the grafted chicks can be attributable in
part to the transferred cells. As the host immune system has not
been neutralized in this model, the antibody production presumably

TABLE 3

Survival of chicks inoculated as 14 to 16 day embryos with whole blood, bone marrow cells or thymocytes from 5 to 9 week old donors.

Lines[a]		Cells	No. of	No. (%) of hosts surviving at		
Donor	Host	Grafted	Embryos	Hatch	1 week	5 weeks
(Intraline combinations)						
1	1	Blood	53	36 (68)[b]	36 (100)[c]	
		Blood	46	23 (50)	18 (78)	16 (70)[c]
1	1	Bone marrow	80	54 (68)	46 (85)	
		Thymocytes	47	41 (87)	41 (100)	
2	2	Blood	65	39 (60)	26 (66)	19 (49)
3	3	Blood	17	16 (94)	16 (100)	
		Blood	45	30 (66)	26 (87)	19 (63)
3	3	Bone marrow	10	7 (70)	6 (86)	
		Thymocytes	19	14 (74)	12 (86)	
4	4	Blood	35	22 (63)	15 (68)	8 (36)
(Interline combinations)						
1	3	Bone marrow	38	17 (45)	12 (71)	0
3	2	Thymocytes	12	4 (33)	3 (75)	0

[a] 1 (DK/OR-1), 2 (DK/OR-2), 3 (DK/OR-3), 4 (DK/OR-4)

[b] Percent of hosts surviving to hatch

[c] Percent of chicks that hatched

involves the cooperative interaction of host and donor cellular elements.

RESULTS

Mortality of Cell Transfer Hosts

When 14-day embryos are administered blood, bone marrow cells or thymocytes from immunocompetent allogeneic donors, a GVHR follows that usually kills the immunologically incompetent hosts. The GVHR-related mortality should be absent in histocompatible hosts. The four DK/OR lines were tested with the GVHR mortality assay of embryonic and chick hosts inoculated with immunocompetent cells from donors of the same line. Each embryo received 0.1 ml of whole blood, 10^7 bone marrow cells or 10^7 thymocytes. Survival counts of

the hosts were made at hatching, 1 week and 5 weeks of age. Two
other series were conducted in which the donors and the hosts were
from different lines. The results are summarized in Table 3.

In the combinations where the donor and host were of different
lines, the mortality was high, runting was frequent and no recipients survived to five weeks of age. In all the intra-line cell
transfers, the survival rate was considerably higher, birds were
rarely runted and appeared healthy at five weeks of age.

Bone Marrow Cell Transfer Experiments

In vivo antibody assay. Bone marrow cells from unimmunized
birds were administered to 14-day embryo hosts, one group receiving
bone marrow cells only, the other a MRBC-bone marrow mixture. Another similar series was conducted but with bone marrow cells from
donors immunized four days earlier with MRBC. The hosts were bled
six days later and the serum tested for anti-MRBC hemagglutinin
activity. The results are summarized in Table 4.

Only in the groups of hosts that received a mixture of MRBC-
bone marrow cells from immunized donors were any significant

TABLE 4

In vivo antibody assay of bone marrow cells from unimmunized and
MRBC-primed 5 to 8 week donors. Embryos were inoculated on the
14th day of incubation and bled six days later for antibody determination.

Donors		Hosts		Mean Antibody
Group	No.	Cells Grafted	No.	Titers $\pm$ s.e.
Unimmunized	1	Bone marrow cells	9	0.5 ± 0.0
Unimmunized	3	Bone marrow cells and MRBC	16	0.5 ± 0.0
Immunized	2	Bone marrow cells	18	0.5 ± 0.1
Immunized	3	Bone marrow cells and MRBC	12	2.2 ± 0.4[a]
Immunized[b]	2	Bone marrow cells and MRBC	6	5.4 ± 1.1[c]

[a] P. of 0.01

[b] Second MRBC injection on day 17 of incubation

[c] P of 0.05

hemagglutinin titers obtained. Moreover, the group that received
a second MRBC stimulation showed an even higher response.

     Baby chick immune enhancement assay. It was reported earlier
that baby chicks grafted as embryos with thymocytes or bone marrow
from antigen-primed donors responded to MRBC immunization with an
enhanced response (27,28). Experiments were conducted to ascertain
the factors that would favor the manifestation of the enhancement
effect associated with bone marrow grafting. Bone marrow cells
from unimmunized donors were administered into 18-day embryo hosts.
One group of hosts received bone marrow cells only; the other, a
mixture of bone marrow cells and MRBC. A similar series was set up
with bone marrow from donors immunized four days earlier with MRBC.
Upon hatching, the recipients were immunized with 0.5 ml of a 1%
MRBC suspension and bled six days later for hemagglutinin titers.
The results are summarized in Table 5.

     Bone marrow from unimmunized donors had only a marginal effect
whereas that from antigen-primed donors produced obvious enhancement of the anti-MRBC responsiveness in newly-hatched chicks. Bone
marrow from donors immunized two days or earlier was less effective.
When the bone marrow suspension included MRBC an even greater

TABLE 5

Hemagglutinin titers of untreated newly-hatched chicks and those
grafted with bone marrow cells from unimmunized or MRBC-primed
donors.

| Donors | | Hosts | | Mean Antibody |
Group	No.	Cells Grafted	No.	Titers $\pm$ s.e.
None	–	None	23	0.9 ± 0.3
Unimmunized	3	Bone marrow cells	12	2.1 ± 0.7
Unimmunized	1	Bone marrow cells and MRBC	8	1.4 ± 0.7
Immunized[a]	1	Bone marrow cells	11	9.2 ± 1.0[b]
Immunized[a]	1	Bone marrow cells and MRBC	7	12.8 ± 0.6[c]
Immunized[d]	2	Bone marrow cells and MRBC	14	4.4 ± 0.6[c]

[a] Primed with MRBC four days earlier
[b] P of 0.01
[c] P of 0.05
[d] Primed with MRBC less than 2 days earlier

enhancement effect resulted. A similar augmenting effect by antigen was observed in the in vivo antibody assay system (see Table 4). When MRBC and bone marrow cells from an immunized donor were inoculated together into 14-day embryo hosts the resulting antibody titer was usually low. Following a second MRBC exposure on the 17th day of incubation, however, a significantly higher response was obtained. Encounter of the grafted bone marrow cells with antigen appears to increase their capacity to respond.

DISCUSSION

The results of the GVH splenomegaly assay and the in vivo antibody assay reported earlier (10,26) and the mortality data of chick hosts grafted with immunocompetent cells reported here, indicate that histoincompatibility within the DK/OR-1 and DK/OR-3 inbred White Leghorn lines is relatively low. No significant splenomegaly was observed and the GVHR-related mortality was considerably less among the embryonic hosts grafted with immunocompetent cells from donors of the same line compared with those receiving allogeneic cells. Although the two lines probably still retain a residuum of minor histocompatibility factors which we have not tested, the overall results of the experiments described here would favor further investigations of these lines.

MRBC-specific antigen responsive cells (ARC), detected with the in vivo antibody assay, seem to be absent in the bone marrow of the unimmunized juvenile donors tested, but after immunization with MRBC, soon appear in small numbers in this organ. The ARC concentration, however, was considerably lower than that reported earlier in the peripheral blood and spleen (29). When mixtures of MRBC and bone marrow cells from immunized donors were cultured in embryonic in vivo hosts, and challenged with MRBC three days later, the resulting hemagglutinin titers were considerably elevated. It appears that exposure of bone marrow cells to MRBC at the time of grafting not only triggered the few ARC present in the cell suspension to hemagglutinin production but more significantly expanded concomitantly the pool of potential ARC in the bone marrow inoculum. Baby chicks grafted as embryos with bone marrow from unimmunized juvenile donors showed only a marginal response to MRBC immunization. Chicks that received bone marrow from immunized donors, however, showed a dramatic enhancement in the MRBC humoral response. The effect was even greater when the bone marrow cell suspension included MRBC. Immunization of the donor appears to increase the relative concentration of anti-MRBC ARC and their precursors in the bone marrow. The increase in the precursor pool may have resulted from recruitment or clonal expansion and differentiation of stem cells in situ, or both. Moreover, after transfer into embryonic hosts, the bone marrow cells appear to be capable of further antigen-stimulated clonal expansion.

The anti-MRBC immune response is probably T cell-dependent like the chicken anti-SRBC response (20,21,28). The ARC activity assayed with the in vivo cell transfer system is functionally like that of the mammalian ASU, a synergistic team of T and B memory cells (30). Following immunization with MRBC, the concentration of ARC is high in the peripheral blood and spleen, low in the bone marrow and negligible in the thymus and the bursa of Fabricius (28, 29). These observations are consistent with the conventional view of the distribution of T cells, B cells and their precursors. T and B cells are abundant in the blood, spleen and other peripheral lymphoid sites. B cells and their precursors occur in the bursa, T cells originate in the thymus, and precursors of both lines and some B cells are present in the bone marrow (31,32,33). Recent information on chickens, however, tend to refute the exclusive dichotomy in the distribution of T cells, B cells and their precursors in these tissues (25,34,35). The limited scope of the data presented here, the known heterogeneity in the cell populations of the thymus, bursa and bone marrow and the inability of our assay system in its present design to distinguish between the contributions of donor and host cells preclude at this time any definitive statements regarding the cell types that are responsible for the precocious responsiveness of chicks grafted with bone marrow from immunized donors.

SUMMARY

The histoincompatibility in the DK-OR-1 ($B^{13}B^{13}$) and DK/OR-3 ($B^{19}B^{19}$) inbred White Leghorn chicken lines was assessed with the Simonsen's spleen assay, GVHR mortality counts and antibody production by transferred cells in embryonic in vivo hosts. The two lines appear to be sufficiently histocompatible for use in cell transfer experiments.

The occurrence of antigen responsive cells (ARC) and precursor cells in bone marrow was assessed with the in vivo culture and baby chick immune enhancement assays. Bone marrow of unimmunized donors possessed very little anti-MRBC immune responsiveness. Bone marrow cells from MRBC-primed donors, however, showed low anti-MRBC activity in the in vivo culture which could be elevated with a second antigen stimulation. Chicks grafted as embryos with bone marrow from immunized donors responded to MRBC immunization in an enhanced manner as compared to the control untreated chicks which responded poorly if at all to the antigen. Immunization appears (a) to increase the pool of potential ARC in the bone marrow of the donor and (b) to augment the responsiveness of bone marrow cells transferred into embryonic hosts.

ACKNOWLEDGEMENTS. Research sponsored by a USPHS grant, A1-12488-02, and a grant-in-aid from the University of Oklahoma Office of Research Administration.

REFERENCES

1. Mitchison, N. A., J. Cell. & Comp. Physiol. 50 (sup. 1): 247 (1957).

2. Trnka, Z., Nature (Lond.) 181: 55 (1958)

3. Sibal, L. R. and Olson, V. H., Proc. Soc. Exp. Biol. Med. 97: 575 (1958).

4. Isacson, P., Yale J. Biol. Med. 32: 209 (1959).

5. Haskova, V. and Svoboda, J., Folia Biol. (Praha). 5: 8 (1959).

6. Sterzl, J., Nature (Lond.). 183: 547 (1959).

7. Seto, F., Transplantation. 5: 1280 (1967).

8. Seto, F., J. Exp. Zool. 177: 343 (1971).

9. Seto, F., Proc. Okla. Acad. Sci. 50: 45 (1970).

10. Seto, F., Exp. Hemat. 2: 219 (1974).

11. Schierman, L. W. and Nordskog, A. W., Science 134: 1008 (1961).

12. Schierman, L. W. and Nordskog, A. W., Transplantation. 3: 44 (1965).

13. Craig, J. V. and McDermid, E. M., Transplantation. 1: 191 (1963).

14. Jaffe, W. P. and Payne, L. N., Immunology. 5: 399 (1962).

15. Mun, A. M., Tardent, P., Errico, J., Ebert, J. D., Delanney, L. E. and Argyris, T. S., Biol. Bull. 123: 366 (1962).

16. Orlans, E. and Rose, M. E., Immunology. 18: 473 (1970).

17. Gilmour, D. G., Theis, G. A. and Thorbecke, G. J., J. Exp. Med. 132: 134 (1970).

18. Toivanen, P., Toivanen, A., and Good, R. A., J. Exp. Med. 136: 816 (1972).

19. McArthur, W. P., Gilmour, D. G. and Thorbecke, G. J., Cell. Immunol. 8: 103 (1973).

20. Hala, K., Folia Biol. (Praha). 20: 262 (1974).

21. Sarvas, J., Makela, O., Toivanen, P., and Toivanen, A., Scand. J. Immunol. 31: 455 (1974).

22. Weber, W. T., Transpl. Rev. 24: 113 (1975).

23. Seto, F., Poultry Sci. 52: 1714 (1973).

24. Simonsen, M., Progr. Allergy. 6: 349 (1962).

25. Coppleson, L. W. and Michie, D., Nature (Lond.). 208: 53 (1965).

26. Seto, F., Proc. Okla. Acad. Sci. 53: 61 (1973).

27. Seto, F., Exp. Hemat. 3: 319 (1975).

28. Seto, F., In Phylogeny of Thymus and Bone Marrow-Bursa Cells. (R. K. Wright and E. L. Cooper eds.). (Elsevier/North-Holland, Amsterdam, 1976).

29. Seto, F., Poultry Sci. 49: 1673 (1970).

30. Shearer, G. M., Cudkowicz, G., Connell, M. S. J.. and Priore, R. I., J. Exp. Med. 128: 437 (1968).

31. Abdou, N. I. and Richter, M., Adv. Immunol. 12: 201 (1970).

32. Cooper, M. D., Peterson, R. D. A., South, M. A., and Good, R. A., J. Exp. Med. 128: 75 (1966).

33. Claman, H. N., Bioscience. 23: 576 (1973).

34. Greaves, M. F., Owen, J. J. T., and Raff, M. C., T and B Lymphocytes: origins, properties and roles in immune responses. 316 pp. (Excerpta Medica, Amsterdam, 1973).

35. Droege, W., Europ. J. Immunol. 6: 279 (1976).

ROLE OF THE MAJOR HISTOCOMPATIBILITY COMPLEX IN RESISTANCE TO MAREK'S DISEASE: RESTRICTION OF THE GROWTH OF JMV-MD TUMOR CELLS IN GENETICALLY RESISTANT BIRDS

Longenecker, B.M.[1], Pazderka, F.[2], Gavora, J.S.[3], Spencer, J.L.[4], Stephens, E.A.[5], Witter, R.L.[6] and Ruth, R.F.[7]

Departments of Immunology[1], Medicine[2] and Zoology[7], University of Alberta, Edmonton, Alberta, Canada; Animal Research Institute[3], Animal Diseases Research Institute (E)[4], Agriculture Canada, Ottawa, Ontario, Canada; U.S. Department of Agriculture[5,6], ARS, Regional Poultry Research Laboratory, East Lansing, Michigan

SUMMARY

B^{21} is associated with resistance to Marek's disease (MD). Forty populations of chickens from all over the world were examined for the presence of the B^{21} allele. B^{21} was found in twelve of these populations and it's presence was confirmed by GVH testing in all ten populations which were tested. The populations in which B^{21} was detected represent the extreme production types of the species and include the progenitor of the species, the Red Jungle Fowl. Our studies suggest that B^{21} may have strong survival value for the species. An allogeneic transplantable lymphoma of MD, the JMV tumor cell line, grows more slowly in MD resistant (B^{21}/B^{21}) chicks than in MD susceptible (B^2/B^2) chicks. This is the first direct evidence that genetic resistance to MD may involve an active (immunological?) restriction of tumor cell growth. JMV cells were further characterized as a transplant of B_1 carrying lymphoblastoid cells, an allele which may be associated with susceptibility to MD.

INTRODUCTION

Possible involvement of the major histocompatibility system in resistance to Marek's disease (MD) was reported by Hansen *et al.* (1967), Brewer *et al.* (1969), Briles and Oleson (1971) and Briles (1974). Hansen *et al.* compared the effects of two *B* alleles, B^{19}

and B^{21}, which had been defined by extensive serologic comparisons
of Hy-Line International's lines of inbred White Leghorns. B^{19}
was associated with relative susceptibility and B^{21} with relative
resistance to MD. Other studies by Hansen and his co-workers indicated that MD-resistant Line N carried a B allele which could
not be discriminated from Hy-Line B^{21} by serologic tests (personal
communication). Since the Hy-Line alleles were defined by antisera absorbed to mono-specificity and the serologic work of others
depended on the use of panels of cross-reactive sera, it was apparent that the identity and non-identity of B alleles drawn from
separate populations could be a source of endless disputation. The
situation was resolved by a combination of serologic mono-specificity with the graft-versus-host (GVH) reaction known as the pock
test (Pazderka *et al.*, 1975a, 1975b). The latter discriminates
between GVH reactions due to B antigen and GVH reactions due to
other antigens (Longenecker *et al.*, 1970,1972,1973). This approach
proved that H-Line B^{21} is identical with Line N B^{21} (Pazderka *et
al.*,1975; Longenecker *et al.*, 1976). This also permitted B^{21} to be
cleanly discriminated from the B^2 allele present in MD resistant
Line 6 and MD susceptible Line 7 (East Lansing) (Pazderka *et al.*,
1975a, 1975b). In 1975 it was generally agreed that the Hy-Line
system should be followed primarily because six of its alleles had
been rediscovered in various populations and three of these rediscoveries had been confirmed by the GVH pock test (Pazderka *et
al.*, 1975a). In the course of this, W.E. Briles and F. Pazderka
separately established that the Hy-Line allele B^{15} was two separate
alleles now designated B^{15} and B^5 (unpublished data). The resolu-
tion of the terminological and geographical problems of the B system
and the demonstration that resistance to MD is co-inherited with
B^{21} evolved together and are a forceful demonstration of the value
of collaboration and cross-communication in B research. Our studies
(Longenecker *et al.*, 1976) have firmly established the association
of B^{21} with MD resistance by employing classical mendelian analysis.
This association has recently been confirmed (Briles *et al.*, 1977).

In this report we examine populations other than Line N in
search of B^{21} as a step toward a panoramic test of the possibility
that B^{21} is always associated with resistance to MD. We also describe the fate of B^2 and B^{21} homozygotes of one of these populations challenged with a transplantable MD tumor (JMV) (Spencer *et
al.*, 1976), we characterize this lymphoma as a transplant of B^1
carrying lymphoblastoid cells which do not yield virus which transform host lymphocytes, and we suggest that B^{21} confers resistance
to this non-infective form of MD, a suggestion which discriminates
resistance to MD lymphoma from resistance to transformation by the
herpesvirus of MD.

MATERIALS AND METHODS

B alloantigen blood typing was done as described previously (Pazderka *et al.*, 1975a, 1975b). The GVH pock assay was done according to Longenecker *et al.*, 1970. Ottawa line XP, which is segregating for B^2 and B^{21} was inoculated with the BC-1 isolate of MDV (suspension of ovarian tumor cells, Spencer *et al.*, 1974) at 21 days, blood typed at 25 days, and on day 80 survivors were killed and examined for gross lesions of Marek's disease. Separate hatches from the line XP were not challenged with MDV but were blood typed as adults and divided into B^{21}/B^{21} and B^2/B^2 sublines. Newly hatched progeny from these sublines were challenged subcutaneously with 650 cells from the low passage JMV tumor transplant (Spencer *et al.*, 1976) originally derived from an MD lymphoma (Sevoian *et al.*, 1964). Mortality was observed up to eighteen days post inoculation. It has been established that death up to this time is due to the growth of the JMV transplant (Spencer *et al.*, 1976; Gavora *et al.*, 1977).

In order to determine the B alloantigens of JMV cells, 8-week old White Leghorns of line 6_3, which is uniformly homozygous for the B^2 allele, were immunized with 10^8 JMV tumor cells taken from other line 6_3 White Leghorns. Line 6_3 (B^2/B^2) White Leghorns were chosen for immunization since we had previously shown (Stephens *et al.*, 1976) that JMV cells do not carry the B_2 alloantigen. The JMV cells were injected intramuscularly in complete Freund's adjuvant. The chickens were re-immunized intraabdominally without adjuvant at the ages of 10, 12, 15, 17 and 21 weeks and bled one and two weeks after the last immunization. These sera were tested for their capacity to agglutinate the erythrocytes of birds of several B genotypes both before and after absorption with erythrocytes from birds of several B genotypes.

RESULTS

Forty populations of chickens which were obtained from all over the world were blood typed for 'B' using alloantisera monospecific for our eight reference B alloantigens (Pazderka *et al.*, 1975a, 1975b). In eight of these populations none of the reference B alleles were detected; the pattern of reactivity with our antisera indicated the existence of still unidentified B alleles in these strains. The B_{21} alloantigen was detected serologically in 12 of the remaining 32 populations and its presence was confirmed by GVH testing in all ten populations which were tested (Table 1). Of the two lines (XN, R-80) not examined with the GVH test, serologically detected B^{21} was associated with resistance in line XN (Longenecker *et al.*, 1976). Line R-80 was not tested for MD resistance. The 12 populations in which B^{21} was detected represent the extreme production types of the species: White Leghorn,

Table 1   Chicken populations in which B^{21} was detected

Origin	Line	Breed	Phenotypic Frequency of B_{21}[a]	Alloantigen Confirmed by GVH
Cornell	N	WL[c]	100	+
Cornell	P	WL	20	+
Wagengingen	W-157	WL	100	+
Wagengingen	W-179	WL	100	+
Ottawa	XR	WL	43	+
Ottawa	XN	WL	54	NT[b]
Ottawa	XP	WL	85	+
Wagengingen	R-80	RIR[d]	45	NT
Vancouver	BA	BA[e]	64	+
Ames	M	FAY[f]	7	+
Saskatoon	FAY	FAY	6	+
San Diego) Toronto)	–	JF[g]	75	+

[a] Alloantigen detected by hemagglutination using monospecific antisera

[b] but B^{21} in line XN is associated with MD resistance (Longenecker *et al.*, 1976)

[c] White Leghorn

[d] Rhode Island Red

[e] Black Australorp

[f] Fayoumi

[g] Jungle Fowl

Rhode Island Red, Black Australop, Fayoumi and the Red Jungle Fowl, the progenitor of the species (Weiss and Biggs, 1972).

Among these populations the XP line was chosen to reconfirm the association of B^{21} with resistance to MD. Table 2 shows the incidence of MD in B^{21}/B^{21}, B^2/B^{21} and B^2/B^2 birds of the XP line (Longenecker *et al.*, 1976). The beneficial effect of the B^{21} allele in this line is obvious (χ^2_{2df} = 38.51; p <0.001). Progeny of the B^{21}/B^{21} and B^2/B^2 sublines which were established from the XP line were challenged at hatching with JMV tumor cells and mortality to 18 days of age was followed. Death occurred in 37.1% of the B^2/B^2 and 13.3% of the B^{21}/B^{21} progeny (Table 3) due to the growth of the tumor transplant. This difference is significant (χ^2_{1df} = 5.5; p <0.025). These results suggest that JMV cells grow less well in a genetically resistant (B^{21}) environment than in a genetically susceptible (B^2) environment. One possible explanation for these results might be that JMV cells share major histocompatibility antigens with B^2/B^2 chicks. Our previous data show that this is not the case (Stephens *et al.*, 1976). Another possibility is that JMV bears the B^{21} alloantigen as well as virally-modified B^{21} alloantigens which might allow preferential immunological recognition of these modified alloantigens by B^{21}/B^{21} individuals (Doherty and Zinkernagel, 1975). In order to examine this possibility, antisera which had been prepared in line 6$_3$ (B^2/B^2) birds against JMV cells were tested for their capacity to agglutinate erythrocytes from birds of various 'B' genotypes. All but one serum agglutinated the erythrocytes of a B^1/B^1 chicken more strongly or more completely than they agglutinated the erythrocytes of five other genotypes: B^2/B^2, B^{13}/B^{13}, B^{14}/B^{14}, B^{15}/B^{15} and B^{21}/B^{21} (Table 4). The exceptional serum did not agglutinate any of the erythrocytes. The weak agglutinations of erythrocytes of genotypes other than B^1/B^1 are not surprising. Immunization of chickens with erythrocytes of B genotype, other than that of the chicken being immunized, produces pan-agglutinating antisera, i.e. antisera which react with all B genotypes which include B alleles not present in the immunized chicken. It is conventional to attribute these serologic cross-reactions to public antigens, i.e. those encoded by cistrons present in more than one allelic complex, and to discriminate between these and private antigens, i.e. those encoded by cistrons unique to one allelic complex. Each B allele encodes at least one private antigen which serves as the definitive serologic antigen by which the allele is identified. The immunization with JMV tumor cells indicates that these cells carry serologic antigens characteristic of allele B^1 in company with public antigens shared with one or more alleles B^2, B^3, B^5, B^6, B^{13}, B^{14}, B^{15} and B^{21}. The only exceptional feature of these tests is the agglutination of erythrocytes from two B^2/B^2 chickens. This type of reaction also occurs when B^2/B^2 chickens are immunized with erythrocytes from a donor who is not a close relative of the immunized B^2/B^2 chicken. The antisera may agglutinate the erythrocytes of other B^2/B^2 non-relatives. Such reactions are due to other blood groups, e.g. A, C, etc., which may be shared by the donor of the immunizing cells and the donor of the test cells, but are not shared with the immunized chicken. Such non-B reactions as well as the reactions with the public antigens of B alleles are eliminated by absorption of the sera with erythrocytes from selected genotypes.

Two of the stronger antisera were analyzed in detail (Table 5). Antiserum #49 was absorbed with B^2/B^2 erythrocytes which removed agglutinins for B^2/B^2, B^2/B^3, B^2/B^6, B^{13}/B^{13} and B^{14}/B^{14} erythrocytes, attributable to presence of shared, non-B antigens. B^3 and B^6 represent new alleles identified in the Black Australorp strain. Absorption with B^1/B^1 erythrocytes removed all remaining activity. Absorption with B^{21}/B^{21} erythrocytes removed agglutinins for B^5/B^5 and B^{21}/B^{21} erythrocytes. Absorption with B^{15}/B^{15} erythrocytes removed agglutinins for B^{15}/B^{15} erythrocytes, leaving weak activity for B^1/B^1 erythrocytes. Finally, the antiserum was tested with erythrocytes taken from a panel of 18 chickens not used in the absorptions (Table 6). Eight of these were B^1 erythrocytes and 10 lacked B_1 antigens. The antiserum agglutinated all B^1 erythrocytes (1.0 $\pm$ 0.0) and none of the others. Assuming this result to be unrelated to B^1, Fisher's exact probability is 2.3 x 10^{-5}, about one chance in 40,000. The second antiserum (#47) was absorbed with B^2/B^3 and B^{21}/B^{21} erythrocytes (Table 5), leaving moderate activity for B^1/B^1 erythrocytes. Tested with the same panel of erythrocytes (Table 6), this gave results slightly more emphatic than those for the first antiserum (2.0 $\pm$ 0.19 for B^1 erythrocytes; 0.0 for all others).

The results strongly suggest that the JMV cells against which the Line 63 B^2/B^2 chickens produced antibody are not derived from Line 63 lymphocytes and that JMV cells bear the B_1 alloantigens.

Table 2   Incidence of Marek's disease in chickens of various B genotypes

'B' Genotype	No. Tested	% MD
B^2/B^2	67	19.4
B^2/B^{21}	148	0.6
B^{21}/B^{21}	65	0

Table 3   Mortality due to growth of the JMV tumor transplant in B^2/B^2 and B^{21}/B^{21} sublines

'B' Genotype	No. Tested	% Dead
B^2/B^2	62	37.1
B^{21}/B^{21}	30	13.3

Table 4 Test of unabsorbed antisera against JMV cells produced in B^2/B^2 chickens

RBC/s B. Phenotype	Antiserum No. 37	38	39	40	41	42	47	48	49	50	51
B^1/B^1	0	+++	+++	+++	+++	+++	+++	+++	+++	+++	+++
B^2/B^2	0	+	+	+	0	+	0	+	+	+	+
B^2/B^2	0	0	+	+	0	+	+	+	+	+	+
B^2/B^3							++		+		
B^2/B^6							+		0		
B^5/B^5							++		+		
B^{13}/B^{13}	0	+	+	+	+	+	+	+	+	+	+
B^{13}/B^{13}							+		+		
B^{14}/B^{14}	0	+	+	+	+	+	+	+	+	+	+
B^{14}/B^{14}							+		+		
B^{15}/B^{15}	0	+	+	+	+	+	0	+	0	+	+
B^{19}/B^{19}							0		0		
B^{21}/B^{21}	0	++	+	++	+	+	++	+	++	+	+
B^{21}/B^{21}	0	++	+	++	+	+	++	+	+	+	+

+++ = strong agglutination   ++ = moderate agglutination   + = weak agglutination

0 = no agglutination   blank = not tested

Table 5　Test of partially absorbed antisera against JMV cells produced in B^2/B^2 chickens

RBC/s Phenotype	Antiserum #47 Absorbed B^2/B^3	Antiserum #49 Absorbed B^2/B^2	Antiserum #49 Absorbed B^2/B^2, B^{21}/B^{21}
B^1/B^1	+++	+++	+++
B^2/B^2		0	
B^2/B^2	0	0	0
B^2/B^3	0	0	
B^2/B^6		0	
B^5/B^5		++	0
B^{13}/B^{13}	0	0	
B^{13}/B^{13}		0	0
B^{14}/B^{14}	0	0	0
B^{14}/B^{14}		0	
B^{15}/B^{15}	0	+	+
B^{21}/B^{21}	+	+	0
B^{21}/B^{21}	+		0

Table 6 Test of absorbed antisera against JMV cells produced
in B^2/B^2 chickens

RBC's Phenotype	Antiserum #47 absorbed with B^2/B^3 and B^{21}/B^{21} RBC's	Antiserum #49 absorbed with B^2/B^2, B^{21}/B^{21} and B^{15}/B^{15} RBC's
B^1/B^1	+	+
B^1/B^1	++	+
B^1/B^1	++	+
B^1/B^2	+++	+
B^1/B^{13}	++	+
B^1/B^{13}	++	+
B^1/B^{14}	++	+
B^1/B^{14}	++	+
B^2/B^2	0	0
B^2/B^2	0	0
B^2/B^{19}	0	0
B^2/B^{19}	0	0
B^{13}/B^{13}	0	0
B^{14}/B^{14}	0	0
B^{14}/B^{14}	0	0
B^{15}/B^{15}	0	0
B^{19}/B^{19}	0	0
B^{21}/B^{21}	0	0

DISCUSSION

Our studies demonstrate that the B^{21} allele, whose alloantigens were detected serologically and confirmed in most cases
using the GVH test, is widespread throughout the species. B^{21} was
demonstrated in several White Leghorn lines and in all five lines
which were tested for B^{21}-associated MD resistance, such an association was demonstrated (Longenecker *et al*., 1976). B^{21} was also
demonstrated in a "heavy" breed (the Black Australorp), an ancient
Egyptian breed (the Fayoumi) and in the progenitor of the species
(the Red Jungle Fowl). Although in most cases the actual fre-
quencies of the B^{21} gene in these populations cannot be estimated,
the fact that B^{21} was found in small samples of unrelated strains
suggests that the B^{21} allele is not indifferent with respect to
its selective value. The rediscoveries of B^{21} can be attributed
only to inheritance from a common ancestor or to parallel mutations. In either case, powerful selective forces must have acted
to maintain the allele in breeds which represent the extreme production types of the species.

One of the White Leghorn lines (XP) which was found to be
segregating for the B^{21} and B^2 alleles was used to establish
homozygous B^{21}/B^{21} and B^2/B^2 sublines. The progeny of the B^{21}
subline which are resistant to MD were found to resist the growth
of JMV tumor cells almost three times better than the progeny of
the B^2 subline which are susceptible to MD. Thus, the JMV tumor
cells appear to grow less well in the B^{21} (genetically resistant)
environment. One possible explanation for these results is that
the B^{21} progeny are better able to reject the JMV cells via immunological mechanisms. The relevant antigens on the JMV cells
could be the membrane-associated tumor specific antigen of MD
(MATSA) (Witter *et al*., 1975), other virus-associated antigens,
the foreign B_1 alloantigens described in this report (Tables 4-6),
or other alloantigens not associated with B. Experiments are in
progress to attempt to distinguish these possibilities but, regardless of the mechanism, it will be important to test further
whether the growth of JMV cells can be used as a rapid method for
the detection of B-associated resistance to MD.

Much controversy has existed in the past as to whether JMV
tumors arise from *de novo* viral transformation of host lymphocytes
or from the growth (transplantation) of JMV cells (Spencer *et al*.,
1967; Kim, 1972; Hong and Sevoian, 1974). Recent studies have
provided evidence that JMV is a cell transplant (Spencer *et al*.,
1976; Stephens *et al*., 1976) and the present study represents an
important confirmation of that work using a cell marker unrelated
to those used previously. Our finding of B_1 on JMV cells is
especially interesting in view of the fact that B^1 was found in
high frequency (Pazderka *et al*., 1975a, 1975b) in one of the most

highly MD-susceptible lines known, Cornell Strain S. Our serological demonstration of B_1 on JMV cells is consistent with the observations of Gavora *et al.* (1977) that Strain-S is by far the most susceptible to the JMV tumor transplant. The estimated dose for day old chicks that would kill fifty per cent of a challenged population (LD50) of Strain-S was only 50 cells compared to 600-10,000 for several other lines of chickens (Gavora *et al.*) indicating that these lines have some resistance to tumor cell growth. It is nevertheless remarkable that tumors arise at all in these strains following the inoculation of so few cells since JMV tumors are cell transplants which have foreign B_1 alloantigens which should have blocked their colonization in B_1 negative hosts. Alternatively, it may be that the B_1 determinants detected by erythrocyte agglutination differ from those B antigens important in the rejection of a tumor cell transplant. If so, the JMV tumors represent the first genetic accident which discriminates the private serologic antigen of a B allele from its major histo-incompatibility determinants. Such an accident, eliminating the signal by which the host would first recognize the JMV tumor as foreign (Doherty and Zinkernagel, 1975), might be all that is needed to provide the circumstances in which tumorigeneisis does not require the complete genome of the tumorigenic virus (Stephens *et al.*, 1976).

REFERENCES

1. Brewer, R.N., Moore, C.W. and Johnson, L.W., Poult. Sci. 48:1790 (abstract) (1969).

2. Briles, W.E. in First World Congress on Genetics Applied to Livestock Production (Gráficas Orbe, Madrid), Vol. 1:299 (1974).

3. Briles, W.E. and Oleson, W.L., Poult. Sci. 50:1558 (abstract) (1971).

4. Briles, W.E., Stone, H.A. and Cole, R.K., Sci. 195:193 (1977).

5. Doherty, P.D. and Zinkernagel, R.M., J. Immunol. 114:30 (1975).

6. Gavora, G.S., Spencer, J.L., Hare, W.C.D. and Morse, P.M., Poult. Sci., in press (1977).

7. Hanson, M.P., Van Zandt, J.N. and Law, G.R.J., Poult. Sci. 46:1268 (abstract) (1967).

8. Hong, C.C. and Sevoian, M., Avian Dis. 18:305 (1974).

9. Kim, S.N., Yoon, J.W., Olmsted, J. and Kenyon, A.M., Fed.
    Proc. 31:260 (abstract) (1972).

10. Longenecker, B.M. Sheridan, S., Law, G.R.J. and Ruth, R.F.,
    Transplantation 6:544-557 (1970).

11. Longenecker, B.M., Pazderka, F., Law, G.R.J. and Ruth, R.F.,
    Transplantation 14:424-431 (1972).

12. Longenecker, B.M., Pazderka, F., Law, G.R.J. and Ruth, R.F.,
    Cellular Immunology 8:1-11 (1973).

13. Longenecker, B.M., Pazderka, F., Gavora, J.S., Spencer, J.L.
    and Ruth, R.F., Immunogenetics 3:401-407 (1976).

14. Pazderka, F., Longenecker, B.M., Law, G.R.J., Stone, H.A.
    and Ruth, R.F., Immunogenetics 2:93-100 (1975).

15. Pazderka, F., Longenecker, B.M., Law, G.R.J. and Ruth, R.F.,
    Immunogenetics 2:101-130 (1975).

16. Sevoian, M., Larose, R.N. and Chamberlain, D.M., Proc. 101st
    Ann. Mtg. Am. Vet. Med. Assoc. pp 342 (1964).

17. Spencer, J.L. and Calnek, B.W., Avian Dis. 11:274 (1967).

18. Spencer, J.L., Gavora, J.S., Grunder, A.A., Robertson, A.
    and Speckman, G.A., Avian Dis. 18:33 (1974).

19. Spencer, J.L., Gavora, J.A., Hare, A.A. and Grunder, A.A.,
    Avian Dis. 20:268 (1976).

20. Stephens, E.A., Witter, R.L., Lee, L.F., Sharma, J.M.,
    Nazerian, K. and Longenecker, B.M., J. Natl. Can. Inst.
    57:865 (1976).

21. Weiss, R.A. and Biggs, P.M., J. Natl. Cancer Inst. 49:1713
    (1972).

22. Witter, R.L., Stephens, A., Sharma, J.M. and Nazerian, K.,
    Jour. Immunol. 115:177 (1975).

ACKNOWLEDGEMENTS

This work was supported by the National Cancer Institute of
Canada and the Medical Research Council. B. M. Longenecker is a
Research Associate of the NCI of Canada.

THE INFLUENCE OF THE MAJOR HISTOCOMPATIBILITY LOCUS ON MAREK'S DISEASE IN THE CHICKEN

H.A. Stone, W.E. Briles, and W.H. McGibbon

Regional Poultry Research Laboratory, U.S.D.A., A.R.S.;
Northern Illinois University, DeKalb, Illinois;
University of Wisconsin, Madison, Wisconsin

INTRODUCTION

In the early to mid 1960's Marek's disease was becoming a severe problem to the poultry industry. This served as a stimulus for our laboratory to initiate research on the disease which eventually evolved to a concerted effort in the late 1960's and early 1970's. Early studies were plagued by an inability to obtain reproducible results from trial to trial. However, a report by Sevoian (1962) established reliable methodology and facilitated the development of long range research programs. In a relatively short period of time, tissue culture propagation was documented (Churchill and Biggs, 1967; and Solomon, et al., 1968), the causative agent, a DNA virus was found (Biggs, et al., 1968; and Nazerian et al., 1968), its infectious characteristics were intensely investigated (Witter, et al., 1969; Purchase and Biggs, 1967; and Biggs, 1968), and a protective vaccine was developed (Churchill, et al., 1969; and Okazaki et al., 1970). Concurrently, genetic studies were being made by a number of investigators throughout the world. A great amount of effort on the genetic control of Marek's disease was made by the Northeastern (NE-60) Regional Cooperative Breeding project of which the Regional Poultry Research Laboratory was a member. The general consensus of opinion was that genetic differences in susceptibility existed in both meat and egg type chickens, but it was a difficult task to markedly alter the susceptibility state. Fortunately, lines did exist at East Lansing (Table 1) as well as other locations which showed extreme differences in Marek's disease susceptibility and lent themselves favorably to the study of genetic control mechanisms.

299

The inevitable conclusion that genetics and immunology would become highly interrelated was first indicated in 1900 by virtue of the rediscovery of Mendel's principles underlying the mechanisms of inheritance (Mendel, 1866) and the discovery by Landsteiner (1900) of the antigenic differences in human blood which might be inherited. Since then, many investigators have studied the principles of inheritance of blood antigens so that today a great deal is known about a number of species.

Of the presently known blood group systems in the chicken, the B locus, or major histocompatibility locus, has been shown to be significantly related to Marek's disease and shows much promise in disease control. The first report of this was by Hansen et al (1967) who showed that progeny with B^{21} had approximately one-half the mortality of progeny with B^{19}.

Concurrently, with the collection of this data, Cole (1968) demonstrated in the Cornell Randombred flock that the Marek's disease susceptibility could be rapidly changed provided the proper genetic material was present. His unselected flock had 51% Marek's mortality in the initial survey. In only 3 generations of selection for resistance and susceptibility on the basis of sire family mortality, lines were developed and respectively designated N and P (Table 2).

Lines N and P are now maintained at East Lansing. The first generation was blood typed by Dr. W. E. Briles in 1972 and produced the results shown in Table 3. These findings led immediately to tests on progeny of the two heterogenous B^1B^{21} N line females when mated to a B^2B^2 P line male. Of 44 progeny produced, Table 4, the incidence of Marek's disease to twenty weeks of age was 92.6% among 27 B^1B^2 chicks and 11.8% among 17 B^2B^{21} chicks.

These results were sufficiently encouraging that a series of PxN (B^2B^{21}) progeny were produced at East Lansing and shipped to Dr. Briles at Northern Illinois University for maintenance until sexual maturity. Matings were then made of (PxN)xP or Px(PxN) to produce progeny segregating for the B^{21} allele. Eggs were shipped to East Lansing, chicks were hatched and exposed to Marek's disease by inoculation and evaluated to 20 weeks of age. Table 5 presents the results obtained. In four consecutive bi-weekly hatches the Marek's disease mortality for the B^2B^2 progeny ranged from 50-100% while in contrast the mortality for the B^2B^{21} was 0.0 to 11.1. Total mortality for combined hatches was 60/97 (61.9%) vs 5/79 (6.3%) for B^2B^2 and B^2B^{21} progeny respectively.

The question arose as to whether or not the response observed in Tables 4 and 5 was entirely due to the B blood group locus or to an accumulation of genetic gain made during the selection of

TABLE 1. Least-squares mean % mortality with Marek's disease[1]

Line	Strain of Marek's disease							
	GA				JM			
	Inoculated		Contact		Inoculated		Contact	
	N^2	%	N	%	N	%	N	%
6	49	2.7	49	0.1	48	11.6	50	0.7
7	49	86.3	49	75.9	46	96.0	50	80.0
15I	50	68.1	48	55.2	49	55.1	49	29.5

[1] See Crittenden et al. Poultry Science 51:242-261.
[2] Number of birds present at 11 days of age.

TABLE 2. Marek's disease mortality in the Cornell N and P lines

Line	Chicks Exposed	Marek's Disease Mortality	Susceptibility	MD oo	Positive oo
N	152	0.0	0.7	0.0	1.1
P	160	80.6	95.0	92.3	97.6

TABLE 3. Red blood cell classifications at the B locus
(W. E. Briles and B. M. Longenecker)

Line	B Blood Group Allele							
	1	2	3	4	5	6	7	21
6							100.0*	
7							100.0	
N	1.0							99.0
P	8.0	74.0	9.0	6.0	3.0	1.0		

*Gene frequency.

$B^1 = B^{13}$

$B^2 = B^{19}$

$B^3 = B^{17}$ — probably no longer in line - in
1976 were $B^{13}B^{19}$ or $B^{19}B^{19}$

$B^4 = B^{15}$

$B^5 = B^5$

$B^6 = B^6$

TABLE 4.   Marek's disease mortality in PxN chicks with differing
           B blood group genotypes

Hatch	Genotype	Number Inoc	MD	% MD
1	B^2B^{1*}	11**	11	100.0
	B^2B^{21}	4	0	0.0
2	B^2B^1	7	6	85.7
	B^2B^{21}	6	0	0.0
3	B^2B^1	5	4	80.0
	B^2B^{21}	5	2	40.0
4	B^2B^1	4	4	100.0
	B B	2	0	0.0
Total	B^2B^1 $B^{13}B^{19}$	27	25	92.6
	B^2B^{21} $B^{19}B^{21}$	17	2	11.8

*
 All chicks were produced by mating a B^2B^2 P line male with a
 B^1B^{21} N line female.
**
 All chicks were inoculated at two weeks of age.

TABLE 5.   Marek's disease mortality in Px(PxN) and (PxN)XP chickens
           with differing B blood group antigens

Hatch no.	Genotype (B^XB^X)	Number chicks	MD	% MD
1	2,2	21	15	71.4
	2,21	21	2	9.5
2	2,2	20	10	50.0
	2,21	14	1	7.1
3	2,2	10	10	100.0
	2,21	10	0	0.0
4	2,2	22	17	77.3
	2,21	18	2	11.1
5	2,2	24	8	33.0
	2,21	16	0	0.0
Total	2,2	97	60	61.9
	2,21	79	5	6.3

W. E. Briles and H. A. Stone (unpublished data)

the lines. Therefore, it was decided to study the influence of the alleles in the Cornell Random bred population maintained in Madison, Wisconsin by Dr. W. H. McGibbon. Matings were made (Table 6) to produce progeny with varying B genotypes for exposure via inoculation at two weeks of age with 2000 tissue culture plaque-forming units of JM Marek's disease virus. The results obtained in five consecutive bi-weekly hatches are shown in Table 7. Chickens of genotypes lacking the B^{21} allele had significantly higher Marek's mortality (50% to 77%) than did those of genotypes with B^{21} (0% to 9.0%). These results suggest that the genetic basis for the rapid acquisition of resistance to Marek's disease in line N may be due to the increase in frequency of the B^{21} allele.

To further substantiate this, matings were again made in the Cornell Randombred flock (Table 8) to produce $B^{21}B^{21}$ and B^2B^2 progeny (simulated N and P lines respectively) for exposure.

TABLE 6. Mating system used to produce chicks with different B blood genotypes (Cornell Randombred stock)

Mating Code	Parent genotypes[1]		Possible progeny genotypes
1A	$B_1^{1}B^{3}$	$B_2^{2}B^{2}$	1,2; 2,3
2A	$B_1^{1}B^{3}$	$B_2^{2}B^{2}$	1,2; 2,3
3A	$B^{1}B^{3}$	$B^{2}B^{2}$	1,1; 1,2; 1,3; 2,3
1B	$B_2^{2}B^{21}$	$B_2^{2}B^{3}$	2,2; 2,3; 2,21; 3,21
2B	$B_2^{2}B^{21}$	$B_2^{2}B^{25}$	2,2; 2,15; 2,21; 21,25
3B	$B^{2}B^{21}$	$B^{2}B^{3}$	2,2; 2,21; 3,21
1C	$B_2^{2}B^{5}$	$B_1^{1}B^{21}$	1,2; 1,5; 2,21; 5,21
2C	$B_2^{2}B^{5}$	$B_1^{1}B^{21}$	1,2; 1,5; 2,21; 5,21
3C	$B^{2}B^{5}$	$B^{1}B^{21}$	1,2; 1,5; 2,21; 5,21
1D	$B_2^{2}B^{2}$	$B_1^{1}B^{21}$	1,2; 2,21
2D	$B_2^{2}B^{2}$	$B_1^{1}B^{21}$	1,2; 2,21
3D	$B^{2}B^{2}$	$B^{1}B^{21}$	1,2; 2,21

[1]Parents maintained at Madison, Wisconsin by Dr. W. H. McGibbon.

Table 7

MD mortality in selected matings of the Cornell Randombred flock by B blood genotypes

Mating Code	B^1B^2	$B^{1-3}B^1$	B^1B^5	B^2B^3	B^2B^{2-3}	B^2B^{25}	B^2B^{21}	B^3B^{21}	B^5B^{21}	$B^{21}B^{25}$
1A	12/16*			19/26						
2A	5/9			9/12						
3A	9/12	12/21		5/7						
1B					14/26		0/9	1/13		
2B						21/24	1/5			1/11
3B					26/26		0/21	0/11		
1C			4/8				0/8		0/8	
2C			2/4				0/10		0/3	
3C			6/6				0/12		0/6	
1D	12/23						3/27			
2D	27/28						5/25			
3D	17/24						0/20			
Total	100/134	12/21	12/18	33/45	40/52	21/24	9/137	1/24	0/17	1/11

* Marek's disease mortality/chicks at risk

Stone, H.A., W.E. Briles and W.H. McGibbon (unpublished data)

TABLE 8.   Mating system used to initiate the development of
Marek's disease resistant and susceptible lines

Parent genotype	Mating code	Possible progeny genotype
$B^{21}B^{21}$ x $B^{21}B^{21}$	1A + 1B	$B^{21}B^{21}$
x B^2B^4	1C, 1D + 1E	B^2B^{21}, B^4B^{21}
x B^4B^{27}	1F	B^4B^{21}, $B^{21}B^{27}$
$B^{21}B^{21}$ x $B^{21}B^{21}$	2A, 2B + 2C	$B^{21}B^{21}$
x B^2B^4	2D + 2E	B^2B^{21}, B^4B^{21}
B^2B^4 x B^4B^4	3A	B^2B^4, B^4B^4
x B^2B^4	3B	B^2B^2, B^2B^4, B^4B^4
x B^4B^{27}	3C	B^2B^4, B^2B^{27}, B^4B^4, B^4B^{27}
x B^2B^{27}	3D	B^2B^2, B^2B^4, B^2B^{27}, B^4B^{27}
B^4B^4 x B^4B^4	4A, 4B, 4C + 4D	B^4B^4
B^2B^{21} x B^4B^{21}	5A, 5B + 5C	B^2B^4, B^2B^{21}, B^4B^{21}, $B^{21}B^{21}$
x B^4B^4	5D	B^2B^4, B^4B^{21}
x B^2B^4	5E	B^2B^2, B^2B^4, B^2B^{21}, B^4B^{21}

(handwritten annotations in left margin near row B^2B^4: "B^{15}", "$B4=B^{15}$")

The results in four consecutive bi-weekly hatches are shown
in Table 9.   Again chickens without the B^{21} allele had significantly
higher Marek's mortality (46% to 100%) than did those with B^{21}
(0% to 7%).   Of particular interest was the 0% mortality found
in the $B^{21}B^{21}$ chickens.

CONCLUSIONS

These results indicate a very strong association between the
Marek's disease susceptibility and the B histocompatibility locus
in chickens of lines N and P.   However, further research is required
before an explanation can be made for this association.

TABLE 9

Marek's disease mortality in selected B blood group genotypes of the Cornell Randombred flock

Family	B^2B^2	B^2B^4	B^2B^{27}	B^4B^4	B^4B^{27}	B^2B^{21}	B^4B^{21}	$B^{21}B^{21}$	$B^{21}B^{27}$
1A									
1B									
1C						0/7	0/8	0/8	
1D						0/12	0/5	0/15	
1E						0/8	1/9		
1F							0/9		0/6
2A									
2C									
2D						0/12	1/9	0/12	
2E						1/9	0/9	0/22	
3A		1/11		2/9					
3B	1/2	2/15		3/5					
3C		4/6		2/3	2/2				
3D	2/4	3/4	1/1		2/2				
4A				25/30					
4B				12/21					
4C				13/15					
4D				2/6					
5A		1/2				1/2	0/2		
5B		2/4				2/6	0/3	0/5	
5C						0/2	0/3	0/3	
5D		4/6					0/8		
5E	3/7	1/1				0/2	0/5		
Genotype	6/13	18/49	1/1	59/89	4/4	4/60	2/70	0/65	0/6
Totals		88/156						6/201	

REFERENCES

1. Biggs, P.M., Immunol. 43: 93 (1968).

2. Biggs, P.M., A.E. Churchill, D.G. Rootes and R.C. Chubb, Perspectives Virol. 6: 211 (1968).

3. Crittenden, L.B., R.L. Muhm and B.R. Burmester, Poul. Sci. 51: 261 (1972).

4. Churchill, A.E. and P.M. Biggs, Nature 215: 528 (1967).

5. Churchill, A.E., L.N. Payne, and R.C. Chubb, Nature 221: 744 (1969).

6. Cole, R.K., Avian Dis. 12: 9 (1968).

7. Hansen, M.P., J.N. Van Zandt, and G.R.L. Law, Poult. Sci. 46: 1268 (1967).

8. Landsteiner, K. Zbl. Bakt. 27: 357 (1900).

9. Mendel, G., Verh. Naturf. Verein Brunn Abh. 4: 3 (1866).

10. Nazerian, K. and B.R. Burmester, Cancer Res. 28: 2454 (1968).

11. Okazaki, W., H.G. Purchase, and B.R. Burmester, Avian Dis. 14: 413 (1970).

12. Purchase, H.G. and P.M. Biggs, Res. Vet. Sci. 8: 440 (1967).

13. Sevorian, M. and D.M. Chamberlain, Vet. Med. 57: 608 (1962).

14. Solomon, J.J., R.L. Witter, K. Nazerian and B.R. Burmester Proc. Soc. Expt. Biol. Med. 127: 173 (1968).

15. Witter, R.L., G.H. Burgoyne, and J.J. Solomon, Avian Dis. 13: 171 (1969).

GENETIC AND CELLULAR CONTROL OF SPONTANEOUS AUTOIMMUNE THYROIDITIS

IN OS CHICKENS

Larry D. Bacon, Roy S. Sundick and Noel R. Rose

Wayne State University School of Medicine

540 E. Canfield, Detroit, Michigan 48201

INTRODUCTION

Starting in 1956 (1) R.K. Cole selected a substrain of pheno-typically hypothyroid chickens from the White Leghorn Cornell C strain (CS), eventually establishing the Obese strain (OS). OS and CS flocks are maintained at Cornell University, Ithaca, New York, by closed matings that purposely avoid inbreeding (2). Three additional sublines of OS, viz., OSA, OSB, and OSC, are produced by sib matings in the authors' laboratory for the purpose of developing inbred OS lines (3).

E. Witebsky, J.H. Kite and G. Wick, in collaboration with Cole, established that spontaneously occurring autoimmune thyroiditis (SAT) was responsible for the hypothyroidism of OS chickens. They showed there was an extensive infiltration of the thyroids by lym-phocytes and that antibodies specific for pooled or autologous chicken thyroglobulin were present in most birds over four weeks of age (4,5). The severity of thyroiditis was greatly reduced in neo-natally bursectomized birds (6,7), but increased in those neonatally thymectomized (8,9). Cole determined that SAT is inherited as a polygenic trait expressed with some degree of dominance (1). Sev-eral reviews summarize these findings with the OS chicken (3,10).

We would like to focus here on some of our recent results that demonstrate an influence of the major histocompatibility (B) locus on SAT, and on studies still underway to define the cellular regula-tion of the autoimmune response.

DELINEATION OF B-LOCUS GENOTYPES

The B-locus genotypes were determined for OS and CS chickens in 1972. Based on previous work (11) with backcross chickens of two partially inbred lines, it was known that graft-vs-host (GVH) splenomegaly and skin-graft rejections could be used to establish B-genotypes that were subsequently verifiable by agglutination reactions. These two transplantation assays were, therefore, used in studies on offspring of matings within OS and CS. Offspring of a family were injected with either sire or dam peripheral blood at 13 days and studied for splenomegaly at 19 days of embryogenesis; other offspring were hatched and grafted at two weeks with wattle tissue from both parents and skin from two full-sibs. The genotypes of grafted offspring were predicted and appropriate combinations selected for immunization. Following immunization, B-locus specific antisera were obtained (12). The specificity of these sera for the B-locus was verified by comparison with antisera provided by J.V. Craig and L.W. Schierman.

In the OS chickens two B-alleles, B^l and B^4, were identified with approximately equal gene frequency. A third allele, B^3, was only rarely observed (f = 0.04) in a heterozygous state. Only one of the frequent alleles of OS, B^l, was identified in CS chickens. The frequency of B^l was similar in both OS and CS. The B^3 allele and another allele, B^2, were present in moderate frequency in CS. F. Pazderka and R.F. Ruth have tested OS and CS birds and suggest that our alleles, B^l, B^2, and B^3, correspond to their B^{l3}, B^5, and B^{l5}, respectively. Serological evidence of W.E. and R. Briles indicate that our B^l, B^3, and B^4 alleles correspond to their B^{l3}, B^{l5}, and B^5. Thus B^l and B^3 correspond with B^{l3} and B^{l5}, but a standard nomenclature for B^2 and B^4 is not yet established.

Adsorption tests indicated that alloantigens B_1 and B_3 in OS and CS birds are identical (12). Two additional tests of immune function also indicate that the B^l genes are identical in these two strains. First, R. Jones in our laboratory has shown that B^lB^l OS birds did not respond to B^lB^l CS birds in one-way mixed lymphocyte culture (13). Second, C. Polley has shown that if B^lB^l bursal cells are reciprocally transferred between OS and CS chemically bursectomized chicks, antibody response to SRBC is fully reconstituted, as is bursa size and germinal center formation in the spleen (also see below) (14).

INFLUENCE OF THE B-LOCUS ON SAT

Two studies clearly show that the B-locus influences SAT. The first was carried out with OS chicks (15). Heterozygous B^lB^4 X B^lB^4 matings were established, primarily using OSA chicks. The inbred offspring had an 0.40 inbreeding coefficient. Groups of chicks were bled and killed at 3, 6, and 10 weeks of age. At all three ages the thyroids of the $B^l B^l$ and $B^l B^4$ chicks had significantly greater lymphocyte infiltration than the $B^4 B^4$ birds. The mean hemagglutinating titer to thyroglobulin was significantly higher in $B^l B^l$ and $B^l B^4$ than in $B^4 B^4$ chicks at six and eight weeks of age. The $B^l B^l$ chicks had significantly higher titers than $B^l B^4$ chicks at six weeks (p < 0.01). Some additional results of chicks from $B^4 B^4$ matings indicated that $B^4 B^4$ birds, particularly of the OSB line, do develop as severe thyroiditis as $B^l B^l$ and $B^l B^4$ birds (15). The B-genotype influence is most pronounced in partially inbred OSA.

Recently some studies were undertaken to ascertain the influence of B-genotype to SAT in $(OSxCS)F_1$ chickens. Randomly selected CS chickens with B^l, B^2, or B^3 genes were mated with several OS $B^l B^4$ or $B^3 B^4$ males in separate breeding pens at Cornell University. The chicks were hatched in our laboratory, their B-blood group determined by hemagglutination, and they were killed at seven weeks of age. As shown in Table 1, more $B^3 B^3$, $B^l B^3$, $B^2 B^3$, and $B^3 B^4$ birds had SAT than $B^l B^l$ or $B^l B^4$ birds, whereas no $B^l B^2$ or $B^2 B^4$ birds had significant disease (16).

Table 1. Thyroiditis in $(OS \times CS)F_1$ chickens.

Genotype	Birds with thyroid pathology >0.4 or $\log_2$ antibody titer >4[a]
	No./Total
$B^2 B^4$	0/16
$B^l B^2$	0/09
$B^l B^l$	5/18
$B^l B^4$	12/26
$B^3 B^3$	7/11
$B^l B^3$	20/33
$B^2 B^3$	13/17
$B^3 B^4$	20/24

[a]The correlation value for antibody titer and pathology index is r_s = 0.79, p < .001.

We have recently suggested five possible ways the B-locus may influence SAT (3).

1. In mice, Ir genes apparently determine immune response to experimentally injected thyroglobulin (17), and they are localized at the K or IA region of the mouse major histocompatibility complex (MHC) (18). Ir genes have been linked to the B-locus of chickens (19,20), and similar genes may be relevant to SAT. Thus, B^3 may determine high, B^l moderate, and B^2 or B^4 low or no response to thyroglobulin.

2. The non-responder chickens may recognize an antigenic determinant of thyroglobulin but preferentially develop suppressor T rather than helper T cells, similar to non-responder strains of mice injected with the well-defined antigen, GAT (21). The most likely candidate for the suppressor gene in OS is the B^4 allele, or one closely linked to it. Thus, OSA B^4B^4 neonatally thymecto-mized birds which develop severe thyroiditis may do so because they lack suppressor T cells (22). The B^2 allele may act as a suppressor in (OS X CS)F_1 chickens.

3. Non-specific regulation of T-cell proliferation by genes at the B-locus may be pertinent. Longenecker et al. (23) have shown that the magnitude of GVH reaction in chickens is controlled by the B genotype. Based on serological tests, B^l and B^3 are comparable to B^{l3} and B^{l5}, and these are associated with high GVH competence. A lymphoproliferative hypothesis would not explain the organ specificity of the autoimmune lesions. However, this might result if the target organs were also altered.

4. Susceptibility to virus infection could explain the B-influence on SAT. It is conceivable that virus infection of the thyroid in OS chickens results in virus-altered B-associated antigens [as in the mouse LCM model (24)] and stimulate an autoimmune response. One could then envision that OS and CS birds differ in their susceptibility to, or support of replication of, this virus. Furthermore, birds of certain B-locus genotypes might have greater immune responses to the virus-altered antigen.

5. Lastly, B-linked genes may influence thyroglobulin itself, since Tomazic and Rose have shown in experimentally induced thyroiditis of mice that the effectiveness of the purified thyroglobulin used for immunization was dependent in part upon the H-2 type of the thyroid donors (25). Further experiments are in progress to choose among these different hypotheses, although they are not mutually exclusive.

CELLULAR REGULATION OF IMMUNE FUNCTION IN OS CHICKENS

Considerable evidence indicates that thymectomy of OS chickens increases the severity of SAT, but has little effect in CS birds (3,22). Two recent results indicate that there are functional differences in T-cell mediated immune responses in OS B^lB^l compared with CS B^lB^l chickens.

M. Jakobisiak conducted intrastrain skin grafts between chicks in our laboratory (26). Each chick received one intrastrain graft and one autograft. Rejection was, therefore, due to minor histocompatibility antigens that were found to be equivalent in the two strains. OS and CS chicks grafted at hatching or at two weeks of age rejected grafts at a similar time. However, neonatal thymectomy of normal CS chicks allowed eight of 13 grafts to survive over 50 days, whereas in OS birds only one of 16 grafts survived. This finding provides evidence for a lack of suppressor T cells, or increased numbers of effector T cells, in the periphery of OS chicks at hatching.

R. Jones has studied *in vitro* mitogen responses using peripheral blood lymphocytes from young adults incubated with phytohemagglutinin (PHA) or Concanavalin A (Con A) (27). Cell proliferation was determined by ^{3}H-thymidine uptake at three time intervals. The maximum stimulation index for each bird was determined and used to compare eight OS B^lB^l with eight CS B^lB^l birds. The OS B^lB^l birds had a significantly lower PHA response (p < 0.01) and lower Con A response than did the CS B^lB^l chickens. Eight OS B^4B^4 birds were comparable to OS B^lB^l birds, and were stimulated significantly lower by PHA and Con A than were the CS B^lB^l birds.

J. Nowak in our group is currently studying F_c receptor-bearing cells in OS B^lB^l and CS B^lB^l chickens. Until the time of hatching, both strains have a similar ontogenic pattern of cells with F_c receptors. From hatching onward, OS chicks have a greater percentage of F_c-bearing mononuclear cells in their spleens than do CS birds. F_c receptor-bearing cells may be relevant to SAT because of their possible role in antibody-dependent cellular cytotoxicity, as has been shown in humans (28). J. Jaroszewski has found that OSA B^4B^4 birds develop severe SAT if given high-titered antisera to thyroglobulin, in contrast to CS B^lB^l birds (29). This result in OS may be due to thyroid abnormalities, but high levels of F_c receptor-bearing lymphocytes may be a major contributing factor.

B. Albini and G. Wick have noted a significant increase in IgM-bearing B cells in OS chickens (30). This finding is in agreement with the recent results of Luster *et al.* (31). Our collaborative work with M. Luster and G. Leslie indicated OS B^lB^l birds have abnormally high levels of IgM, but low to undetectable levels of IgA, in contrast to control CS B^lB^l chicks of the same age (32). These results may suggest the presence of extensive abnormalities in thymus regulatory functions.

C. Polley in our laboratory has conducted reciprocal bursal cell transfers between OS B^lB^l and CS B^lB^l birds as described previously. Recipients were chemically bursectomized at hatching and reconstituted with 5 x 10^6 bursa cells from four-day-old hatchmates. Chemically bursectomized six-week-old OS control birds had much reduced thyroid infiltrations and no antibody to thyroglobulin. Whereas thyroiditis was fully reconstituted in OS recipients by either OS or CS bursa cells, neither type of donor cell conveyed disease to CS chicks (14). These results suggest that bursa cells themselves determine neither resistance nor susceptibility to SAT.

DISCUSSION AND CONCLUSIONS

The major histocompatibility complex (*MHC*) of the chicken, the *B*-locus, clearly influences the development of spontaneous autoimmune thyroiditis. This *B*-locus control is demonstrated in the non-inbred OS, but becomes much more obvious when one examines a partially inbred population such as OSA. Undoubtedly, many genetic traits play a role in the pathogenesis of this autoimmune disease so that the association with the *MHC* is obscured in randomly bred birds. This observation may explain why it has been difficult to find a linkage of human chronic thyroiditis with a particular *HLA* haplotype, even though another thyroid disease, Graves' disease, is significantly linked with *HLA-B8* (33). Only by examining somewhat isolated populations in Newfoundland were Farid and his colleagues able to uncover a significant relationship to the haplotypes *HLA-B8*, *HLA-Bl*, *Wl5*, and *W27* (34).

Independent of the *B*-locus effect, OS chickens show functional differences in their T-cell mediated immune responses. The most likely explanation of the abnormality is a disturbance in the orderly timing in thymus maturation during embryogenesis, resulting in premature peripheralization of helper or effector T cells before suppressor T cells. After hatching, the major ongoing function of the thymus seems to be one of supplying suppressor function. The other immunological abnormalities of OS chickens, such as IgA deficiency, can best be viewed as further indicators of a fundamental defect in thymus-based regulation.

The pathogenic effects of autoimmunization depend upon an intact bursa and probably upon the presence of high levels of circulating autoantibody to thyroglobulin. Yet adaptive reconstitution of non-susceptible CS birds with OS or hybrid B cells, or passive transfer of preformed antibody, rarely produces disease in CS recipients. Obviously, other elements are required for expression of disease. Among the plausible explanations for the resistance of

CS chickens to thyroiditis are the (a) presence of suppressor (T) cells, (b) lack of suitable numbers of F_c-bearing mononuclear cells capable of cooperating with antibody, and (c) abnormalities in the thyroid gland itself. Direct evidence that the thyroid function of OS birds differs from that of CS has been found in our recent investigations (3,22,35, and 36). Even before the onset of any demonstrable autoimmune reaction and apparently independent of the maternal transfer of thyroglobulin antibodies (35), the thyroids of OS chickens take up greater amounts of iodine and have a higher ratio of mono- to di-iodotyrosine than those of comparable CS birds (3). Thus, these investigations distinguish several genetic factors that contribute to the inheritance of SAT in OS chickens.

SUMMARY

B-locus genotypes have been defined in Obese strain (OS) chickens that spontaneously develop autoimmune thyroiditis (SAT), and in White Leghorn Cornell C strain (CS) chickens from which the OS was selected. The B-locus influences SAT, and some possible mechanisms are discussed. Thymic abnormalities in OS, as contrasted with CS birds, are also discussed and may play a role in SAT, as may an intrinsic defect in the thyroid gland itself.

ACKNOWLEDGEMENTS

This work was supported by NIH research grants CA-02357, CA-16426, and AM-20028-01. The skilled technical assistance of Ms. S. Kirchberger and Ms. H. Pietraszkiewicz is gratefully acknowledged. We thank Ms. Linda Harbison for her contribution to the preparation of this manuscript.

REFERENCES

1. Cole, R. K., Genetics, 53: 1021 (1966).

2. Cole, R. K., Kite, J. H., Jr., Wick, G. and Witebsky, E.,
   Poultry Sci., 49: 839 (1970).

3. Rose, N. R., Bacon, L. D. and Sundick, R. S., Transplant.
   Rev., 31: 264 (1976).

4. Witebsky, E., Kite, J. H., Jr., Wick, G. and Cole, R. K.,
   J. Immunol. 103: 708 (1969).

5. Kite, J. H., Jr., Wick, G., Twarog, B. and Witebsky, E.,
   J. Immunol., 103: 1331 (1969).

6. Cole, R. K., Kite, J. H., Jr. and Witebsky, E., Science,
   169: 1357 (1968).

7. Wick, G., Kite, J. H., Jr., Cole, R. K. and Witebsky, E.,
   J. Immunol., 104: 45 (1970).

8. Wick, G., Kite, J. H., Jr. and Witebsky, E., J. Immunol.,
   104: 54 (1970).

9. Welch, P., Rose, N. R. and Kite, J. H. Jr., J. Immunol.,
   110: 575 (1973).

10. Wick, G., Sundick, R. S. and Albini, B., Clin. Immunol.
    Immunopathol., 3: 272 (1974).

11. Bacon, L. D., Ph.D. Dissertation, Kansas State University,
    Manhattan, Kansas (1969).

12. Bacon, L. D., Kite, J. H., Jr. and Rose, N. R., Transplan.,
    16: 591 (1973).

13. Jones, R. F. and Bacon, L. D., Fed. Proc. (abstract), 36:
    1191 (1977).

14. Polley, C. R., Bacon, L. D. and Rose, N. R., Fed. Proc.
    (abstract), 36: 1207 (1977).

15. Bacon, L. D., Kite, J. H. Jr. and Rose, N. R., Science, 186:
    274 (1974).

16. Bacon, L. D., Fed. Proc. (abstract), 35: 713 (1976).

17. Vladutiu, A. O. and Rose, N. R., Science, 174: 1137 (1971).

18. Tomazic, V., Rose, N. R. and Shreffler, D. C., J. Immunol., 112: 965 (1974).

19. Günther, E., Balcarová, J., Hálá, K., Rude, E. and Hraba, T., Europ. J. Immunol., 4: 548 (1974).

20. Benedict, A. A., Pollard, L. W., Morrow, P. R., Abplanalp, H. A., Maurer, P. H. and Briles, E. W., Immunogenetics, 2: 113 (1975).

21. Benacerraf, B., Kapp, J. A., Debre, P., Pierce, C. W. and de la Croix, F., Transplant. Rev., 26: 21 (1975).

22. Sundick, R. S., Livezey, M., Brown, T. and Bagchi, M., Fed. Proc. (abstract), 35: 521 (1976).

23. Longenecker, B. M., Pazderka, F. and Ruth, R. F., Transplan., 14: 424 (1972).

24. Doherty, P. C. and Zinkernagel, R. M., J. exp. Med., 141: 502 (1975).

25. Tomazic, V. and Rose, N. R., Immunology, 30: 63 (1976).

26. Jakobisiak, M., Sundick, R. S., Bacon, L. D. and Rose, N. R., Proc. Nat. Acad. Sci., 73: 2877 (1976).

27. Jones, R. F., Bacon, L. D. and Rose, N. R., in preparation.

28. Calder, E. A., McLeman, D. and Irvine, W. J., Clin. exp. Immunol., 15: 467 (1973).

29. Jaroszewski, J., Sundick, R. S. and Rose, N. R., Submitted for publication.

30. Albini, B. and Wick, G., Nature new Biol., 249: 653 (1974).

31. Luster, M. I., Leslie, G. A. and Cole, R. K., Nature, 263: 331 (1976).

32. Luster, M. I., Bacon, L. D., Rose, N. R. and Leslie, G. A., in preparation.

33. Grumet, F. C., Konishi, J., Payne, R. and Kriss, J. P., Clin. Res., 21: 439 (1973).

34. Farid, N. R., Barnard, J., Kutas, C., Noel, E. P. and Marshall, W. H., Int. Arch. Allergy Appl. Immunol., 49: 837 (1975).

35. Sundick, R. S. and Wick, G., Clin. exp. Immunol., 18: 127 (1974).

36. Sundick, R. S. and Wick, G., J. Immunol., 116: 1319 (1976).

SYNGENEIC INBRED LINES OF CHICKENS AND THEIR USE IN IMMUNOGENETICS

Phillip R. Morrow and Hans Abplanalp

Department of Avian Sciences
University of California
Davis, California   95616

INTRODUCTION

The chicken has seen wide use in immunology and has, among other things, the distinction of giving the B lymphocyte its letter, from the unique bursa of Fabricius. The use of rodent species has, however, dominated immunogenetics.

The use of inbred lines of chickens has been limited in the past because reasonably viable lines were hard to come by and their actual homozygosity was often difficult to establish. This paper will document the development and use of several inbred lines of White Leghorn chickens at the University of California at Davis.

HISTORY AND BREEDING OF THE DAVIS INBRED LINES

The lines described in this paper originated from a population of Single Comb White Leghorn chickens developed at the Department of Poultry Husbandry of the University of California, Berkeley. This flock, called the Production Line (P), had been under selection for high egg production since 1932.

In 1952, two new populations were extracted from the P line. One was reproduced using random selection of breeders and was called the Random Line (R), while in the Index Line (I), parents were selected based on an index for egg production.

In 1956, 20 males from the R line were each mated to one or
two full sisters, giving 33 full-sib matings. Also, 35 males
from the I line were each mated to full sisters to give 54 additional matings. In 1957, 104 new full-sib lines were started (39
from the R line, 65 from the I line) and 88 were begun in 1958,
for a total over three years of 279 lines. Each line was subjected
to continuous full-sib mating with one generation per year. The
only selection, applied throughout, has been for large family size.
This has permitted the mating of several males and females each
generation. Lines were lost as inbreeding progressed, until only
six remained in 1970. These had the letter codes C, H, I, K, M and
N₀ Three of these (H, K and M) were discarded in 1971. The remaining three lines (C, I and N) seem to be viable.

The strategy of producing inbred lines in this case is different from that most commonly used (1-3) which is to take a small
number of birds, produce an expanded progeny population and begin
full-sib matings thereafter. It may be that the broader sample of
genetic variation available under the present inbreeding scheme
resulted in a better chance of arriving at a combination of genes
which could survive the homozygosity due to inbreeding. Any other
method may have a limited amount of genetic variation available from
the beginning due to the founder principle (4). Also, the amount of
variation carried into the inbreeding system will depend on the
degree of expansion and the number of initial full-sib matings.

Many workers have found continued segregation for blood
group loci in highly inbred lines of chickens (2, 5-9). It is
possible that this could be in part, a reflection of the inbreeding
scheme used, since the Davis inbreds show striking homozygosity, as
discussed below.

HOMOZYGOSITY OF THE DAVIS INBRED LINES

The calculated inbreeding coefficient (F) of the three Davis
lines is now .98 or greater (10). In order to obtain an indication
of actual homozygosity, tests of red blood cell systems and histocompatibility were made.

Blood typing of ten red cell systems was performed in cooperation with Dr. and Mrs. Briles at Northern Illinois University, De
Kalb, Illinois, beginning in 1970. The allele designations were
made based on the Briles' reagents, and do not imply identity with
alleles having the same number codes in other unrelated populations,
especially for the B locus.

Table 1 is a summary for the three surviving lines in the four consecutive generations, 1970 to 1973. Each of the lines has become fixed for one allele at each of the ten loci. Line C was still segregating for the A9-E1 and A2-E2 pairs at the linked A and E loci in 1970 and 1971, however the most frequent linkage (A9-E1) became fixed in 1972. Line I was segregating for the B and C systems in 1970 and 1971. These both apparently became fixed in 1972. Line N was homozygous for all ten systems from the time blood typing began in 1970.

Table 2 shows the three discarded lines (H, K and M). Two of them (H and M) also appear to have been fixed for all ten loci from 1970. The most important observation is that all three of these lines had the B8 allele, which the surviving lines do not now have. While this may be additional evidence for B locus effects on fitness, the surviving lines indicate viable homozygosity at the B locus can be attained without direct selection.

Because the reagents used in Briles' laboratory were not developed from these Davis inbred lines, it was possible that residual segregation was occurring at blood group loci which was not detected by these tests. For this reason two additional blood tests were performed.

In the first test, four birds from each of the three inbred lines C, I, and N were used for within-line isoimmunizations. Each recipient was given three injections (3 cc. each) at three-day intervals of a fifty percent suspension of washed red blood cells in saline of a single donor from the same line. Sera were then collected from these twelve birds. When tested against their donor cells, all failed to show any signs of agglutination.

In a second test, cross-line immunizations were made using two males from each of the three inbred lines (11). These were all injected with a red cell suspension containing equal amounts of red cells from six individuals from each of seven inbred lines at Davis (C, I and N, plus four other lines). The red cells of the donor birds were washed and pooled into seven line groups, and equal amounts of these cell suspensions were then mixed each day injections were made. Again three injections (3 cc. each) were given at three-day intervals. The recipients were thus ex-posed to a wide variety of foreign red cell antigens. Complete identity of the members within each of the inbred lines would mean the red cell antigens possessed by the immunized birds for a given line would be the same as those of any other individual from the same line. In that case the line reagents should not agglutinate the red cells from other birds of the same line. Any agglutination would indicate polymorphism for a red cell antigen. Although the

TABLE 1

Summary of blood typing results for the surviving highly inbred lines.
(numbers shown under each blood group system designate the particular allele(s) present.

line	year	# of Individual typed	# of families	BLOOD GROUP SYSTEMS									
				A	E	B	C	D	H	I	K	L	P
C	1970	11	4	4,2	1,2	6	2	3	1	2	2	-*	10
	1971	21	4	4,2	1,2	6	2	3	1	2	2	1	10
	1972	21	1	4	1	6	2	3	1	2	2	1	10
	1973	7	1	4	1	6	2	3	1	2	2	1	10
I	1970	18	3	4	7	2,8	2,3	3	2	4	3	-	3
	1971	35	6	4	7	2,8	2,3	3	2	4	3	1	3
	1972	7	1	4	7	2	2	3	2	4	3	1	3
	1973	14	2	4	7	2	2	3	2	4	3	1	3
N	1970	8	1	4	7	4	2	1	2	2	2	-	3
	1971	4	2	4	7	4	2	1	2	2	2	1	3
	1972	7	1	4	7	4	2	1	2	2	2	1	3
	1973	7	1	4	7	4	2	1	2	2	2	1	3

* Locus L was not typed in 1970.

TABLE 2

Summary of blood typing results for the discontinued highly inbred lines. (numbers shown under each blood group system designate the particular allele(s) present).

line	year	# of individuals typed	# of families	A	E	B	C	D	H	I	K	L*	P
H	1970	3	2	4	7	8	5	1	1	2	2	–	3
	1971	10	1	4	7	8	5	1	1	2	2	1	3
K	1970	8	2	7	1	8,4	3	1	2	2	2,3	–	3
	1971	5	3	7	1	8	3	1	2	2	2,3	1	3
M	1970	3	1	4	7	8	3	1	1	4	3	–	2
	1971	5	1	4	7	8	3	1	1	4	3	1	2

(Columns A–P grouped under heading: BLOOD GROUP SYSTEMS)

* Locus L was not typed in 1970.

test does not specify the locus or loci segregating, it is a general
indication of the homogeneity of a line.

The antisera collected from the two recipient males of
each line agglutinated red cells from birds of the other lines
at titrations of 1:16 (serum to saline) or higher. The two line
reagents were then tested against red cells of individuals from
their own line at a 1:1 dilution.

For lines C and I, none of the red cell samples taken from
five males and five females were agglutinated by the respective
antisera. In line N the two line reagents agglutinated some
samples. It was found, however, that red cells of one of the
immunized males were agglutinated in the presence of his own
serum. In addition, freshly collected and washed red cells were
observed to agglutinate in saline without antiserum.

Two females from line N were then used as recipients for
cross-line immunizations using donor cells from lines C and I only.
The resulting antisera failed to show agglutination with red cells
from ten line N birds, including cells from the female recipients.
Titers of 1:16 or higher were obtained against red cells from the
donor lines. Although the unusual agglutinations in line N cannot
be explained, the female antisera do not reveal any hidden segregation. These tests thus support the reliability of the blood typing
results, indicating lines C, I and N to be homozygous at the major
blood group loci. Also, these antisera are used each generation
to insure the purity of the lines.

Two types of histocompatibility tests were also performed.
In 1974, wattle to shank transplants (12) were made between males
within the three lines. Of seventeen homografts in line I, sixteen
survived to the last inspection at 4 weeks post-grafting. Ten males
inspected six months later all still had viable wattle tissue on
their shanks. In line N, twenty of twenty-one homografts survived
4 weeks, and the 12 males remaining at 6 months all had viable
grafts. Three of the line C grafts were rejected before 4 weeks had
elapsed. This may have been a technique problem, since these were
the first transplants performed and some control autografts on the
same birds were lost. Six months later the six remaining birds of
line C all had viable grafts.

Graft-versus-host (GVH) studies were also performed within lines
(13). Addition of buffy coat cells from four adult inbred donors
onto the CAMs of five embryos of the same line consistently failed
to show any spleen enlargement. Also, no lesions on the CAM were
found (14), indicating no segregation of major (B locus) or minor
(non-B locus) histocompatibility loci within any of the lines.

This indicates the inbreds are homozygous for the major and most minor histocompatibility genes.

Table 3 is a condensed version of Table 1, showing the alleles carried by the three inbred lines at ten of the blood group loci. The B and C systems are histocompatibility loci (15), and there is evidence that the A locus antigens may be present on lymphocytes (16). This table also shows a number code for each line. These are to facilitate computerization of records for all lines at Davis. Thus the terms "line 2" and "line C" are synonymous, and so on.

USES IN IMMUNOGENETICS

In collaboration with other workers, these lines have been useful in the following areas:

Immune Response Genes. B locus linked immune response genes have been described (17, 18).

Complement activity. Total hemolytic complement activity is associated with the B locus (19), and this may eventually be shown to be due to different levels of a single component, with the structural gene in the MHC, as in the mouse (20, 21).

Allotypes. Genetically controlled markers on the heavy chain of the chicken 7S immunoglobulin show multiple specificities which are inherited together (22, 23).

Antigen characterization. Strong isoantisera raised between lines using red blood cells are being used for biochemical studies (24).

Adoptive transfer. Syngeneic lines must be used in reconstitution experiments to avoid allogeneic reactions. Mechanisms regulating suppression are now under study (25).

Cell cooperation and the MHC. Work is in progress to determine the role of the B locus in the interactions between the different cells of the immune system.

SUMMARY

Inbred lines of chickens are widely used in immunology and immunogenetics. The actual homozygosity of such lines should be confirmed, preferably by blood typing and histocompatibility tests. In addition, the history and breeding of inbred lines may have an effect on the level of homozygosity attained. Lines which are shown to be essentially syngeneic can be used in a variety of ways.

TABLE 3

Alleles present in Davis inbred lines.

Line		A	E	B	C	D	H	I	K	L	P
		BLOOD GROUP SYSTEMS									
002	C	4	1	6	2	3	1	2	2	1	10
003	I	4	7	2	2	3	2	4	3	1	3
007	N	4	7	4	2	1	2	2	2	1	3

REFERENCES

1. Pease, M. and Dudley, F., Rept. Proc. 10th World's Poultry Congress. 2:45-49 (1954).

2. Hala, K., Hasek, M., Hlozanek, I., Hort, J., Knizetova, F., Mervartova, H., Folia Biol. (Praha). 12:407-421 (1966).

3. Hala, K., Vilhelmova, M., Hasek, M., Kratochvilova, J., Plachy, J., Benda, V. and Karakoz, I., Folia Biol. (Praha). 20:378-385 (1974).

4. Mayr, E., Animal Species and Evolution, 453 pp. (Belknap Press, Cambridge, 1970).

5. Briles, W.E., Allen, C.P., and Millen, T.W., Genetics. 42: 631-648 (1957).

6. Gilmour, D.G., Heredity. 12:141-142 (1958).

7. Gilmour, D.G., Genetics. 44:14-33 (1959).

8. Hasek, M., Knizetova, F. and Mervartova, H., Folia Biol. (Praha) 12:335-341 (1966).

9. Briles, W.E. in XIIth Europ. Conf. Anim. Blood Groups and Biochem. Polymorph. (G. Kovacs and M. Papp, Eds.) (The Hague and Akademiai Kiado, 1972).

10. Wright, S., Amer. Natur. 56:330-338 (1922).

11. Briles, W.E., World's Poultry Sci. Journ. 27:120-131 (1971).

12. Purchase, H.G., Poultry Science 46:1017-1019 (1967).

13. Longenecker, B.M., Sheridan, S., Law, G.R.J. and Ruth, R.F., Transplantation. 9:544-577 (1970).

14. Longenecker, B.M., Pazderka, F., Law, G.R.J. and Ruth, R.F., Cellular Immunology. 8:1-11 (1973).

15. Schierman, L.W. and Nordskog, A.W., Science 134:1008-1009 (1961).

16. Wong, S.Y., Pazderka, F., Longenecker, B.M., Law, G.R.J. and Ruth, R.F., Immunological Communications 1:597-613 (1972).

17. Benedict, A.A., Pollard, L.W., Morrow, P.R., Abplanalp, H.A., Maurer, P.H. and Briles, W.E., Immunogenetics. 2:313-324 (1975).

18. Benedict, A.A., Pollard, L.W. and Maurer, P.H., Immunogenetics 4:199-204 (1977).

19. Chanh, T.C., Benedict, A.A. and Abplanalp, H., J. Exp. Med. 144:555-561 (1976).

20. Lachmann, P.J., Grennan, D., Martin, A., and Demant, P., Nature. 258:242-243 (1975).

21. Curman, B., Ostberg, L., Sandberg, L., Malmheden-Eriksson, I., Stalenheim, G., Rask, L., and Peterson, P.A., Nature. 258:243-245 (1975).

22. Wakeland, E.K. and Benedict, A.A., Immunogenetics. 2:531-541 (1975).

23. Wakeland, E.K., Benedict, A.A. and Abplanalp, H.A., J. Imm. 118:401-404 (1977).

24. Kubo, R.T. and Abplanalp, H., in this conference.

25. Morgan, E., Tempelis, C. and Abplanalb, H, in this conference.

Tumor Immunity

INDUCTION IN B2/B2 CHICKENS OF IMMUNITY TO TRANSPLANTABLE CARCINOGEN-INDUCED FIBROSARCOMAS MEDIATED BY T-CELL MONOCYTE COOPERATION: ROLE OF DELAYED HYPERSENSITIVITY TO UNRELATED ANTIGENS

Michael A. Palladino and G. Jeanette Thorbecke

Department of Pathology, New York University Medical
Center, 550 First Avenue, New York, N. Y. 10016

In previous studies (1) we described the induction with dime-
thylbenzanthracene (DMBA) of fibrosarcomas in B2/B2 (SC) and B15/B21
(FP) chickens (Hyline International, Johnston, Iowa). Tumors taken
from SC chickens (SCFSI-III) proved to be readily transplantable in
SC but not in FP chickens. These transplantable tumors do not contain demonstrable tumor virus products (1) but do show genetic
markers (1), allowing conclusive demonstration of tumor cell proliferation upon transplantation rather than propagation by virus
infection of host cells such as is the case, for example, with
Rous sarcoma (2). Because of these properties, the carcinogen-
induced fibrosarcomas provide an excellent tool for the study of
tumor immunity in histocompatible chickens.

Single tumor cell suspensions ($\geq$ 90% viable) are readily obtained by incubation, with stirring, of minced tumor in Dulbecco's
PBS (0.165 M, pH 7.2) containing 0.2% bovine serum albumin,
0.0025 mg/ml of collagenase and 0.005 mg/ml trypsin (Worthington
Biochemicals, Freehold, N. J.). When tumor cell doses as low as
5×10^4 cells are injected into normal 2- to 10-week old SC chickens,
tumor growth is seen within 2 to 3 weeks after injection in virtually 100% of recipients. The three tumors show comparable growth
rates as indicated in Fig. 1.

Induction and demonstration of tumor immunity. Injection of
mitomycin-treated cells, either subcutaneously or intravenously
(i.v.) caused a resistance to challenge with 10^6 cells of the same
tumor line 2 weeks later in a high percentage of animals. Spleen
cells of such chickens did not transfer immunity in Winn assays
(not in Tables) carried out in wing webs of 2- to 4-week old
normal recipients, using simultaneous injection of spleen cells
and 10^6 SCFS cells. Thus, a more effective way of immunizing
SC chickens to SCFS was sought by injecting untreated tumor cells

331

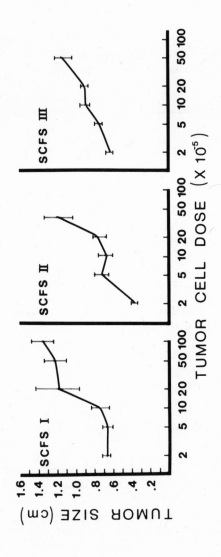

Figure 1. Growth of 3 different SCFS tumor lines in 4- to 10-week old recipients measured 2 weeks after injection in the wing web of 2×10^5 to 1×10^7 live tumor cells.

together with bacterial adjuvants. Complete Freund's adjuvant
(CFA) was found ineffective, but admixture of C. parvum (CP) (10^9
killed bacteria) or Bacillus Calmette Guerin (BCG, TMC1011, 2 X 10^7
live bacteria; kindly provided by Drs. G. B. Mackaness and R. J.
North of the Trudeau Institute, Saranac Lake, N. Y.), particularly
in animals which had previously been injected with these agents,
proved to be a much more effective method of immunization. Table I
shows the results obtained with those groups of animals which had
received a prior i.v. injection of the same agent used to inject
either with the tumor cells or into a 10- to 14-day growing tumor.
The incidence of progressive tumor growth as judged 4 to 6 weeks
after wing web injection of 10^6 SCFS was quite low in such recipients. A marked reduction in progressive tumor growth incidence was
also obtained with two 10-day spaced injections of BCG or CP into
the tumor site (not in Table). Animals which had not been preinjected with these agents and which had received only a single
injection of BCG into the tumor site showed much less initial
tumor growth inhibition and little tendency to reject the tumors
by 4 to 6 weeks (not in Table).

CP-preinjected, agammaglobulinemic chickens also showed the
initial tumor growth inhibition on the side where CP was injected
with the tumor cells. However, the ability to reject tumor on the
side where 10^6 tumor cells had been injected without CP was less
in the BX than in the normal chickens (Table 1, 35% vs. 100%).
This was considered due to the impaired health of BX as compared
to normal chickens of this age (> 12 weeks). In other studies,
similar observations were made when the ability of BX and normal
chickens to give delayed hypersensitivity reactions were compared
(3). In those studies it was found that the reactivity of BX
chickens could be improved by weekly injections of chicken Ig preparations. When the animals which had rejected tumor growth on
both sides were rechallenged in one wing web with 10^7 cells of the
same SCFS tumor line and on the other side with 10^7 cells of one
of the other SCFS lines, tumor growth was minimal for the original
immunizing tumor but much more marked for the other tumor line in
every experiment. However, progressive growth for the other tumor
line was rarely seen in such animals (2 of 29) indicating a certain
degree of cross-reactivity between SCFS lines.

Spleen cells from chickens which had been immunized with live
tumor cells and either CP or BCG were active in suppressing growth
of simultaneously injected tumor cells of the immunizing tumor line
(Table 2). This immunity was readily demonstrable with spleen cell
to tumor cell ratios as low as 5:1 (not in Table). Cells from normal chickens or from chickens injected with either CP or BCG alone
did not inhibit tumor growth in such Winn tests. Crossreactivity
between the three different SCFS lines was not evident when the
immunity was studied in the Winn assay (Table 2).

Cellular collaboration in the expression of tumor-specific
immunity. The use of the Winn test allowed us to study in detail

TABLE 1

EFFECT OF C. PARVUM AND BCG PRETREATMENT ON GROWTH OF 10^6 SCFS CELLS IN L AND R WING WEBS OF NL AND AGAMMAGLOBULINEMIC SC CHICKENS

TYPE OF CHICKEN	PREINJECTION i.v., DAY -7	(NO.)	INJECTED WITH TUMOR CELLS OR INTO TUMOR (L SIDE)	TUMOR SIZE (cm) ± S.E. AT 10-14 DAYS		PROGRESSIVE GROWTH %	
				L	R	L	R
NL	2×10^7 BCG	(4)	-	1.03 ± .04	.85 ± .06	100	100
NL	2×10^7 BCG	(9)	2×10^7 BCG (Day 0)	.27 ± .06	.49 ± .09	0	11
NL	2×10^7 BCG	(7)	2×10^7 BCG (Day 10)	.62 ± .05	.53 ± .04	14	14
NL	10^9 CP	(6)	10^9 CP (Day 0)	.23 ± .11	.69 ± .07	0	0
NL	10^9 CP	(9)	10^9 CP (Day 14)	.62 ± .04	.56 ± .04	0	11
BX	10^9 CP	(7)	-	.68 ± .26	.60 ± .20	87	87
BX	10^9 CP	(20)	10^9 CP (Day 0)	.16 ± .05	.69 ± .07	25	65

TABLE 2

SPECIFICITY OF TUMOR IMMUNITY IN SPLEEN CELLS FROM SC CHICKENS
AFTER CP- OR BCG-INDUCED REJECTION OF SCFS TRANSPLANTS (WINN ASSAY)

PRETREATMENT OF DONORS*	SPLEEN TO TUMOR CELL RATIO IN WING WEB**	TUMORS PRESENT/TOTAL TEST SITES[✝]		
		SCFSI	SCFSIII	SCFSII
None	10-20	7/7	13/14	
CP alone	20	21/21		
CP + SCFSI	10#	0/4		4/4
BCG + SCFSI	10-20	2/16	8/8	
BCG + SCFSIII	10-20	5/5	0/22	

*Donors received 10⁹ CP alone (i.v., day -5 or day -42) or were treated to induce tumor immunity with CP or BCG i.v. + CP or BCG again either on day of SCFS injection or into 10-day growing SCFS tumor.

**10⁶ tumor cell used/site.

✝Determined on day 14 after tumor cell injection.

#Nylon wool nonadherent immune spleen cells were used in this experiment.

the cell types required for the in vivo expression of tumor immunity
to SCFS. While immune spleen or peripheral blood leukocytes, when
used in a Winn assay performed on normal recipients, could support
tumor immunity, thymus cells from such animals could not. Immune
spleen cells from BX donors also transferred tumor immunity into
normal as well as into BX recipients (not in Tables). Incubation
of immune spleen cells with rabbit anti-chicken T cell serum and
guinea pig C abolished the tumor immunity while NRS and C treatment
did not decrease the immunity expressed by untreated immune spleen
cells (Table 3).

Nylon wool fractionation of immune spleen cells showed all
immunity to be restricted to the nonadherent T cell fraction. The
nylon wool adherent fraction containing mostly B cells and macrophages did not inhibit tumor growth at all (results of a typical
experiment in Table 3). It is known that transfer of delayed
hypersensitivity (DH) can be accomplished when normal but not when
irradiated recipients are used (4, 5). Results of such experiments
suggested a cooperation between immune T cells and normal monocytes
in the expression of DH reactions (6, 7). A similar cooperation
between cells has been suggested to occur in the expression of adoptive tumor immunity (8). We therefore performed experiments to determine whether recipient chickens which had been pretreated to
inhibit monocyte-macrophage activity could support the adoptive
tumor immunity. The results summarized in Table 4 show clearly that
tumor immunity of immune nylon wool nonadherent spleen cells could
not be expressed in irradiated recipients or in recipients pretreated
with silica. Additional evidence that the silica had acted through
inactivation of macrophages was obtained by demonstrating protection
against the silica effect of pretreatment with PVNO (poly (2-vinyl
Pyridine-N-oxide), Polysciences, Warrington, Pa.), a lysosome sta-
bilizing agent (9). Moreover, pretreatment of recipients with
trypan blue, another macrophage inhibiting agent (10) was shown
to interfere with the expression of adoptive tumor immunity in a
separate experiment (not in Table). The ability of irradiated recipients to allow expression of tumor immunity could be reconstituted
by 1) i.v. injection of 2 X 10^8 spleen or bone marrow cells from unimmunized BX donors 48 hours prior to tumor cell + immune nylon wool
nonadherent spleen ("T") cell injection (Table 5), 2) wing web injection of 10^6 spleen cells from BX donors simultaneous with tumor cells
and immune T cells (not in Table); 3) wing web injection of purified
peripheral blood monocytes simultaneous with tumor cells and immune
T cells (Table 5). Peripheral blood monocytes which had been cultured for 5 days in vitro in a medium containing 10% normal chicken
serum and which had been washed free of nonadherent cells were harvested with 0.001 M EDTA (pH 7.0) and injected into wing webs.
These cells did not cause any inhibition of tumor growth when injected without immune T cells. Thus, cooperation between tumor immune
T cells and normal monocytes apparently mediated the tumor growth
inhibition. Attempts to demonstrate direct cytotoxicity of tumor

TABLE 3

T-CELL NATURE OF SCFS IMMUNE SPLEEN CELLS MEDIATING
ADOPTIVE IMMUNITY IN WINN TESTS

EXPT. NO.	PRETREATMENT* OF DONOR CELLS	SPLEEN TO TUMOR CELL RATIO	TUMOR GROWTH IN WING WEB**	
			SIZE $\pm$ S.E. (cm)	INCIDENCE
1	-	0	$.83 \pm .05$	8/8
	Unfractionated	5-20	$.06 \pm .05$	3/12
	N. W. Nonadherent	5-20	$.04 \pm .01$	1/10
	N. W. Adherent	5-20	$.91 \pm .04$	8/8
2	NRS + C	20	ND	1/8
	R anti-T + C	20	ND	8/8

*Expt. 1: Nylon wool (N.W.) fractionation: 45 mins at 37° C incubation on column.
Expt. 2: Immune spleen cells were incubated for 60 min at 37°C at 10⁷ cells/ml with 1:75 NRS
or R antiserum to chicken T cells and 1:18 guinea pig C.
**Determined on day 8 (Expt. 2) or 14 (Expt. 1); tumor size not determined (ND) in Expt. 2.

TABLE 4

EFFECT OF γ-IRRADIATION OR MACROPHAGE INACTIVATION ON THE
EXPRESSION OF ADOPTIVE IMMUNITY TO SCFSI IN CHICKENS

PRETREATMENT OF RECIPIENTS	IMMUNE SPL CELLS* ADDED TO SCFSI IN WING WEB	TUMOR SIZE ON DAY 7		
		cm $\pm$ S.E. (n)	p vs IMMUNE CONTROL	p vs TUMOR ALONE
None	–	.59 $\pm$ .02 (20)	p$\ll$.001	
None	+	.21 $\pm$ .03 (18)		p$\ll$.001
γ-Irradiation**	+	.54 $\pm$ .03 (12)	p$\ll$.001	NS
silica✝	+	.68 $\pm$ .02 (8)	p$\ll$.001	NS
PVNO + silica✝	+	.29 $\pm$ .05 (14)	NS	p$\ll$.001

*Spleen cell donors immune to SCFSI + C. parvum; injections in wing web on day 0 consisted of 10^6 SCFSI + or – 10^7 nylon wool nonadherent spleen cells.

**760 R, day –1.

✝Total of 2 x 3 mg silica i.v. (days –1 and 0) + or – 150 mg/kg PVNO subc. on day –2.

TABLE 5

RECONSTITUTION OF THE ABILITY OF IRRADIATED RECIPIENTS TO SUPPORT EXPRESSION OF
ADOPTIVE TUMOR IMMUNITY TO SCFS IN THE WING WEB WINN TEST

1260 R γ-IRRADIATION*	METHOD OF RECONSTITUTION CELLS, INJECTED, DAY	10^7 IMMUNE SPL CELLS** IN WING WEB (DAY 0)	TUMOR GROWTH (cm) $\pm$ S.E. (INCIDENCE)† EXPT. 1	EXPT. 2
–	–	–	.83 ± .05 (8/8)	.97 ± .04 (5/5)
–	–	+	.06 ± .03 (3/12)	.08 ± .04 (3/10)
+	–	+	.46 ± .08 (12/14)	.72 ± .07 (10/10)
+	2×10^8 BX Spleen, i.v., day -2	+	.02 ± .02 (1/16)	
+	2×10^8 BX BM, i.v., day -2	+	.01 ± .00 (1/18)	
+	10^6 Monocytes#, w.w., day 0	+		.11 ± .06 (3/10)
–	10^6 Monocytes#, w.w., day 0	–		.94 ± .08 (5/5)

*Total of 1260 R γ-irradiation on days -3 and -2 (Expt. 1) or on days -2 and -1 (Expt. 2).

**Immune spleen cells, obtained from donors injected with SCFSI + C. parvum, were used unfraction-
ated (Expt. 1) or as nylon wool nonadherent spleen cells (Expt. 2).

†Tumor growth determined day 7 (Expt. 1) or day 10 (Expt. 2).

#Adherent peripheral blood monocytes cultured for 5 days prior to injection into wing web (w.w.).

immune spleen cells on SCFS cells in vitro have so far failed. This
would appear to agree with the lack of tumor growth inhibition in
vivo by immune T cells alone. However, T cell cytotoxicity in vitro
has thus far not been clearly demonstrated with chicken spleen cells
in any system examined and these negative results can therefore not
be interpreted.

Tumor growth inhibition by local delayed hypersensitivity reactions to unrelated antigens. In view of reports that local DH reactions to bacterial antigens in tumors may cause tumor growth inhibition (11-14) and also because the properties of the adoptive tumor-
specific immunity followed those of adoptive DH, the role of DH reactions to unrelated antigens in the tumor was also examined in our
system. It was considered possible that the initial tumor growth
inhibition demonstrated in Table 1 could have been caused by a local
DH to CP or BCG in the tumor. Thus, animals were preimmunized
either to human γ-globulin (HGG) emulsified in CFA or to CP. The
corresponding antigen was then injected with the tumor cells into
the wing web in a group of immunized and also in a group of control
chickens. The dose of 10^7 CP or 200 μg HGG used for the wing web
injections did not affect growth in chickens immunized to give DH
reactions. DH reactions were always measured in the wattles as described previously (15). Results of a typical experiment are represented in Table 6. In one of the other two similar experiments performed to date, a complete regression of tumor growth was observed
in 50% of the animals. It should be noted that there was an additional nonspecific effect of preinjection with 10^9 CP i.v. noted in
the experiment in Table 6. It appeared that tumor growth between
14 and 21 days after injection was much slower in such CP pretreated
animals than in HGG pretreated or control chickens.

Adoptive DH reactions to 10^7 CP at tumor injection sites also
inhibited tumor growth (Table 7). This was readily demonstrated in
normal but not in irradiated recipients. Thus, the adoptive tumor
immunity and DH reactions appeared to act through a similar effector
cell mechanism.

In previous studies with bacterial antigens it was suggested
that antigenic crossreactivity between bacteria and tumor cells was
causing the "bystander" inhibition of tumor growth (16, 17). Such
a crossreactivity does not seem likely in the present studies since
the antigen HGG mediated an effect entirely comparable to that of
CP or BCG. Additional studies (not in Tables) have shown that injection of mitomycin-treated allogeneic spleen cells together with
SCFS cells also delay tumor growth.

Summary. Immunity to carcinogen-induced transplantable fibrosarcoma (SCFS) was induced in histocompatible C. parvum or BCG
pretreated chickens by injection of SCFS cells with C. parvum or
BCG into wing webs. Splenic T cells from such chickens, which had
rejected subsequent SCFS transplants, demonstrated tumor immunity
in Winn assays with specificity for the immunizing SCFS line. Recipients could not support expression of tumor immunity when pretreated with silica, γ-irradiation or trypan blue, and their

TABLE 6

INHIBITORY INFLUENCE OF A LOCAL DELAYED HYPERSENSITIVITY REACTION
ON GROWTH OF SCFSI IN SC CHICKENS

PRETREATMENT OF RECIPIENTS	(NO.)	ADDED TO 10^6 SCFSI IN WING WEB	TUMOR SIZE (cm) $\pm$ S.E. ON DAY*		
			7-10	14	21
None	(5)	200 μg HGG	.49 $\pm$ .07	1.05 $\pm$ .08	1.46 $\pm$ .04
200 μg HGG + CFA**, day -10	(5)	None	.45 $\div$ .03	.98 $\pm$ .08	$\geqq$ 1.50
200 μg HGG + CFA**, day -10	(5)	200 μg HGG	.09 $\pm$ .04	.50 $\pm$ .08	1.13 $\pm$ .06
None	(5)	10^7 CP	.50 $\pm$ .07	1.13 $\pm$ .03	$\geqq$ 1.50
10^9 CP, i.v., day -5	(5)	None	.51 $\pm$ .03	.85 $\pm$ .08	1.03 $\pm$ .24
10^9 CP, i.v., day -5 + 10^7 CP, i.v., day 0	(10)	None	.31 $\pm$ .07	1.03 $\pm$ .05	1.16 $\pm$ .13
10^9 CP, i.v., day -5	(5)	10^7 CP	.12 $\pm$ .05	.50 $\pm$ .05	.63 $\pm$ .20

*100% tumor incidence in all recipients at 5 weeks.
**Strong positive DH upon wattle testing at termination of experiment.

TABLE 7

RETARDATION OF SCFSI TUMOR GROWTH IN WING WEB BY SIMULTANEOUS INJECTION OF C. PARVUM SENSITIZED SPLEEN CELLS* AND C. PARVUM

PRETREATMENT OF RECIPIENTS	(NO.)	ADDED TO 10^6 SCFSI IN WING WEB	TUMOR GROWTH ON DAY 9	
			SIZE $+$ S.E. (cm)	INCIDENCE (%)
None	(4)	None	.68 $\pm$ .03	100
None	(4)	10^7 CP	.53 $\pm$ .05**	100
None	(12)	2-5 x 10^7 Spl Cells	.63 $\pm$ .04	100
None	(12)	10^7 CP + 2-5 x 10^7 Spl Cells	.31 $\pm$ .06**/	75
1260 R, day -2, -1	(6)	2 x 10^7 Spl Cells	.69 $\pm$ .03	100
1260 R, day -2, -1	(6)	10^7 CP + 2 x 10^7 Spl Cells	.71 $\pm$ .04/	100

*Donors of spleen cells received i.v. injection of 10^9 C. parvum (CP) 5 days prior to transfer.
**Statistically significant difference p< .02.
/Statistically significant difference p< .001.

competence was restored by normal monocytes. Local delayed reactions to unrelated antigens, such as HGG or C. parvum, inhibited tumor growth according to a similar mechanism. It is concluded that in the chicken cooperation between immune T cells and normal monocytes results in tumor growth inhibition when occurring in the tumor site both when the antigen resides on the tumor cell itself and when an unrelated extraneous antigen is injected along with the tumor cells. Such locally occurring reactions also appear effective in inducing tumor-specific immunity in the chicken.

References
1. Lerman, S. P., Palladino, M. A. and Thorbecke, G. J., J. Natl. Cancer Inst. 57:295 (1976).
2. Ponten, J., J. Natl. Cancer Inst. 29:1147 (1962).
3. Palladino, M. A., Grebenau, M. D. and Thorbecke, G. J., manuscript in preparation.
4. Coe, J. E., Feldman, J. D. and Lee, S., J. Exp. Med. 123:267 (1966).
5. Lubaroff, D. M. and Waksman, B. H., J. Exp. Med. 128:1425 (1968).
6. Volkman, A. and Collins, F. M., Cell. Immunol. 2:552 (1971).
7. McGregor, D. D. and Logie, P. S., Cell. Immunol. 18:454 (1975).
8. Simes, R. J., Kearney, R. and Nelson, D. S., Immunology 29:343 (1975).
9. Rios, A. and Simmons, R. L., Transplantation 13:343 (1972).
10. Hibbs, J. B., Transplantation 19:77 (1975).
11. Klein, E., Holtermann, O., Milgrom, H., Case, R. W., Klein, D., Rosner, D., and Djerassi, I., Med. Clin. N. Amer. 60:389 (1976).
12. Zbar, B., Bernstein, I. D. and Rapp, H. J., J. Natl. Cancer Inst. 46:831 (1971).
13. Tuttle, R. L. and North, R. J., J. RES 20:209 (1976).
14. Ashley, M. P., Kotlarski, I. and Hardy, D., Immunology 32:1 (1977).
15. Palladino, M. A., Gilmour, D. G., Scafuri, A. R., Stone, H. A. and Thorbecke, G. J., Immunogenetics, in press.
16. Borsos, T. and Rapp, H. J., J. Natl. Cancer Inst. 51:1085 (1973).
17. Bucana, C. and Hanna, M. G., J. Natl. Cancer Inst. 53:1313 (1974).

Acknowledgments. These studies were supported by Grant #CA-14462 from the National Cancer Institute, USPHS, and by Contract #CB64043, Department of Health, Education and Welfare. MAP is a Fellow under USPHS Training Grant 5TOI-GM00127.

ROLE OF TUMOR ANTIGEN IN VACCINE PROTECTION IN MAREK'S DISEASE

J. M. Sharma

U.S. Department of Agriculture, ARS, Regional
Poultry Research Laboratory
3606 East Mount Hope Road
East Lansing, Michigan 48823

INTRODUCTION

Recently, we have observed that chickens vaccinated with the
herpesvirus of turkey (HVT) develop lymphoproliferative lesions
(1) and a cell mediated immune response to the Marek's disease
tumor associated surface antigen (MATSA) (2). The purpose of this
presentation is to consider these observations in view of the
overall mechanism of vaccine protection in Marek's disease (MD)
and to speculate on the possible role MATSA immunity may play in
protection. Furthermore, additional data are presented that
confirm earlier observations on the presence of MATSA in HVT
infected chickens.

Marek's disease is the only known naturally occurring
malignancy that can be prevented by vaccination. The disease is
caused by a herpesvirus which is ubiquitous and under field
conditions, infects almost all chickens at a young age. In
susceptible chickens the disease is manifested by progressive
paralysis that usually results in death. Vaccination with HVT
prevents clinical manifestations of the disease, although vaccinated
chickens remain susceptible to infection with MD virus (MDV) and
develop persistent viremia both with the vaccine virus and with
MDV. The mechanism by which vaccines provide protection against
MD is not clearly understood. Although there is evidence that
immunosuppression in the T cell system abrogates protection by
vaccination (3,4), the characteristics of the protective immunity
and the nature of the immunizing antigen(s) are not known.

MATSA, has been specifically associated with transformation
by MDV (5,6). The cells of lymphoblastoid cell lines developed

345

from MD lymphomas and a certain proportion of cells in lymphomas in vivo contain MATSA. We and others have observed that chickens infected with MDV generate effector cells that are specifically cytotoxic to MATSA-bearing cells of MD cell lines (7,8).

Because lymphoproliferative lesions were observed in HVT infected chickens (1), we theorized that the proliferative cells may contain an antigen serologically related to MATSA and if so, an immune response to this antigen may develop in vaccinated chickens which could protect against subsequent lymphoma formation by MDV.

EXPERIMENTAL DESIGN

Chickens were the F_1 progeny of a cross between inbred lines 15 and 7 maintained at this laboratory (9). Parent stock was housed in isolation under specific pathogen free conditions and was not exposed to MDV or HVT. Progeny chickens, free from antibodies to MDV or HVT, were also held under isolation in Horsfall Bauer cages for the entire length of the experiment.

Chickens were inoculated intraabdominally with $2x10^4$ plaque forming units of FC126 isolate of HVT or with 10^4 plaque forming units of clone 111S of the JM isolate of MDV. At 7 and 8 days after inoculation, samples of virus-inoculated and uninoculated control chickens were examined for: a) lesions in peripheral nerves and gonads and b) cell mediated cytotoxic response to MATSA in an in vitro cytotoxic assay.

All sampled chickens were necropsied. Sections of vagus nerve, brachial and sciatic plexuses and of gonads were examined histologically. Microscopic nerve lesions were given a score of 1, 2, 3, or 4, based on increasing intensity of lymphoid cell infiltration as described in (10).

For cell mediated immune response to MATSA, single spleen cell suspensions from test chickens were incubated at 37° C for 4 hours with ^{51}Cr-labeled MSB-1 target cells, and the specific release of ^{51}Cr in the spleen cell + ^{51}Cr-labeled MSB-1 cell mixture was quantitated as described in detail elsewhere (8). The MSB-1 cell line is an in vitro propagating line of T lymphoblasts (11) derived from cell suspension of a MD lymphoma (12). The cells of this line are considered transformed by MDV because they contain MDV genome (13) and MATSA (6). In the above cytotoxic assay, the killing of MATSA-bearing MSB-1 cells has been considered a measure of anti-MATSA immunity (7,8). In some cases, cells of the TLT line (provided by K. Nazerian of this laboratory) were used as targets. This line was derived from a lymphoid leukosis tumor (14). The MATSA-free cells of TLT line are lymphoblastoid in nature and are productively infected with RNA tumor virus.

RESULTS AND DISCUSSION

Results given in Table 1 indicated that chickens infected with HVT had detectable lesions. The lesions consisted of lymphoid cell infiltration in peripheral nerves and occasionally in gonads. The infiltrating cells in the HVT lesions were morphologically similar to the proliferative cells seen routinely in MDV lesions (15). Some cells in the HVT lesions appeared transformed because they were blastoid in nature with abundant basophilic cytoplasm. As expected, MDV-infected chickens also had lymphoproliferative lesions.

Cell mediated cytotoxic response to MSB-1 cells was clearly detectable in chickens inoculated with HVT or with MDV. This response was specific to MSB-1 cells because effector cells cytotoxic for MSB-1 cells did not react with target cells of line TLT which lacked MATSA. Circumstantial evidence strongly implicates MATSA in the cell mediated cytotoxic response detected in vitro: Firstly, MSB-1 cells and MDV-induced lymphoma cells contain serologically related MATSA (6). Cells with morphologic characteristics of transformed cells were also noted in HVT induced lesion. These cells may also contain MATSA, although a direct proof for this is lacking; secondly, effector cells generated by MDV or HVT infection do not react with cells that lacked MATSA (Table 1, ref. 8) and thirdly, several unrelated, non-MATSA-inducing replicating and non-replicating antigens (avian adenovirus, complete Freund's adjuvant, sheep erythrocytes and Brucella abortus) do not generate MSB-1 specific effector cells during the time period of peak cytotoxic activity in MDV or HVT infected chickens (unpublished). Additionally, the specific cytotoxic activity seen in MDV infection is probably not an enhanced expression of natural cytotoxicity present in certain animals against some target cells because the MSB-1 specific effector cell in the MDV immune system is a T lymphocyte readily susceptible to lysis with anti-thymocyte antibody and complement (unpublished). The natural killer cells in the mouse are Fc-receptor-bearing prethymic cells (16) that are relatively resistant to anti-T cell serum (17).

Results on pathologic and cell-mediated immune responses of chickens inoculated with HVT noted in Table 1 were confirmed in several repeat experiments reported elsewhere (2). Because HVT inoculated chickens developed MD like lesions and cell mediated immune response against MATSA, it seems likely that HVT may be a transforming virus and that infection with HVT results in the appearance of a MATSA which is immunologically related to MATSA present on cells transformed by MDV. Although our results strongly suggest that HVT may transform cells, unequivocal proof firmly establishing the presence of transformed cells in HVT infected chickens in pending.

Table 1. Lesion response and cell-mediated immune response to MATSA-bearing MSB-1 and MATSA-lacking TLT target cells in chickens exposed to HVT and MVD.

Treatment	Days after inoculation	% specific release of ^{51}Cr from target cells[a]						Lesions[b]	
		MSB-1			TLT			+/tested	Mean lesion score
		Effector cells from bird No.			Effector cells from bird No.				
		1	2	3	1	2	3		
HVT	7	7.1	11.9	20.8	0	1.3	2.1	2/4	0.5
MDV		17.3	17.5	24.4	0.6	0.7	0	3/4	1.2
HVT	8	6.1	8.8	4.7	0.1	0.3	0	3/3	1.0
MDV		6.0	7.3	4.8	0	1.4	0.5	3/3	1.3

[a] Spleen cells from test chickens and target cells were reacted using triplicate cultures per sample. Specific release of ^{51}Cr was calculated by the following formula:

$$\% \text{ specific release} = \frac{\text{CPM in target cells mixed with spleen cells from infected chickens} - \text{CPM in target cells mixed with spleen cells from uninoculated control chickens}}{\text{CPM in target cells mixed with detergent (maximum release)} - \text{CPM in target cells mixed with spleen cells from uninoculated control chickens}} \times 100$$

[b] Positive lesions consisted of microscopic lymphoid cell proliferation in peripheral nerves (vagii, brachial and sciatic plexuses) or in gonads. Lesions in each chicken were given a score of 1-4 on the basis of increasing intensity of lymphoproliferation. Lesions scores of all chickens in a group were averaged to obtain the mean lesion score. Uninoculated chickens had no detectable lesions.

The detection of MATSA immunity in HVT inoculated chickens is of most interest. Likely, this immunity may play an important role in vaccine protection against MD.

Figure 1 outlines some of the events that occur after MDV infection in vaccinated and unvaccinated chickens and provides a theoretical explanation of how MATSA immunity may influence the outcome of infection.

When an unvaccinated susceptible chicken contacts MDV, (Figure 1 - top panel), the virus replicates rapidly initiating lytic and proliferative phases of infection (18) and high titers of virus can be readily recovered from almost all tissues. Rapidly progressing infection results in general immunosuppression of humoral and cellular immune systems (for references see 19). Although the susceptible chicken develops detectable immune response to MATSA and to other viral antigens (referred to here as membrane antigens, MA), the virus load and associated cellular transformation advance at an uncontrollably rapid rate and result in a progressive clinical disease.

Vaccination with live HVT (Figure 1 - middle panel) results in infection with the vaccine virus. HVT initiates cellular transformation and generates MATSA. Because immune functions in HVT infected chickens remain intact (20), the host mounts a vigorous immune response to MATSA and to MA of HVT. HVT-induced transformation remains restricted, possibly because of anti-MATSA immunity. In the vaccinated chicken, response to a subsequent challenge with virulent MDV is modified in several ways: replication and possibly spread of MDV is restricted by existing MA immunity thus the MDV load is kept to a minimum although MDV is not completely eliminated and low levels of virulent virus persist in the vaccinated, challenged host (1,21); immune systems of the host are spared; existent MATSA immunity prevents progression of transformation by MDV and any transforming events that are initiated by MDV generate additional MATSA immunity; and, because MDV persists in the host albeit at a low level, additional MA immunity is probably also generated thus contributing to the maintenance of reduced virus load. The end result is the survival of the host.

Perhaps the best indication of the protective role of MATSA is provided by the observation that immunization with membrane fractions of cultured cells productively infected with HVT also prevents MD (22,23). The membrane fractions lack infectious virus and MATSA but apparently contain MA. Thus, chickens vaccinated with HVT membrane fractions (Figure 1 - bottom panel) will not become infected with HVT and hence will not develop MATSA immunity but will respond immunologically to MA present on cell fractions. Upon challenge with MDV, the existing MA immunity will restrict

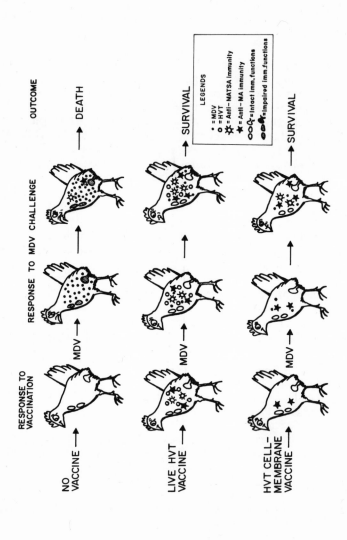

Fig. 1.   Proposed mechanism of vaccine protection in MD.   See text for explanation.

replication of MDV, and associated destructive events. The integrity of the immune systems is retained. Because viremia with MDV is not completely eliminated in chickens pretreated with membrane fractions (23), the chicken remains susceptible to the emergence of transformed cells. The existent anti-MA immunity which lacks anti-MATSA component will be ineffective in controlling progression of transformed clones. In this vaccination system, the host apparently develops MATSA immunity in response to transformation initiated by MDV and this immune response is probably the most important factor in protecting against the clinical manifestations of the disease.

The theoretical explanation for vaccine action presented above is consistent in principle with that proposed by Payne et al (24) except that recognition of MATSA immunity in vaccinated birds in our studies allows for a possible direct role of the tumor antigen in vaccine protection. Recently we have noted that chickens vaccinated with apathogenic or attenuated MDV also develop a cytotoxic immune response against MSB-1 cells (unpublished). Whether the cytotoxic response detected by the in vitro tests employed by us represents a measure of protection in vivo remains to be determined. Because susceptible chickens that succumb to MD also develop MATSA immunity detectable during the early stages of infection (8), mere presence of this immunity at a certain stage of infection cannot be considered a marker for resistance although development of MATSA immunity may be an important requisite for resistance.

SUMMARY

Chickens vaccinated with HVT developed lymphoproliferative lesions and a cell-mediated immune response to MATSA. These observations are considered in view of the overall mechanism of vaccine protection in MD. A mechanism of vaccine action is proposed that suggests that MATSA immunity in vaccinated chickens may play an important role in protection.

REFERENCES

1. Witter, R. L., Sharma, J. M., and Offenbecker, Linda, Avian Dis.,
    20: 676 (1976).

2. Sharma, J. M. (Submitted)

3. Purchase, H. G. and Sharma, J. M., Nature, 248: 419 (1974).

4. Else, R. W., Vet. Rec., 95: 187 (1974).

5. Powell, P. C., Payne, L. N., Frazier, J. A. and Rennie, M.,
    Nature, 251: 79 (1974).

6. Witter, R. L., Stephens, E. A., Sharma, J. M. and Nazerian, K.,
    J. Immunol., 115: 177 (1975).

7. Powell, P. C., Bibl. Haemat., 43: 348 (1976).

8. Sharma, J. M. and Coulson, B. C., J. Nat. Cancer Inst.,
    (In the press).

9. Stone, H. A., Technical Bulletin No. 1514. Agricultural
    Research Service, United States Department of Agriculture,
    (1975).

10. Sharma, J. M., Witter, R. L., Burmester, B. R., Inf. and
    Immun., 8: 715 (1973).

11. Nazerian, K. and Sharma, J. M., J. Nat. Cancer Inst., 54: 277
    (1975).

12. Akiyama, Y. and Kato, S., Biken J., 17: 105 (1974).

13. Lee, L. F., Nazerian, K. and Boezi, J. A. in Oncogenesis and
    Herpesvirus II pp. 199 (de The, Epstein, eds.) (International
    Agency for Research on Cancer, 1975).

14. Siegfried, L. M. and Olson, C., J. Nat. Cancer Inst., 48: 791
    (1972).

15. Payne, L. N. and Biggs, P. M., J. Nat. Cancer Inst., 39: 281
    (1967).

16. Herberman, R. B., Bartram, S., Haskill, J. S., Nunn, M.,
    Holden, H. T. and West, W. H. (Submitted).

17. Nunn, M. E., Djeu, J. Y., Glaser, M., Lavrin, D. H. and
     Herberman, R. B., J. Nat. Cancer Inst., 56: 393 (1976).

18. Payne, L. N. and Rennie, M., J. Nat. Cancer Inst. 51: 1559
     (1973).

19. Nazerian, K., Lee, L. F., and Sharma, J. M. Prog. Med.
     Virol., 22: 123 (1976).

20. Schierman, L. W., Theis, G. A. and McBride, R. A., J. Immunol.
     116: 1497 (1976).

21. Purchase, H. G. and Okazaki, W., Avian Dis., 15: 391 (1971).

22. Kaaden, O. R., Dietzschold, B. and Ueberschar, S., Med.
     Microbiol., 159: 261 (1974).

23. Lesnik, F. and Ross, L. J. N., Int. J. Cancer, 16: 153 (1975).

24. Payne, L. N., Frazier, J. A. and Powell, P. C., Int. Rev. Exp.
     Pathol., 16: 59 (1976).

IMMUNE RESPONSES AND PREVENTION OF LYMPHOID LEUKOSIS TUMORS IN CHICKENS FED AN ANDROGEN ANALOG

Carlos H. Romero[1] and Fred R. Frank[2]

USDA, ARS, Regional Poultry Research Laboratory,
3606 East Mount Hope Road, East Lansing, MI 48823[1]
The UpJohn Company, Kalamazoo, Michigan 49001[2]

Lymphoid leukosis (LL) can be controlled by several methods (2,8), one of which is by elimination of target cells for LL transformation residing in the bursa of Fabricius (8). Although the identity of the target cell within the bursa microenvironment remains unknown, removal of the bursa by surgical procedures up to 4 months of age (7) or by destruction of the lymphoid cells in the bursa by either the infectious bursal agent (9), or the lymphotoxic agent cyclophosphamide (10), or testosterone derivatives (1) prevents the development of LL tumors. However, these procedures cannot be used under field conditions because of their negative effects on liveability, productivity, and the immune response.

Mibolerone (17β-hydroxy-7α, 17-dimethylestr-4-en-3-one) is an androgen analog that when fed to chickens at µg levels during the first weeks of life induces a slow but progressive involution of the bursa of Fabricius (4). We have investigated the potential of the androgen analog in the prevention of lymphoid tumors induced by LL viruses (in preparation). Also, we needed to know the effect of the early bursa regression on the immunocompetence of chickens that had been fed the androgen analog. The immunocompetence of chickens fed mibolerone was studied by measuring the humoral antibody response to inert antigens and infectious agents; by quantitating the number of antibody-producing cells in the spleen; by stimulation of peripheral blood leukocytes with phytohemagglutinin (PHA); by the ability to resist challenge with avian pathogens after vaccination; and by the lack of increase in the rate of shedding in hens infected with LL viruses. A transfer technique was used to assay the presence of stem cells in the spleens of chickens 2 to 20 weeks of age that had been fed the androgen analog (13). The present report is a summary of studies intended to be published in more detail elsewhere.

Prevention of LL tumors: Chickens of the cross of inbred lines 15 and 7 from the U.S. Regional Poultry Research Laboratory (RPRL) free from infection by LL viruses (LLV's) but highly susceptible to LL tumor development were experimentally infected at 1 day and 2 weeks of age with a tumorigenic dose of RAV-1 and RAV-2 and were allocated to 2 dietary treatments. One diet contained 1.5 µg of the androgen analog per gram of basal feed and was administered during the first 7 to 8 weeks of life of the chickens. The second diet consisted of only basal feel and was administered throughout the experiments. In test to assess the effect on naturally occurring LL tumors, commercial White Leghorns chickens naturally infected with field LLV's were allocated to 4 dietary treatments. The androgen analog was administered at 1.0, 1.5, and 2.0 µg per gram of basal feed during the first 7 weeks of life, and the 4th diet consisted of only basal feed. Regression of the bursa of Fabricius was monitored by killing 6 chickens in each dietary treatment at 7 weeks of age. Regression proceeded as expected; i.e., in the RAV-1 experiment bursa weights of chickens fed the basal feed averaged 3.412 gm and bursa weights of chickens fed the androgen analog averaged 0.143 gm, a reduction of more than 20 times the bursa weight. The experiments were ended when chickens were 5 (RAV-1), 6 (RAV-2), and 7 (field LLV's) months old. All chickens tested were necropsied.

The androgen analog prevented the development of LL tumors in chickens infected with RAV-1, RAV-2, and field LLV's at all doses tested. Although LL tumor mortality in chickens fed the basal feed and infected with the above viruses was 71.8, 42.3 and 25.0 percent respectively, tumor mortality in chickens fed the androgen analog and infected with the same viruses was 2.8, 0.0, and 0.0 percent (Table 1). Although the exact mechanism of tumor prevention by the androgen analog is not yet known, mibolerone may act (a) by inducing a rapid maturation and migration of bursal cells to the peripheral lymphoid organs, (b) by eliminating the target cells from the bursal follicles, or (c) simply because the number of follicles remaining in the regressed bursa is not large enough for transformation and consequent disease to take place. In this respect, the chicken immune system may be able to eliminate the smaller number of transformed lymphoid cells from the bursas of mibolerone-fed chickens.

Table 1.   Prevention of LL tumors in chickens fed mibolerone

Mibolerone	LLV	No. at risk	No. survivors	No. other neoplasms	No. with LL	% LL tumors
+	RAV-1	72	68	2	2	2.8
−	RAV-1	71	17	3	51	71.8
+	RAV-2	28	27	1	0	0.0
−	RAV-2	26	15	0	11	42.3
+	Field LLV's	37	35	2	0	0.0
−	Field LLV's	16	12	0	4	25.0

LL antibody and viremia: Serum neutralization (3) tests on plasmas of 18-week-old chickens that had been fed mibolerone and were infected with LLV's indicated that induction of bursa regression by the androgen analog did not affect the development of LL neutralizing antibodies. Likewise, mibolerone-fed chickens that became viremic as a consequence of horizontal infection with LLV's or due to experimental infection lost the viremia as antibodies developed in a manner similar to that of chickens fed a basal diet. Titrations of infected plasmas by phenotypic mixing (6) showed that LL viremic-mibolerone-fed chickens carry loads of virus similar to those carried by chickens fed the basal diets. Finally, hens that had been fed the androgen analog and that were infected with LLV's did not shed LLV's or group-specific (gs) antigen in the albumen of unincubated eggs at a rate higher than that of hens fed the basal diet. Thus, mibolerone prevents the development of LL tumors without interfering with the natural cycle of infection of LLV's

Mibolerone and humoral antibody: Chickens of the 15 and 7 cross from the RPRL were fed mibolerone at a dose of 1.0 µg per gm of feed during the first 7 weeks of life (1.0 µg/7 wk regimen) or 4.0 µg per gm of feed from days 29 to 49 (4.0 µg/3 wk regimen) or were fed the basal diet. At 8 and 10 weeks of age, all chickens were injected via the wing wein with 1 ml of saline containing both 5×10^8 sheep erythrocytes and a 1:50 dilution of the standard Brucella abortus tube antigen. One week after each antigenic stimulation, sera were collected and tested for the primary and secondary antibody response by a microagglutination technique (15). Mibolerone-induced bursa regression did not affect the antibody-forming capacity of chickens subjected to both mibolerone regimens. The levels of serum antibody for the primary and secondary responses were comparable with those of chickens fed a basal diet (Table 2). However, the primary antibody response to B. abortus in chickens fed the 1.0 µg/7 wk regimen was less than that of chickens fed the 4.0 µg/ 3 wk regimen or fed basal diet alone. The difference was significant at 0.05 probability but not at 0.01 probability levels when tested by analysis of variance.

Table 2. Humoral antibody responses in chickens fed mibolerone

Mibolerone	Antibody to sheep erythrocytes			Antibody to B. abortus	
	Responders/ total	Primary response $\log_2 \pm$ SE	Secondary response $\log_2 \pm$ SE	Responders/ total	Primary response $\log_2 \pm$ SE
1.0 µg/7 wk	8/8	10.8+0.49	12.3+0.53	8/8	5.0+0.78
4.0 µg/3 wk	8/8	10.9+0.29	12.0+0.33	8/8	8.5+1.05
Basal diet	8/8	10.6+0.32	11.8+0.25	8/8	8.25+0.37

Mibolerone and antibody-producing cells: In efforts to quantitate the number of antibody-producing cells in the spleen of chickens fed the androgen analog, 6 to 8 chickens from each dietary treatment in the humoral antibody trial were used. The spleens were aseptically removed 1 week after primary and secondary stimulation and after preparing single cell suspensions they were assayed for production of hemolytic plaques; a modified indirect Jerne's plaque assay was used (11). The spleen of chickens that had been fed the androgen analog contained many antibody-producing cells as detected by the hemolytic plaque assay. The differences among the three treatment groups were not significant in the number of antibody-producing cells for the primary response (Table 3). However, when spleens were taken after the secondary response, those of chickens fed mibolerone at either the 1.0 µg/7 wk regimen or the 4.0 µg/3 wk regimen contained higher numbers of antibody-producing cells than those of chickens fed the basal diet (Table 3). The differences, though, were not statistically significant at the 0.05 probability level by analysis of variance.

Table 3.   Number of antibody-producing cells in the spleens of chickens fed mibolerone

Mibolerone	Primary response[1]		Secondary response[1]	
	No. chickens	IgPFCx10^3/ spleen Mean $\pm$ SE	No. chickens	IgPFCx10^3/ spleen Mean $\pm$ SE
1.0 µg/7 wk	6	14.8$\pm$3.6	8	37.6$\pm$7.5
4.0 µg/3 wk	6	22.6$\pm$4.2	8	39.7$\pm$9.0
Basal diet	7	17.5$\pm$4.2	8	18.6$\pm$2.7

[1] Assays were for total numbers of antibody (Ig) plaque forming cells (PFC). No. of PFC are the grand means of duplicate assays per spleen x 10^3.

Mibolerone and PHA stimulation of leukocytes: The stimulation of peripheral leukocytes and spleen cells by PHA is considered to be an in vitro correlate of cellular immunity, which in turn is an expression of thymus function (14). We, then needed to determine whether chickens that had been fed the androgen analog and had regressed their bursae had a normal response when peripheral leukocytes were assayed in a blastogenesis assay (5). Seven chickens from each dietary treatment in the humoral antibody trial were bled for peripheral blood leukocytes at 9 weeks of age and tested for ^{3}H thymidine incorporation after culture in the presence of PHA. The mean stimulation indexes (SI) of leukocytes derived from chickens fed the 1.0 µg/7 wk regimen and basal diet were higher than the SI of leukocytes derived from chickens fed the 4.0 µg/3 wk regimen. However, statistical differences were not significant at the 0.05 probability when both the PHA counts and the SI were subjected to analysis of variance (Table 4). These results reflected the integrity of the thymus function in chickens fed mibolerone at the levels tested.

Table 4. PHA stimulation of peripheral leukocytes from chickens fed mibolerone.

Mibolerone	No. chickens	Background counts[1] + SE	PHA counts[2] + SE	Stimulation index[3]
1.0 µg/7 wk	7	1120 + 245	37820 + 3867	34
4.0 µg/3 wk	7	1300 + 198	19590 + 6283	15
Basal diet	7	834 + 245	31842 + 4960	38

[1,2] Values are the grand means of the means of duplicate[1] or triplicate[2] + standard error 1-ml cultures per chicken pulsed for 16 hours (48 - 64 hours of culture) with 1 µCi of ^{3}H thymidine.

[3] Stimulation index = $\dfrac{\text{Average PHA counts}}{\text{Average background counts}}$

Mibolerone and vaccination immunity: Because vaccination immunity against specific avian pathogens is most likely dependent on the functional integrity of cell systems derived from both thymus and bursa of Fabricius, we needed to know whether regression of the bursa of Fabricius induced by feeding the androgen analog would in any way interfere with the development of immunity provided by vaccination against specific avian pathogens. A series of vaccination-challenge trials were set up to test for vaccination immunity against avian encephalomyelitis virus, Pasteurella multocida, Marek's disease virus, Newcastle disease virus, infectious bronchitis virus, infectious laryngotracheitis virus, and fowl pox virus. The experimental designs correspond to those published in the Federal Register of the United States Government and also described in Methods for Examining Poultry Biologics and for Identifying and Quantifying Avian Pathogens, National Academy of Sciences, Washington D.C. The results of these trials showed that chickens fed the androgen analog at a rate of 1.0 to 2.0 µg per gram of feed during the first 7 weeks of life were fully immunocompetent as judged by their ability to resist challenge after vaccination against the virulent avian pathogens mentioned above. Chickens fed the androgen analog were protected against the development of lesions, clinical signs, or mortality.

Mibolerone and stem cells: The androgen analog, then, induces a rapid regression of the bursa without interfering with the immunocompetence of the chicken. We then asked whether chickens remained immunocompetent because the androgen analog induced a more rapid maturation and migration of the bursal stem cells that

could be recovered in the spleen in the form of postbursal stem
cells. We, therefore, examined the spleens taken from chickens 2
to 20 weeks of age for the presence of postbursal stem cells by
procedures similar to those of Toivanen et al. (13). Test
chickens were fed either a basal diet (normal donors) or a diet
containing 1.0 µg of the androgen analog per gram of feed
(mibolerone donors) or they were fed a basal diet and treated with
4 mg of cyclophosphamide (CY donors) daily for 4 days starting
on the day of hatching. At 2, 4, 6, 8, 11, 13, 15, 17, and 20 weeks
of age, spleens from 5 to 25 chickens from each group were removed
and examined for post bursal stem cells by transferring cell
suspensions into CY-treated syngeneic recipient chickens of the
line 6 subline 1 from the RPRL (12). Groups of CY-treated
recipients were left untransplanted (no donors), and untreated
chickens (normal controls) served as positive controls for humoral
antibody responses. The immunocompetence of the recipient chickens
was tested 5 weeks after the cell transfer by antigenic stimuli
with sheep erythrocytes and B. abortus. Spleens of chickens fed
the androgen analog failed to reconstitute the immunological
capability of CY-treated recipients in a manner similar to that
of spleen cells from normal donors, (Fig. 1, & 2). Spleens of
CY-treated donors did not contain postbursal stem cells. Postbursal stem cells were detected in the spleens of chickens fed the
basal diet as early as 2 weeks of age; activity was highest after
the 13th week of age.

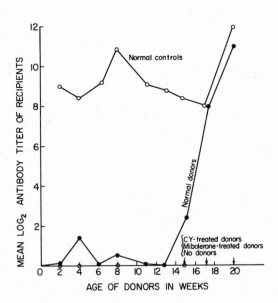

Fig. 1. Restoration of the humoral antibody response to Brucella
abortus with stem cells from the spleen.

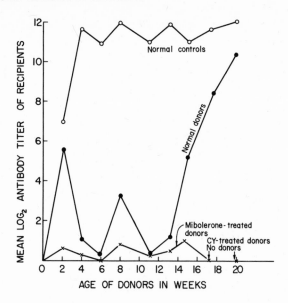

Fig. 2   Restoration of the humoral antibody response to sheep erythrocytes with stem cells from the spleen.

Possible explanations for the absence of postbursal stem cells in the spleens of chickens fed the androgen analog are: (a) The bursal stem cells matured to a stage beyond that of the post-bursal stem cell and were not detected by the present stem cell assay; (b) the stem cells lost their homing ability, failed to colonize the spleen, and died out; (c) the cells derived from the stem cells did not respond to sheep erythrocytes and B. abortus because of a unique antigenic competition; (d) the androgen analog was toxic for the stem cells; or (e) migration was delayed beyond 20 weeks. Of these possibilities, the first alternative appears most likely because we found that the spleens of chickens fed the androgen analog contain immunocompetent cells when assayed by a hemolytic plaque assay.

We have then, shown that the androgen analog mibolerone when fed to growing chickens at μg levels prevents the development of LL tumors by virtue of inducing early bursa regression. The chickens remain fully immunocompetent to both inert and infectious antigens. However, they do not seem to have post bursal stem cells in their spleens.

REFERENCES

1.   Burmester, B. R., Poult. Sci., 48: 401 (1969).

2.   Crittenden, L. B., Avian Dis., 19: 281 (1975).

3.   Ishizaki, R. and Vogt, P. K., Virology, 30: 375 (1966).

4.   Kakuk, T. J., Frank, F. R., Weddon, T. E., Burmester, B. R.,
     Purchase, H. G. and Romero, C. H. Avian Dis., Accepted for
     publication (1977).

5.   Lee, L. F., Avian Dis., 18: 602 (1974)

6.   Okazaki, W., Purchase, H. G. and Burmester, B. R., Avian
     Dis., 19: 311 (1975).

7.   Peterson, R. D. A., Purchase, H. G., Burmester, B. R.,
     Cooper, M. D. and Good, R. A. J. Natl. Cancer Inst., 36:
     585 (1966).

8.   Purchase, H. G. and Burmester, B. R., in Diseases of Poultry
     (M. S. Hofstad, B. W. Calnek, W. M. Reid, Ed.) (Iowa State
     University Press, Ames, in press).

9.   Purchase, H. G. and Cheville, N. F., Avian Path., 4: 239 (1975).

10. Purchase, H. G. and Gilmour, D. G., J. Natl. Cancer Inst.,
     55: 851 (1975).

11. Romero, C. H., Purchase, H. G., Frank, F., Burmester, B. R.,
     Kakuk, T. J. and Chang, T. S., Avian Dis., Accepted for
     publication (1977).

12. Stone, H. A., USDA Technical Bulletin No. 1514 (1975).

13. Toivanen, P., Toivanen, A., Linna, T. J. and Good, R. A.,
     J. Immunol., 109: 1071 (1972).

14. Weber, W. T., Exp. Cell Res., 46: 464 (1967).

15. Wegman, T. G. and Smithies, O., Transfusion, 6: 67 (1967).

Immunoglobulins

GENETIC POLYMORPHISM OF CHICKEN 7S IMMUNOGLOBULINS

E. K. Wakeland, J.M. Foppoli and A.A. Benedict

Dept. of Microbiology, University of Hawaii

Honolulu, Hawaii 96822

INTRODUCTION

We have previously described five 7S immunoglobulin (Ig) heavy (H) chain allotypic specificities which are inherited among highly inbred chicken lines as codominant genetic traits segregating at an autosomal locus (1-4). These allotypes have been divided into two groups by structural analysis: a) Specificities CS-1.1 and CS-1.2 are present in the Fd portion of the 7S Ig H chain probably in a region analogous to the C_{H1} domain of mammalian γ chains; and b) specificities CS-1.3, CH-1.4, and CS-1.5 are located in a region of the 7S Ig H chain which is sensitive to papain digestion (2,3).

Genetic studies have demonstrated that specificities in the Fd portion are inherited in association with specificities in the papain sensitive region (1). Analysis of the distribution of these specificities among the 7S Ig of inbred lines which carry specific phenogroups has demonstrated that both of the specificities forming a phenogroup are on the same molecules (5). Thus, these specificities represent combinations of intracistronic genetic markers, probably occurring in two regions of the 7S Ig H chain constant region structural gene.

Extensive phenotypic polymorphisms among chicken serum proteins have been described previously by several investigators (6-8). McDermid et al. (6) reported that sixteen alloantisera prepared against washed bacterial

agglutinates in chickens each had a unique pattern of
reactivity with a panel of outbred chicken sera.
The specificities detected by these alloantisera were
not localized to specific serum proteins. David et al.(7)
suggested that chicken Ig genes were extremely polymorphic on the basis of the high frequency of birds which
were negative for all of his specificities in closed
flocks. Finally, Ivanyi (8) also found several allotype negative birds and a variety of cross reactions
with his alloantisera in European flocks.

GENETIC POLYMORPHISM OF THE CS-1 GENE

We have recently completed a survey of 48 inbred
chicken lines derived from five sources in the United
States and Europe (9). These lines were typed for six
structurally defined 7S Ig allotypic specificities.
Usually, 20 to 30 individual sera from each inbred line
were typed, and a line was defined as homozygous for
7S Ig allotypes if all of the individual sera had the
same allotypic phenotype. Only 28 inbred lines were
homozygous for CS-1 specificities by this criterion.

As shown in Table 1, ten distinct alleles of the
CS-1 gene were detected in this survey (9). The first
six alleles were detected in lines which were homozygous
for CS-1 specificities. The last four alleles were only
observed in CS-1 polymorphic lines.

These data reveal several properties of the genetic
polymorphism of the CS-1 gene. First, the Fd and papain
sensitive regions each contain a series of mutually
exclusive allotypic specificities. Thus, each CS-1 gene
allele contains no more than one specificity from each
region. If the Fd region is assumed to contain three
specificities (CS-1.1, 1.2, and 1.-), while the papain
sensitive region contains four (CS-1.3, 1.4, 1.5, 1.-),
then a total of twelve possible allelic combinations
would be theoretically expected. In this survey, only
seven of the twelve possible combinations were observed,
indicating that some disequilibrium exists between these
intracistronic markers. Also, only line IS-GH contained
an allele which was negative for all of our specificities.
Thus, all but 7 birds of the more than 600 chickens typed
during this survey could be unambiguously classified with
alloantisera to the six 7S Ig specificities we have defined. These results indicate that the genetic polymorphism of the CS-1 gene is only slightly more extensive
than that observed for the Ig-1 gene of inbred mice (10).

Table 1. CS-1 gene alleles observed in a survey of 48 inbred lines.

Chicken Line[a]	Allele	Allotypic Specificities					
		Fd Region		Papain Sensitive			
		1	2	3	4	5	6[b]
UCD 2	$CS-1^a$	+	−	−	+	−	−
UCD 3	$CS-1^b$	+	−	+	−	−	−
UCD 7	$CS-1^c$	−	+	−	−	−	−
RH-C	$CS-1^d$	−	−	+	−	−	−
RPRL 6_1	$CS-1^e$	+	−	−	+	−	+
RPRL $15I_4$	$CS-1^f$	−	−	+	−	−	+
IS-W	$CS-1^g$	−	−	−	−	+	+
IS 9	$CS-1^h$	−	−	−	−	−	+
RPRL-N	$CS-1^i$	+	−	−	−	−	−
IS-GH	$CS-1^j$	−	−	−	−	−	−

[a]The sources of these inbred lines were listed previously (9).
[b]This specificity has not been localized to a specific region of the 7S Ig H chain.

However, the ten alleles which we currently detect represent the minimum number of alleles necessary to explain the data.

One final point can be made concerning the evolutionary origin of some of the CS-1 gene alleles. Allotypic surveys in mice and humans have detected alleles which are most easily explained by intracistronic recombination (11-13). For example, Lieberman and Potter (11) suggested that an unusual Ig-1 allele which was detected in a wild mouse probably arose via intracistronic recombination between two alleles represented among inbred lines. Similar conclusions were reached by Natvig et al. (12,13) concerning unusual human IgG_1 proteins, and thus some precedent exists for intracistronic recombination among Ig structural genes.

Our results suggest that intracistronic recombination may have played a significant role in the generation of the genetic polymorphism of CS-1 gene alleles. As shown in the diagram below, any attempt to explain the evolutionary relationship of the $CS-1^b$, $CS-1^d$,, $CS-1^i$, and $CS-1^j$

alleles by single step mutations requires the supposition
of two identical, independent mutational events. However,
this relationship would result if intracistronic recombination between specificities in the Fd and papain sensitive regions occurred during the evolution of these
alleles.

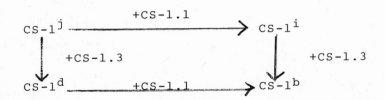

A similar relationship can be drawn between the CS-1^h,
CS-1^f, CS-1^d, and CS-1^j alleles, which suggests that intracistronic recombination may play a significant role
in the production of genetic polymorphism in the CS-1
gene

CS-1 GENE PSEUDOALLELES AND POSSIBLE POSITIONAL EFFECTS

     Several laboratories have recently reported the de-
tection of inappropriate or "latent" allotypic specificities at low, fluctuating levels in the sera of normal
individuals. This phenomenon has been described in man,
mice, and rabbits; and can involve allotypes localized
to the V_H, C_H, or C_k structural gene products (14-18).
These results indicate that Ig structural genes are
pseudoallelic in some individuals. Several theories
have been put forward to explain these data; and although
they differ in detail, they all basically advocate the
inheritance of a series of allelic regulatory genes which
control the activation of specific subsets of Ig structural genes (19,20). The regulatory gene hypothesis
suggests that all the structural gene alleles are pseudoalleles and that inheritance studies are detecting the
transmission of allelic regulatory genes which activate
specific sub-populations of the Ig structural genes
present in each individual.

     During our survey of chicken allotypic specificities,
several inbred lines were found to contain low levels of
inappropriate or "unexpected" allotypes (21). These preliminary findings have been confirmed and expanded in
an accompanying report in this volume (22). In essence,
the results indicate that some inbred chicken lines

contain at least two copies of the 7S Ig H chain structural gene. However, when two CS-1 pseudoalleles are
present within a single line, apparently one of them is
utilized for the production of the majority of the 7S
Ig, while the second is only expressed at very low levels.
This is similar to the "latent" allotypes of mammalian
species and can be explained by a regulatory gene
hypothesis.

Alternate Mechanism for Latent Allotypes

These data may also be interpreted as indicative
of positional requirements for the proper expression
of Ig structural genes. Several features of the organization of Ig structural genes support the importance of
chromosomal position on proper expression. First, the V_H
and C_H genes have been maintained in close linkage during
their evolution (reviewed in 23). Tartof has suggested
that the tight linkage of V_H and C_H genes may be necessary for the translocation and splicing events (24).
The extremely tight linkage between C_H region genes (i.e.,
no recombinants among mice in over 5,000 test progeny,
25) suggests that the position of these genes is highly
conserved and thus critical to their proper expression.
Tight linkage of C_H structural genes is observed in
humans, mice, rabbits, and chickens (26,27) and thus
this type of organization has been highly conserved
during the evolution of the Ig gene complex.

The role of positional requirements in the expression
of Ig structural genes could be postulated to be the result of the mechanism of V_H and C_H joining. Thus, the
manner in which V_H and C_H region genes are brought into
close proximity could involve the interaction of specific
regions of the chromosome. This highly speculative model
would suggest that the C_H region genes being predominantly
expressed are those which occupy a specific position in
the chromosome, while C_H structural genes in other
positions are fused with V_H structural genes and expressed much less frequently. Thus, "latent" or "unexpected"
allotypes would result from homologous but unequal crossover events which moved the structural genes(s) in the
"preferential" region of one chromosome into a less
favorable position in a recombinant chromosome. Homologous but unequal crossover events have been designated
by several investigators as a major factor in the evolution of Ig structural genes (28-30).

SUMMARY

A survey of 48 inbred lines derived from five sources in the United States and Europe revealed considerable genetic polymorphism of the CS-1 gene. A minimum of ten alleles were detected as unique combinations of CS-1 specificities. The relationship of some of the alleles would indicate that intracistronic recombination may have played a role in the production of some of the polymorphism.

REFERENCES

1. Wakeland, E.K. and Benedict, A.A., Immunogenetics, 2:531(1975).

2. Wakeland, E.K. and Benedict, A.A., J. Immunol., 117: 2185(1976).

3. Wakeland, E.K. and Benedict, A.A., in Advances In Experimental Medicine and Biology, Vol. 64, pp. 431-437(Plenum Press, New York, 1975).

4. Wakeland, E.K., Benedict, A.A. and Abplanalp, H.A., J. Immunol., 118:401(1977).

5. Stormant, C., Amer. Naturalist, 89:105(1955).

6. McDermid, E.M., Petrosky, E. and Yamazaki, H., Immunol. 17:413(1969).

7. David, C.S., Kaeberle, M.L. and Nordskog, A.W., Biochem. Genet. 3:197(1969).

8. Ivanyi, J., J. Immunogenetics 2:69(1975).

9. Wakeland, E.K., Foppoli, J.M. and Benedict, A.A., submitted for publication.

10. Herzenberg, L.A. and Herzenberg, L.A., in Handbook of Experimental Immunology, p. 13.1. (F.A. Davis, Philadelphia, 1973).

11. Lieberman, R. and Potter, M., J. Exp. Med., 130: 519(1969).

12. Natvig, J.B., Michaelson, T.E., Gedde-Dahl, T., Jr. and Fisher, T., J. Immunogenetics, 1:33(1974).

13. Natvig, J.B., Michaelson, T.E. and Nielson, J.C.
     Scand. J. Immunol., 3:127(1974).

14. Strosberg, A.D., Hamers-Casterman, C., Van Der
     Loo, W. and Hamers, R., J. Immunol., 113:1313(1974).

15. Bosma, M. and Bosma, G., J. Exp. Med. 139:512(1974).

16. Mudgett, M., Fraser, B. and Kindt, T.J., J. Exp.
     Med., 141:1448(1975).

17. Rodkey, L.S., Farnsworth, V., Goodfleisch, R. and
     Hood, L., Fred. Proc. 35:629(1976).

18. Rivat, L., Gilbert, D. and Ropartz, C., Immunology,
     24:1041(1973).

19. Hood, L., Fed. Proc. 35, 2185(1976).

20. Wang, A., Fed. Eur. Biochem. Soc.(Symp.), 36:19
     (1975).

21. Wakeland, E.K., in Ph.D. Dissertation, (Univ. of
     Hawaii, 1976).

22. Foppoli, J.M., Wakeland, E.K. and Benedict, A.A.,
     in this conference.

23. Mage, R.G., Lieberman, R., Potter, M. and Terry,
     W.D., in The Antigens, p. 300(Academic Press,
     New York, 1973).

24. Tartof, K.D., in Annual Review of Genetics, Vol. 9,
     p. 355(Annual Reviews Inc., California, 1975).

25. Wiegert, M., F.A.S.E.B. Symposium: Idiotypes As A
     Molecular and Cellular Probe, 1976.

26. Hood, L., Campbell, J.H. and Elgin, S.C.R., in
     Annual Review of Genetics, Vol. 9, p. 305 (Annual
     Reviews Inc., California, 1975).

27. Pink, J.R.L. and Ivanyi, J., Eur. J. Immunol., 5:
     506(1975).

28. Ohno, S. Evolution By Gene Duplication (Springer-
     Verlag, Heidelberg, 1970).

29.   Hood, L. and Prahl, J.   Advance Immunol. 14:291
      (1971).

30.   Gally, J.A. and Edelman, G.M., in Annual Review
      of Genetics, Vol. 6, p. 1(Annual Reviews Inc.,
      California, 1972).

This work was supported by United States Public
Health Service Grant AI05660.

A NOTE ON UNEXPECTED CHICKEN 7S IMMUNOGLOBULIN ALLOTYPES

James M. Foppoli, Edward K. Wakeland[1], and A. A. Benedict

Dept. of Microbiology, University of Hawaii

Honolulu, Hawaii 96822

INTRODUCTION

Allotypes have been detected on both chicken low molecular weight (7S) (1-3) and high molecular weight (17S) (2,4) immunoglobulins (Ig), and their inheritance is similar to allotype inheritance in mammals. The expression of the 7S heavy (H) chain allotypes and their segregation ratios are indistinguishable from those expected for codominant alleles at a single autosomal locus (3,5,6). In addition, genetic analysis of the inheritance of 7S and 17S Ig allotypes is consistent with the presence of alleles at two closely linked loci (7).

Immunoglobulin allotypes have been assumed to be inherited in a simple Mendelian fashion as codominant alleles, but recently this has been questioned. A number of observations suggest the possibility that allelic regulatory genes may be controlling the expression of sets of redundant variable and constant region structural genes. These data include: (a) the analysis of Ig levels in patients with hypogammaglobulinemia's and their relatives (8-10); (b) intermittent expression of a "wrong" Gm allotype in hamsters transplanted with a human lymphoid tumor line (11); (c) the detection of allotypic specificities in supernates of human mixed lymphocyte cultures (12) and PHA stimulated lymphocytes (13) from patients who lack the allotype in their serum; (d) concurrent expression of three alleles at both the a and b loci in individual heterozygous rabbits (14,15) and two IgG constant region alleles in congenic mice homozygous for Ig allotypes (16); and (3) the great sequence variation between the constant regions of b4, b6

[1]Present address: University of Texas School of Medicine, Dallas

and b9 kappa light chain molecules in the rabbit (17,18).

During the course of studies on the chicken 7S Ig allotypes (19) fluctuating low levels of "wrong" allotypes were observed in two inbred lines thought to be homozygous for allotypes. Low levels, detectable only in undiluted sera by radioimmunoassay (RIA), of an allotypic specificity (CS-1.2) were found in sera of UCD 2 birds (see the report by Wakeland, et al. on nomenclature of 7S Ig allotypes for characterization of inbred lines) in which anti-CS-1.2 antibody was generated. In the present report, data are given on an unexpected allotypes detected in inbred chicken line RPRL 15I$_4$.

SPECIFICITIES IN CHICKEN LINES STUDIED

Six allotypic specificities, designated CS-1.1 through CS-1.6, have been demonstrated on chicken 7S Ig (3,5,6). CS-1.1, CS-1.2, CS-1.3, CS-1.4, and CS-1.6 have been localized to the 7S Ig H chains (5,20). The distribution of all six allotypes have been determined for 47 inbred lines (21), and based on these data, 10 alleles have been defined at the CS-1 locus which controls the synthesis of 7S Ig H chains (21).

The UCD 2 and RPRL 15I$_4$ inbred lines are homozygous for the alleles designated by Wakeland, et al. (21) as CS-1^a and CS-1^f, respectively. Allelic designations are based on the formation of phenogroups which are unique combinations of alloantigens present on different regions of the H chains (3,5,22,23). Birds having the CS-1^a allele express phenotypically CS-1.1 and CS-1.4, while those with the CS-1^f allele have specificities CS-1.3 and CS-1.6 (5,20).

DETECTION OF AN UNEXPECTED ALLOTYPE IN 15I$_4$ SERA

Employing double diffusion in agar gels, the CS-1.1 specificity was not detected in 15I$_4$ sera; however, in the dinitrophenylated alloantibody (DAA) RIA (5) undiluted 15I$_4$ sera specifically inhibited binding of anti-CS-1.1 and specific alloantigen (UCD 2 ^{125}I-7S Ig). As shown in Fig. 1, low levels of inhibitory activity were detected in 22 out of 22 sera from 60-day-old chickens. Inhibition values ranged from 36 to 56% with a mean of 43%.

The presence of the unexpected allotype in 15I$_4$ sera may represent either low levels of the CS-1.1 determinant(s) or CS-1.1 cross-reacting determinants. To distinguish between these two possibilities, the inhibition curves formed by either 15I$_4$ sera or pooled 15I$_4$ 7S Ig were compared to the homologous inhibition curves [inhibition of UCD 2 (CS-1.1) and anti-CS-1.1]. Quantitative comparisons were made on the basis of the dilution or concentration

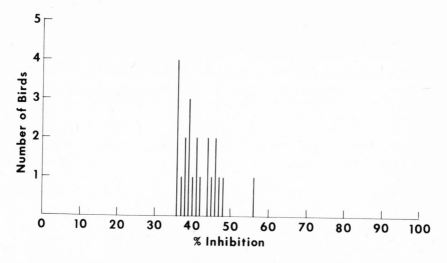

Figure 1.   Inhibition of binding of anti-CS-1.1 anti-serum with UCD 2 ^{125}I-7S Ig by undiluted sera from individual RPRL 15I$_4$ birds.   Each value is the mean of duplicate samples.

of inhibitor required to achieve 50% inhibition (I_{50}).   Regression coefficients of the linear portions of the inhibition curves were compared so that changes in binding avidity of the alloantibody for the inhibitors could be detected.   As shown in Figs. 2 and 3, and tabulated in Table 1, the inhibition slopes were not

Table 1.   Comparison of CS-1.1 inhibitory activity in UCD 2 and RPRL 15I$_4$ sera and 7S Ig.

| Inhibitor | | | I_{50} [a] | |
Line	Preparation	Dilution	Concentration (µg)	Slope [b]
RPRL 15I$_4$	serum	1:2.8	–	−27.0 ± 0.9
UCD 2	serum	1:29,000	–	−28.5 ± 0.9
UCD 2	pooled 7S Ig	–	0.015	69.1 ± 3.1
RPRL 15I$_4$	7S Ig-pool 1	–	2.5	68.3 ± 2.7
RPRL 15I$_4$	7S Ig-pool 2	–	6.6	67.9 ± 0.6

[a]Amount of inhibitor to give 50% inhibition.
[b]Linear regression coefficient calculated using all points on the linear portion of inhibition curves, ± standard error.

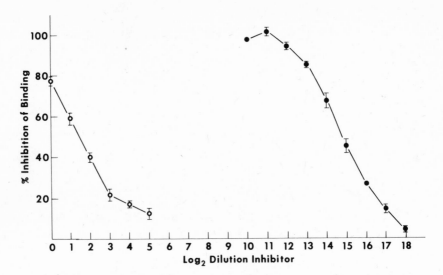

Figure 2. Inhibition of binding of anti–CS-1.1 antiserum with UCD 2 ^{125}I-7S Ig by RPRL 15I$_4$ serum (O——O)
and UCD 2 serum (●——●) from individual birds. Each
point is the mean of triplicate samples, and the brackets refer to the ranges.

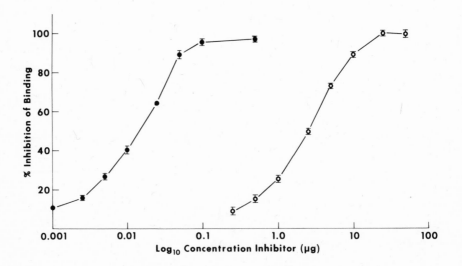

Figure 3. Inhibition of binding of anti–CS-1.1 antiserum
with UCD 2 ^{125}I-7S Ig by RPRL 7S Ig (O——O) and UCD 2 7S
Ig (●——●). Each point is the mean of triplicate samples,
and the brackets refer to the ranges.

significantly different either between $15I_4$ and UCD 2 sera or
their 7S Ig preparations. UCD 2 sera and 7S Ig were approximately
10,000 and 310 times better inhibitors than the respective $15I_4$
preparations. Based on identical slopes of the $15I_4$ and UCD 2 inhibition curves, the determinants on the $15I_4$ molecules probably
are the same as the CS-1.1 determinants and are not cross-reacting
determinants. Furthermore, the quantitative differences suggest
that the $15I_4$ CS-1.1 allotype is associated with a population of
Ig molecules found in low concentrations.

DETECTION OF TWO POPULATIONS OF 7S IG

It is assumed that CS-1.3 and CS-1.6 specificities are on the
same $15I_4$ 7S Ig molecules, similar to the formation of other phenogroups (22). If CS-1.1, -1.3, and -1.6 are present on the same
molecules, than adsorption of ^{125}I-labelled alloantigen with anti-
CS-1.3 or with anti-CS-1.6 will also remove the CS-1.1 specificity.
In such a case, direct binding will be the same with anti-CS-1.1,
-1.3, or -1.6 antisera with unadsorbed and adsorbed $15I_4$ ^{125}I-7S Ig
preparations. On the other hand, if CS-1.1 and the phenogroup CS-
1.3, 1.6 are on separate molecules, then adsorption with anti-CS-
1.6 or -1.3 will selectively remove CS-1.3, 1.6 molecules and
thereby enhance the relative concentration of CS-1.1 molecules. In
this case, direct binding of adsorbed $15I_4$ ^{125}I-7S Ig by anti-CS-
1.1 antiserum will be increased and binding of either anti-CS-1.3
or -1.6 will be decreased. Based on such adsorption experiments
CS-1.1 and CS-1.3, 1.6 were found on separate molecules.

CS-1.1 molecules represent about 0.3% of the Ig population in
$15I_4$ sera as calculated from comparison of I_{50} 7S Ig concentrations
shown in Table 1. The average concentration of CS-1.1 molecules
is 6.9 µg/ml using an average value of 2.3 mg/ml total 7S Ig as
determined by radial immunodiffusion. The levels of CS-1.1 activity remained relatively constant over a 30-day period; however,
in preliminary experiments CS-1.1 bearing molecules have not been
detected in all adult $15I_4$ birds.

SUMMARY

Low concentrations of allotypic specificity CS-1.1 were detected in the serum of $15I_4$ chickens previously believed to lack
this specificity. The average concentration of CS-1.1 bearing
molecules is approximately 7 µg/ml and 4 mg/ml in $15I_4$ and UCD 2
chickens, respectively. The CS-1.1 alloantigen in $15I_4$ chickens
has the same specificity as the line of chickens (UCD 2) in which
it was initially defined, and it is present on a population of
molecules distinct from those which carry the major allotypes in
$15I_4$ chickens.

The presence of two 7S Ig populations in $15I_4$ chickens may be interpreted as evidence either for 7S Ig subclasses with shared allotypes or for a pseudoallelic organization of genes controlling expression of 7S Ig H chains. In the case of pseudoallelic gene organization, the ten alleles as previously defined (21) probably are distributed at a minimum of two closely linked loci.

At this time the evidence favors pseudoallelism. This interpretation stems from the following observations: (a) CS-1.1 molecules cannot be detected in all adult $15I_4$ birds; (b) low levels (<0.01% of normal inhibitory levels) of another specificity (CS-1.2) was found in sera of some UCD 2 (CS-1^a) birds, a line in which anti-CS-1.2 antibody had been generated; and (c) there is no evidence that the two 7S Ig populations in $15I_4$ chickens have unique antigenic determinants — a criterion for definition of a subclass.

The results presented here differ from those reported in mice (16) and in rabbits (14,15) in that detectable levels of the unexpected allotype were not transitory or sporadic but persisted throughout the period of observation. It can be argued that regulation of Ig expression in chickens is different from that found in mammals, or that unexpected ("latent") allotypes (15) may persist in rabbit and mouse sera below levels of detection. Nevertheless, we believe our results to be consistent with a regulatory gene hypothesis (14) although other explanations can be made (21). In any event, the 7S Ig allotype nomenclature should be extended to include a second locus controlling the synthesis of 7S Ig H chains and designated as CS-2.

ACKNOWLEDGEMENTS

This work was supported by United States Public Health Service Grant AI 05660. We are grateful to Dr. Hans Abplanalp, University of California, Davis, for supplying UCD sera and birds, and to Mr. Howard Stone, Regional Poultry Research Laboratory, U.S.D.A., East Lansing, for supplying line $15I_4$ sera and birds.

REFERENCES

1. David, C. S., Genetics, 71: 649 (1972).

2. Ivanyi, J., J. Immunogenet., 2: 69 (1975).

3. Wakeland, E. K. and Benedict, A. A., Immunogenetics, 2: 531 (1975).

4. Pink, J. R. L., Eur. J. Immunol., 4: 679 (1974).

5. Wakeland, E. K. and Benedict, A. A., J. Immunol., 117: 2185
    (1976).

6. Wakeland, E. K. and Benedict, A. A., in Advances in Experi-
    mental Medicine and Biology, Vol. 64, pp. 431-437 (Plenum
    Press, New York, 1975).

7. Pink, J. R. L. and Ivanyi, J., Eur. J. Immunol., 5: 506 (1975).

8. Yount, W. J., Hong, R., Seligmann, M., Good, R. and Kunkel,
    H. G., J. Clin. Invest., 49: 1957 (1970).

9. Rivat, L., Ropartz, C., Burtin, P. and Cruchaud, A., Nature
    (Lond.), 225: 1136 (1970).

10. Litwin, S. D. and Fudenberg, H. H., Proc. Nat. Acad. Sci.
    (Wash.), 69: 7 (1972).

11. Pothier, L., Borel, H. and Adams, R. A., J. Immunol., 113:
    1984 (1974).

12. Rivat, L., Gilbert, D. and Ropartz, C., Immunology, 24: 1041
    (1973).

13. Rivat, L., Gilbert, D. and Ropartz, C., Immunology, 19: 6 (1970).

14. Strosberg, A. D., Hamers-Casterman, C., Van der Loo, W. and
    Hamers, R., J. Immunol., 113: 1313 (1974).

15. Mudgett, M., Fraser, B. and Kindt, T. J., J. Exp. Med., 141:
    1448 (1975).

16. Bosma, M. and Bosma, G., J. Exp. Med., 139: 512 (1974).

17. Rodkey, L. S., Farnsworth, V., Goodfliesch, R. and Hood, L.,
    Fed. Proc., 35: 629 (1976).

18. Strosberg, A. D., Janssens, L. and Zeeuws, P., Fed. Proc.,
    35: 629 (1976).

19. Wakeland, E. K., in Ph.D. dissertation, (University of Hawaii,
    1976).

20. Unpublished data.

21. Wakeland E. K., Foppoli, J. M. and Benedict, A. A., this
    conference.

22. Wakeland, E. K., Benedict, A. A. and Abplanalp, H. A., J. Immunol., 118: 401 (1977).

23. Stormant, C., Amer. Naturalist, 89: 105 (1955).

CHICKEN HIGH MOLECULAR WEIGHT IMMUNOGLOBULIN (IgM) ALLOTYPES:

LOCALIZATION ON THE HEAVY CHAINS AND PROPOSED NOMENCLATURE

James M. Foppoli and Albert A. Benedict

Dept. of Microbiology, University of Hawaii

Honolulu, Hawaii 96822

INTRODUCTION

The polymorphic nature of chicken serum proteins has been recognized for a number of years (1,2), but reports of allotypic antigens associated with IgG (7S Ig) and IgM (17S Ig) did not appear until recently (3,4). The structural and genetic analyses of chicken 7S Ig allotypes have progressed rapidly (5-9), and at least ten alleles have been defined at the locus controlling the synthesis of 7S Ig heavy (H) chains (CS-1 locus) (10). The use of two sensitive radioimmunoassays has facilitated the analysis of 7S Ig allotypes (7,8).

Although the inheritance of chicken 17S Ig allotypes has been analyzed (4,5), only limited structural characterization has been attempted (11). These allotypes have been detected either by immunoelectrophoresis (2) or by gel immunodiffusion (2,4,11). Based on these analyses, three specificites have been designated; namely, M1[a] (5) [previously referred to as C-M1 (4)], M1[b] (11), and M1[c] which cross reacts with M1[b] (11). The M1[a] specificity has been detected on 17S Ig 7S subunits (11), but further structural localization has not been reported.

In view of the importance of allotypes in elucidating the arrangement, expression and inheritance of Ig genes and since the Ig molecule reflects the product of at least 4 genes, assignment of allotypic specificities to class specific H chains or to L chains is desirable whenever possible. It is often assumed that the presence of an allotypic specificity on an Ig of only one class is sufficient to assign the allotype to its H chain. This is not always

381

the case, as has been shown with certain Ms specificities on rabbit IgM (12,13).

In this paper we deal with the following aspects of 17S Ig
allotypes: (a) structural localization of two specificities utilizing a new radioimmunoassay; (b) a survey of 47 inbred chicken lines
for these two allotypes; (c) designation of three alleles at the
locus controlling the synthesis of 17S Ig H chains; and, (d) a
suggested system of nomenclature.

A NEW 17S ALLOTYPE

To discover additional 17S allotypes, UCD 2, 3, and 7 chickens
were immunized with Salmonella O antigen. Their antisera were
precipitated with 18% Na_2SO_4, and the precipitated 7S and 17S Ig
were separated by gel filtration through Sephadex G-200. The 17S
fractions were reacted with Salmonella O antigen (14), the resulting agglutinates were washed, emulsified in Freund's complete
adjuvant (FCA) and given intramuscularly to jungle fowl (Gallus
gallus).

A double antibody radioimmunoassay (RIA) was developed using
^{125}I-17S Ig to detect alloantibody activity in immunized jungle
fowl. The assay is based on the fact that the major antibody produced following immunization of chickens with antigen in FCA is
7S Ig (15). Rabbit anti-chicken 7S Ig Fc is used to precipitate
alloantibody (7S)-alloantigen (17S) complexes. The binding assay
procedure is summarized as follows:

    1. Mix 25 µl of ^{125}I-17S Ig and 25 µl of
        alloantiserum dilution.
    2. Incubate for 8 hr at 4° C.
    3. Add 50 µl of rabbit anti-chicken Fc.
    4. Incubate for 2 hr at 37° C.
    5. Centrifuge at 10,000 rpm for 5 min.

Antiserum from one jungle fowl (2446) bound UCD 3 ^{125}I-17S Ig
following the fourth injection of Salmonella complexes (Fig.1). This
specificity, designated CM-1.4, was present on UCD lines 2, 3 and
7 17S Ig, but absent on the 7S Ig of these lines.

Using anti-M1[a] antiserum supplied by Dr. Ivanyi and UCD 3
^{125}I-17S Ig the binding curve for M1[a] 17S Ig allotype was determined (Fig. 1). Evidence that anti-CM-1.4 and anti-M1[a] antisera
were recognizing different determinants is given as follows: (a)
anti-CM-1.4 was raised in a jungle fowl which is M1[a] positive; (b)
these specificities have different distributions in inbred lines
(Table 3); and (c) anti-M1[a] and anti-CM-1.4 antisera do not cross

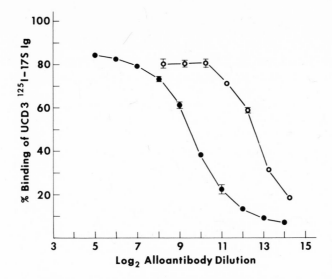

Figure 1. The percent binding of UCD 3 ^{125}I-17S by anti-CM-1.4 (●——●) and anti-M1^a (O——O) antisera.

react in immunodiffusion. The ability of each alloantibody to bind an excess of 80% of the alloantigen is evidence that both specificities are on the same molecules. The dilutions required to bind 50% of the labelled antigen for anti-CM-1.4 and anti-M1^a antisera were 1:700 and 1:6,000, respectively.

STRUCTURAL ANALYSIS

UCD 3 17S Ig preparations were treated in the following ways to determine the effect on the expression of CM-1.4 and M1^a specificities: (a) alkylation with 0.15 M iodoacetamide (IA) for 1 hr followed by dialysis against borate buffer (pH 8.3); (b) reduction with 0.1 M 2-mercaptoethanol (ME) for 1 hr, alkylation with 0.15 M IA, and dialysis against borate buffer (7S subunits); (c) reduction with 0.1 M ME, alkylation with 0.15 M IA, dialysis against 1 M propionic acid for 48 hr, and dialysis against borate buffer ("reassociated subunits"); (d) isolation of H chains by recycling reduced and alkylated 17S through Sephadex equilibrated in 1 M propionic acid.

The results of using these preparations to inhibit the binding of either anti-CM-1.4 or anti-M1^a antiserum to UCD 3 ^{125}I-17S Ig are shown in Fig. 2 and Table 1. Based on the calculated linear regression coefficients (Table 1), anti-CM-1.4 antiserum bound all preparations, except the isolated H chains, with equal avidity. The binding avidity of H chains decreased 21% relative to intact 17S Ig. This difference probably reflects a change in the conformation of the CM-1.4 specificity on the H chains in the absence of L chains. The efficiency of inhibition on both a molar and a weight basis is decreased for the 7S subunits, "reassociated subunits", and H chains compared to the intact or alkylated 17S Ig preparations. In addition, these preparations lose the ability to precipitate with anti-CM-1.4 antiserum in Ouchterlony plates; this may reflect a decrease in effective antigen valence, preventing lattice formation.

Unlike the CM-1.4 inhibition curves, the inhibition curves formed with 7S subunits, "reassociated subunits", and H chains with M1[a] specificity were biphasic (Fig. 3, Table 2). The antiserum may be multispecific and thus recognize allotypic determinants in two distinct regions of the 17S Ig molecule, as had been noted with some rabbit IgA allotypes (17). Perhaps both determinants are modified, but one is altered to a greater extent than the other. Whatever the reason, the regression coefficients decreased 50% (upper portion of inhibition curve) following reduction

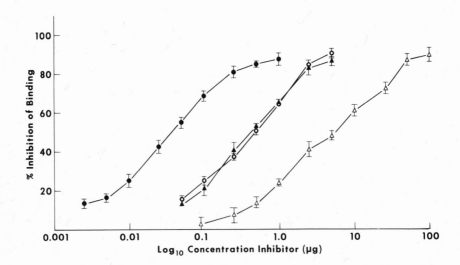

Figure 2. The percent inhibition of binding of anti-CM-1.4 with UCD 3 ^{125}I-17S Ig by UCD 3 17S Ig (●——●), 7S subunits (O——O), "reassociated 7S subunits" (▲——▲), and H chains (△——△).

Table 1. Localization of CM-1.4 allotype on UCD 3 17S subunits
and H chains by binding inhibition analysis.

Inhibitor	I_{50}[a]			Relative I_{50}[c]	
	µg	nM[d]	Slope[b]	Weight	Molar
17S Ig	0.038	0.042	43.5 ± 4.2	1.0	1.0
Alkylated 17S	0.042	0.047	42.7 ± 2.2	1.1	1.1
7S subunits	0.475	2.9	41.0 ± 1.4	12.5	69.0
"Reassociated 7S subunits"	0.415	2.5	42.4 ± 1.3	10.9	59.5
H chains	9.2	147	34.3 ± 1.4	242	3,500
L chains	>100	>4200	(-)	>26,000	>100,000

[a]Amount to inhibit 50% binding.
[b]Linear regression coefficients calculated using all of the points
on the linear portion of the inhibition curve.
[c]Intact 17S Ig is assigned an I_{50} value of 1.
[d]Molar concentrations were calculated using the following (16): 17S
Ig, 890,000; 7S Ig, 166,000; H chains, 62,600; L chains, 23,900.

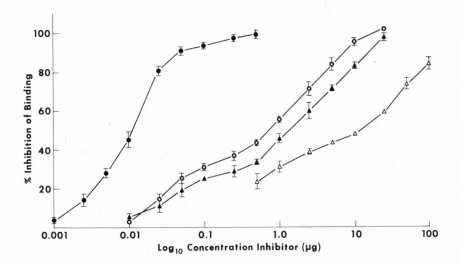

Figure 3. The percent inhibition of binding of anti-M1[a] with
UCD 3 [125]I-17S Ig by UCD 3 17 S Ig (●—●), 7S subunits (▲—▲),
"reassociated 7S subunits" (O—O), and H chains (△—△).

Table 2. Localization of M1[a] allotype on UCD 3 17S subunits and H chains by binding inhibition analysis[a].

Inhibitor	I_{50}			Relative I_{50}	
	µg	nM	Slope	Weight	Molar
17S Ig	0.011	0.012	75.6 ± 8.4	1.0	1.0
Alkylated 17S Ig	0.012	0.013	74.2 ± 6.2	1.1	1.1
7S subunits	1.37	8.3	39.9 ± 0.6[b] 27.2 ± 4.2[c]	124	688
"Reassociated 7S subunits"	0.74	4.5	37.3 ± 0.5[b] 20.3 ± 3.6[c]	67.3	370
H chains	20.2	322	36.8 ± 2.4[b] 20.5 ± 1.2[c]	1836	26,833
L chains	>100	>4200	(-)	>9000	>350,000

[a]All footnotes are the same as in Table 1.
[b]Based on the upper portion of the curve (see Fig. 3).
[c]Based on the lower portion of the curve (see Fig. 3).

and alkylation, and isolation of the H chains. Considering the lower part of the inhibition curves, the decrease in the regression coefficients was more pronounced; that is, the decrease was 64% for the 7S subunits, and 73% for both "reassociated subunits" and H chains. Except for the alkylated control, the relative effi- ciency of inhibition on both a molar and weight basis was greatly decreased. The H chains and 7S subunits were approximately 27,000 and 700, respectively, less efficient as inhibitors on a molar basis.

The M1[a] 7S subunits, "reassociated subunits", and H chains were still capable of precipitation with alloantibody; therefore, the antiserum may be recognizing more than a single antigenic determinant, so that decreasing the valency of the antigen did not significantly affect lattice formation.

POLYMORPHISM

Allotypic markers are useful to study the extent of Ig poly- morphism. In rabbits, 4 alleles have been defined at the n locus controlling IgM synthesis (18,19). At least 3 additional rabbit IgM allotypes have been reported (Ms locus), but their relation- ship to the n specificities is not known (12,13,20). Based on two alloantisera, two alleles at the Ig-6 locus (IgM) have been de- fined in mice (21). In humans, one allotypic specificity has been reported, Mm1 (22), which implies the presence of at least two alleles.

Table 3. Designation of CM-1 gene alleles observed among inbred lines.

Prototype line[a]	Allele[b]	Alloantigen	
		CM-1.4	M1[a]
UCD 3	CM-1^a	+	+
RH WA	CM-1^b	−	−
IS W	CM-1^c	−	+

[a]UCD – University of California, Davis; IS – Iowa State;
RH – Reaseheath. See reference (10) for description.
[b]The CM-1 locus controls the synthesis of 17S Ig H chains.
Alleles are designated by lower case letter superscripts.

Table 4. Distribution of CM-1 alleles among lines homozygous for 17S Ig allotypic specificities.

Allele	Lines[a]	
CM-1^a	IS –	DW, SP, 8, 9
	UCD –	2, 3, 7, 11, 13, 22, 50, 51, 53, 54, 56, 58, 59, 60, 70, 71, 72, 74, 75, 77, 80, 82
	RPRL –	6_1, 6_3, 7_1, 7_2, 15I, $15I_4$, $15I_5$, 100, N, P
	PRC –	R
	RH –	C, CA, CB
CM-1^b	RH –	WA, WB

[a]See reference (10) for description.

In accord with the nomenclature proposed for the chicken 7S Ig allotype locus (CS-1) (8,9), we tentatively designate the 17S Ig H chain allotype locus as CM-1. The use of lower case superscript letters as alleles at the CM-1 locus is in accord with mouse (23) and chicken 7S Ig allotypes (10).

Four 17S Ig allotypic specificities have been detected in chickens (4,11). Two of these alloantigens, CM-1.4 and M1[a], have been studied with respect to their distribution in 47 inbred lines of chickens. These lines are described by Wakeland et al. in this conference (10). Based on these data three alleles are defined. The allelic designations and corresponding phenotypes are shown in Table 3, and the distribution of these alleles among chickens homozygous at the CM-1 locus are shown in Table 4. Further analysis using Ivanyi's specificities M1[b] and M1[c] (11) probably will uncover additional alleles at the CM-1 locus. If so, perhaps chicken 17S allotypes may be more polymorphic than mammalian IgM allotypes.

SUMMARY

An alloantiserum recognizing a genetic marker (CM-1.4) on chicken 17S Ig was generated by immunizing jungle fowl with Salmonella O-anti-Salmonella O (UCD 3) agglutinates.

Specificities CM-1.4 and M1[a] were present on 7S subunits and H chains based on their ability to inhibit in RIA the binding of alloantibody (anti-CM-1.4 or anti-M1[a]) to UCD 3 ^{125}I-17S Ig. CM-1.4 appears to be fully expressed on 7S subunits but is altered on H chains. In contrast, anti-M1[a] bound both 7S subunits and H chains with decreased avidity indicating that the M1[a] specificity was altered in both preparations.

Since CM-1.4 and M1[a] are present on 17S Ig H chains, and absent from 7S Ig, they probably represent allotypic markers in the constant region of 17S Ig H chains.

Having assigned two 17S Ig allotypic specificities to H chains, we propose that the locus controlling their expression be called CM-1. Based on the distribution of the CM-1.4 and M1[a] allotypes in inbred lines of chickens, 3 alleles are defined at the CM-1 locus.

ACKNOWLEDGEMENTS

We wish to thank J. Ivanyi for generously supplying the anti-M1[a] alloantiserum, Drs. Hans Abplanalp and H. A. Stone, for providing inbred chicken lines and sera, and Drs. A. W. Nordskog, K. Morrison and J. R. L. Pink for supplying sera from inbred chicken lines. This work was supported by United States Public Health Service Grant AI 05660.

REFERENCES

1. Skalba, D., Nature, 204: 894 (1964).

2. McDermid, E. M., Petrosky, E. and Yamazaki, H., Immunology, 17: 413 (1969).

3. David, C. S., Genetics, 71: 649 (1972).

4. Pink, J. R. L., Eur. J. Immunol., 4: 679 (1974).

5. Pink, J. R. L. and Ivanyi, J., Eur. J. Immunol., 5: 506 (1975).

6. Wakeland, E. K. and Benedict, A. A., in Advances in Experimental Medicine and Biology, Vol. 64, pp 431-437 (Plenum Press, New York, 1975).

7. Wakeland, E. K. and Benedict, A. A., Immunogenetics, 2: 531 (1975).

8. Wakeland, E. K. and Benedict, A. A., J. Immunol., 117: 2185 (1976).

9. Wakeland, E. K., Benedict, A. A. and Abplanalp, H. A. J. Immunol., 118: 401 (1977).

10. Wakeland, E. K., Foppoli, J. M. and Benedict, A. A., this conference.

11. Ivanyi, J., J. Immunogenetics, 2: 69 (1975).

12. Kelus, A. S., in Gamma Globulins, Proceedings of the Third Nobel Symposium, pp 329-339 (Almquist & Wiksell, Stockholm, 1967).

13. Kelus, A. A. and Pernis, B., Eur. J. Immunol., 1: 123 (1971).

14. Kelus, A. S. and Gell, P. G. H., Progr. Allergy, 11: 141 (1967).

15. Yamaga, K. and Benedict, A. A., J. Immunol., 115: 759 (1975).

16. Benedict, A. A. and Yamaga, K., in Comparative Immunology, pp 353-357 (Blackwell Scientific Publications, 1976).

17. Knight, K. L., Lichter, E. A. and Hanly, W. C., Biochem., 12: 3197 (1973).

18. Gilman-Sachs, A. and Dray, S., Eur. J. Immunol., 2: 505 (1972).

19.   Gilman-Sachs, A., Eskinazi, D. P. and Dray, S., Fed. Proc.,
      36: 1278 (1977).

20.   Sell, S., Science, 153: 641 (1966).

21.   Warner, N. L., Goding, J. W., Gutman, G. A., Warr, G. W.,
      Herzenberg, L. A., Osborne, B. A., Van Der Loo, W., Black,
      S. J. and Loken, M. R., Nature, 265: 447 (1977).

22.   Wells, J. V., Bleumers, J. F. and Fudenberg, H. H., Proc.
      Nat. Acad. Sci. USA, 70: 827 (1973).

23.   Herzenberg, L. A. and Herzenberg, L. A., in Handbook of
      Experimental Immunology, pp 13.1 (F. A. Davis., 1973).

COMPARISON OF THE MICROENVIRONMENT OF CHICKEN AND RABBIT ANTIBODY ACTIVE SITES

Edward W. Voss, Jr. and Robert M. Watt

Department of Microbiology, University of Illinois

Urbana, Illinois   61801

INTRODUCTION

Comparative phylogenetic studies are a valid experimental approach to evaluate relative properties of biological and biochemical systems. Such studies serve to identify evolutionary trends and selective pressures for features which enhance species survival. Phylo-immunochemical studies, for example, have revealed both conserved features of antibodies and tolerated changes to varying degrees and/or nature (1). Comparative immunoglobulin structural analyses at the polypeptide chain level have been the subject of significant amounts of investigation (2), but such studies at the antibody active site level (especially non-mammalian) are relatively lacking in quantity and detail. To this end, we have attempted to study the relative nature of chicken and rabbit IgG anti-hapten antibodies, with emphasis on the highly sensitive fluorescyl hapten system (3, 4).

MATERIALS AND METHODS

Immunogen Preparation. Fluorescyl and dinitrophenyl conjugated procine gamma globulin were prepared and analyzed as previously described (4, 5).

Immunization. All species (i.e., chicken, rabbit, horse, and shark) were immunized with 1 mg/kg body weight of hapten conjugated protein, emulsified in complete Freund's adjuvant (6, 7, 8).

Antibody Purification. IgG antibodies were purified by immunoadsorption as previously described (9). Antibodies from all
species examined were analyzed for purity by immunoelectrophoresis
and polyacrylamide gel electrophoresis.

Assays. Equilibrium dialysis was performed with either ^{3}H-
ε-DNP-L-lysine or ^{3}H-N-acetyl-fluoresceinamine as previously described (3). Fluorescence quenching was performed with ε-DNP-L-
lysine (10) or fluorescein disodium salt (FDS) (3).

Isoelectric Focusing. Isoelectric focusing was performed
using a 110 ml electrolysis column (LKB Instruments) and described
by Vesterberg et al. (11). Isoelectric focusing in the pH range
3-10, stabilized by 20-46% sucrose gradient was carried out for
72 hours at 300 V. Proteins were radioiodinated (^{125}I) by the
chloramine-T oxidation procedure (12).

Fluorescence Lifetime. The fluorescence lifetime of fluorescein, (1 μM in 100 mM KPO_4 buffer, pH 8.0, and at various concentrations of tryptophan) was determined on the cross-correlation
fluorometer described by Spencer and Weber (13). Exciting light
was selected to be 490 nm, while emission was monitored through a
Corning 3-69 glass filter. The excitation modulation frequency
was 30 MHz. Lifetimes measured by phase and modulation at 4° C
were virtually identical, differing by no more than 0.1-0.3 nsecs,
and hence values given are an average of the two.

Deuterium Oxide Studies. In studies designed to measure the
comparative fluorescence properties of antibody fluorescyl ligand
in D_2O and H_2O, the following general protocol was used. To 1.5
ml of D_2O)(99.8% sealed under argon, Koch Isotopes) or H_2O (glass
distilled and passed through the Millipore MQ2 system) was added
20 μl purified antibody containing bound ligand (this will be
referred to as buffered D_2O). The amount of antibody used depended on the concentration of fluorescyl ligand remaining bound
to the high affinity population. This was determined by measuring
the A_{278nm}/A_{500nm} ratio of each purified antibody preparation.
Generally, a final concentration of 50-100 μg/ml of purified IgG
antibodies were used in the fluorometric assays (Aminco-Bowman
spectrophotofluorometer equipped with an X-Y recorder and circulating temperature control bath) in a final concentration of 95.3% D_2O.

In some studies the antibody protein was dialyzed against
frequent changes of 99.8% D_2O.

Circular Dichroic Spectra. Circular dichroism (CD) was measured on a Jasco J-40A spectro-polarimeter calibrated with a 0.6%
aqueous solution of D-10 camphor sulfonic acid. Spectra were recorded at a sensitivity of 1 m$^{\circ}$/cm in 10 mm quartz cells. Data are
presented in terms of ellipticity as a function of wavelength (nm).

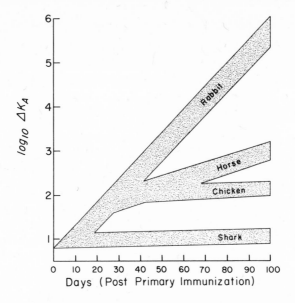

Figure 1.   Correlation between species and time-dependent affinity maturation of the IgG immune response.   Results are based on analyses of purified IgG antibodies from 50 rabbits, 50 chickens, 2 horses, and 6 sharks (equally divided between anti-DNP and anti-fluorescein). K_A is the average intrinsic association constant as measured by equilibrium dialysis.

RESULTS

Comparative Maturation of the IgG Immune Response.   Figure 1 depicts results compiled over several years with IgG antibodies purified to both the DNP and fluorescyl hapten systems.   Figure 1 is based on results gathered from groups of animals (i.e., pooled sera) as well as individual animals (the width of the lines indicates variations observed within a species).   The results show that the rabbit IgG humoral immune response relative to the other three species, generates the greatest degree of maturation in terms of the magnitude of increase in the average intrinsic association constant (ΔK_A).   These results are characteristic of the IgG response to either DNP or fluorescein.   It has been previously demonstrated that the immunoadsorption procedures employed yield purified antibodies representative of the total hapten-specific IgG populations within the antisera (14).   Horse and chicken IgG responses to either hapten show restricted maturation, while the 7S shark antibody shows minimal maturation (8).

The chicken humoral IgG antibody response is represented on a limited phylogenetic scale depicting comparative rates and degrees of time-dependent affinity maturation in figure 1 (15). We have found that secondary and tertiary immunizations do not change the characteristics of the chicken response over a 350 day period.

Comparative Heterogeneity Indices and Isoelectric Focusing Patterns. As implied in figure 1, rabbits generate significant populations (qualitatively and quantitatively) of high affinity IgG anti-hapten molecules, while chickens show a relative absence of high affinity IgG molecules. Rabbit IgG populations generally show a more significant reduction in the Sips distribution index with time (16), relative to values compiled for the chicken IgG response (15). This comparison suggests that chicken IgG antibodies to a hapten should be generally more homogeneous than a comparable population of purified rabbit IgG anti-hapten antibodies. Isoelectric focusing patterns shown in figure 2 support this concept. Figure 2A shows that purified chicken IgG antibodies to the fluorescyl hapten group are quite homogeneous, relative to normal chicken IgG (figure 2B) or purified rabbit anti-fluorescyl and anti-dinitrophenyl IgG antbodies shown in figure 3.

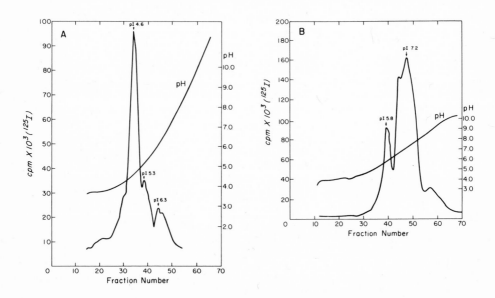

Figure 2. Isoelectric focusing patterns of radioiodinated chicken antibodies. A. Purified anti-fluorescyl IgG antibodies. B. Purified normal chicken IgG.

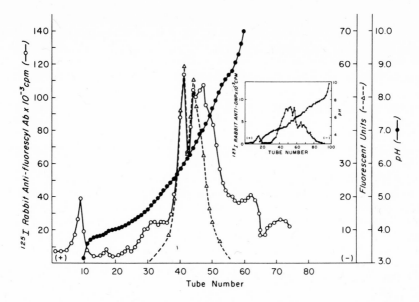

Figure 3.   Isoelectric focusing patterns of radioiodinated (^{125}I) purified rabbit anti-fluorescyl IgG antibodies.   Insert. Profile of purified rabbit anti-DNP IgG antibodies.

Relative Presence of Extremely High Affinity Molecules. Based on the above measurements of average intrinsic association constants and heterogenity indices it was inferred that high affinity sub-populations in rabbits are present in significant amounts and tend to predominate as the response progresses with time. Chicken antibodies on the other hand generally lack high affinity molecules or possess them in only very low percentages throughout the response. Based on a feature of the immunoadsorption procedure utilized in these studies, it is possible to measure the presence and proportion of extremely high affinity IgG molecules in the system. This is made possible by the observation that upon elution of IgG antibodies with high concentrations of ligand (e.g., 0.1 M FDS) and subsequent passage over a double-layer anion exchange column (Dowex 1-X8 and DEAE), antibodies possessing affinities > $10^9 M^{-1}$ will not release ligand to the Dowex resin. Measurements of bound ligand in the rabbit response shows that the percentage of IgG molecules retaining ligand progresses from 0 to 50% (or greater in some instances) as time elapses, while the percentage of high affinity chicken IgG molecules remains between 0 and 15% throughout the response. The population of rabbit IgG retaining ligand

can be demonstrated in isoelectric focusing experiments as shown
in figure 3 by assaying for the residual fluorescence of bound
fluorescyl ligand. (The population shown is antibody purified
from a late primary bleeding.) In contrast, this population is
difficult to detect in representative chicken patterns as shown
in figure 2. This is due to the small percentage of chicken
molecules possessing ligand bound to exceptionally high affinity
sites.

Fluorescyl Ligand as Environmental Probe. When fluorescein
is bound to the active site of anti-fluorescyl IgG molecules, a
significant reduction in the quantum yield of fluorescence can be
measured. Fluorescein bound to either chicken or rabbit IgG antibody molecules shows a similar reduction of ∿90% in the quantum
yield. Thus, in this respect the sites from the two species are
similar. Figure 4 shows that when fluorescein is reacted with L-
tryptophan significant quenching is observed. Further, the upward
curvature in the Stern-Volmer plot (figure 4) indicates that both
static and dynamic components of quenching are present. Of the
amino acids, only tyrosine and tryptophan show quenching upon
interaction with fluorescein. However, quantitatively the latter
is significantly more efficient and may represent a mechanism of
quenching within the antibody active site.

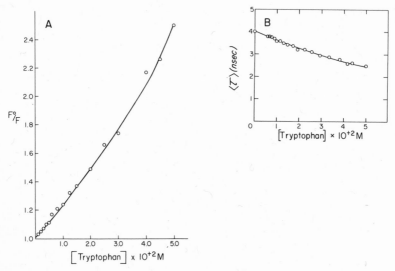

Figure 4. A. Stern-Volmer plot showing fluorescence
quenching of fluorescein by L-tryptophan. F is fluorescence of
ligand in presence of L-tryptophan. F_o is fluorescence of ligand
in buffer.

B. Fluorescence lifteime of fluorescein as a
function of L-tryptophan concentration. <τ> is the average of
fluorescence lifetimes measured by phase and modulation.

Fluorescein, which absorbs maximally at 493 nm, experiences a red spectral-shift to ∿500-505 nm when bound to the active sites of both purified rabbit and chicken IgG antibody molecules. A similar spectral-shift to higher wavelengths can be observed when the ligand is dissolved in methanol or ethanol (relative dielectric constants of 31.2 and 25.8 respectively). Thus, as with the reduction in the quantum yield of ligand fluorescence similar spectral shifts indicate that the sites of chicken and rabbit anti-fluorescyl IgG antibodies are relatively similar.

Fluorescence lifetime measurements (figure 4B) revealed a decrease in the lifetime of fluorescein as a function of tryptophan concentration. Static quenching does not effect the lifetime of a fluorophore as only those molecules non-complexed with the quencher fluoresce, while dynamic quenching represents a new mechanism for dissipation of the excited state and hence results in a decrease in the measured fluorescence lifetime. The curvature seen in the Stern-Volmer plot and the inequality of F_o/F with τ_o/τ at a given tryptophan concentration constitutes proof that indeed both mechanisms of quenching are present (17). Fluorescein bound to rabbit and chicken anti-fluorescyl IgG active sites showed fluorescence lifetimes of ∿ 2 nsec.

Finally, when anti-fluorescyl antibodies were titrated with fluorescein (5 μM), the fluorescence of tryptophanyl residues within the protein was quenched. A normal gamma globulin control for both non-specific binding and radiationless transfer from tryptophan to fluorescein supported the observation that tryptophanyl residues of anti-fluorescyl antibodies were specifically quenched by fluorescein.

Comparative Analysis of High Affinity Populations. Since the previous studies (figure 1) indicated that the rabbit was capable of producing a large population of high affinity anti-hapten molecules (i.e., $K_A > 10^9 M^{-1}$) and chicken only a relatively small percentage of such molecules, it was of interest to measure the comparative nature of these ligand-bound subpopulations. These populations are difficult to characterize in classical ligand binding assays (e.g. equilibrium dialysis and fluorescence quenching) because of certain inadequacies of these procedures to measure high affinity sites and the further complication of ligand inhibited sites.

To characterize these sub-populations in the rabbit and chicken systems, the fluorescence of bound fluorescein was compared in buffer (0.02 M Tris, pH 8.0) and buffered D_2O (95-99%). Deuterium oxide is believed to influence proton transfer reactions (18).

In both systems a significant enhancement of fluorescence
was observed in D_2O.   The percentage of enhancement varied somewhat between individual preparations of antibody from both species,
but in general the degree of enhancement was greater with fluorescein bound to chicken antibodies relative to rabbit antibodies.
Further fluorescence enhancement in D_2O is significantly greater
with ligand in low affinity sites than in high affinity sites.
Similar concentrations of deuterium oxide did not cause fluorescence
enhancement of free fluorescein, fluorescyl conjugated proteins,
nor fluorescein bound to BSA (19).   Thus, the effect was specific
for fluorescein bound to the active site of either chicken or
rabbit IgG anti-fluorescyl antibodies.

Analysis of these antibodies in equilibrium dialysis and
spectral shift assays showed that deuterium oxide did not cause
release of bound ligand.   Further, circular dichroism studies
(figure 5) showed that there was no perturbation of the induced
dichroism of bound fluorescein in D_2O and, therefore, no detectable
conformational change of the antibody.

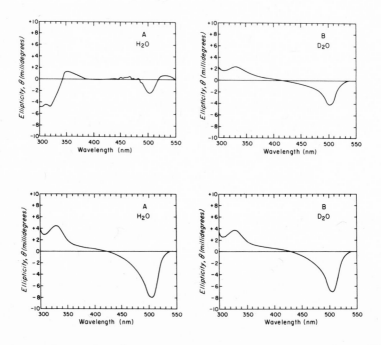

Figure 5.   Induced CD spectra.   Top.   Spectra of purified
chicken anti-fluorescyl IgG molecules in buffer (H_2O) and D_2O.
Bottom.   Spectra of purified rabbit anti-fluorescyl IgG molecules
in buffer (H_2O) and D_2O.

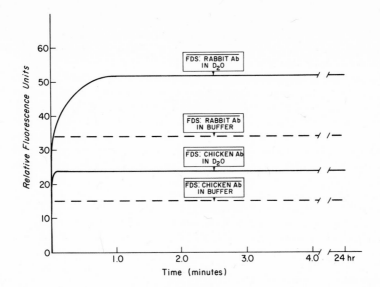

Figure 6.   Comparative equilibration kinetics of D_2O on the fluorescence of fluorescyl ligand bound to chicken and rabbit IgG antibodies at 20°.

Figure 6 shows that when the kinetics of the deuterium oxide effect on the fluorescence of bound fluorescein is studied, the chicken system equilibrates in 2 sec at 20°. At the same temperature, the rabbit system requires 120 sec to reach maximum fluorescence enhancement. When the experiments are repeated at 5°, the rate of D_2O equilibration in the chicken system remains the same, while the rabbit system requires 20 min to show maximum enhancement.

DISCUSSION

By employing two significantly different hapten systems to study comparative maturation of the IgG immune responses, we have shown that the chicken and rabbit responses are typically dissimilar. Figure 1 compared the chicken responses to three other species (i.e. rabbit, horse and shark) with respect to the rate and degree of time dependent affinity maturation. These results suggest that chicken has limited potential and capacity to elicit high affinity IgG molecules to either hapten system. Comparing rabbit and chicken heterogeneity indices, compiled from ligand binding assays, isoelectric focusing results (figures 2 and 3) and the percentage of high affinity ligand occupied sites, it can be concluded that the chicken IgG response can be characterized as being predominantly low affinity with restricted heterogeneity.

In experiments based exclusively on the fluorescein:anti-fluorescyl IgG system it was shown that by comparative quantitation of fluorescence quenching of bound fluorescyl ligand, spectral shift analyses and fluorescence lifetime measurements, the general environments of the active sites of chicken and rabbit antibodies are similar. These results suggested that tryptophan within the active site were involved in the fluorescence quenching observed (figure 4). This was further substantiated with the observation that fluorescein bound to the active site of purified anti-fluorescyl ligand quenched the fluorescence of excited tryptophanyl residues within the immunoglobulin protein. Results generally indicated that the mechanism of quenching by tryptophan is complex (i.e. involving both static and dynamic interactions).

Studies designed to measure the effect of deuterium oxide on the fluorescence of antibody bound ligand, suggested that the chicken and rabbit sites were different. Ligand bound to a selective high affinity chicken antibody population was enhanced to a greater degree than ligand similarly bound to high affinity rabbit antibodies. To this degree, the chicken site resembled low affinity rabbit sites. Further, the D_2O equilibration (kinetic) studies showed that D_2O exchanged very rapidly with H_2O and/or protons within the chicken site. The rate ($\sim$ 2 min), of exchange was independent of temperature (i.e. at 5° and 20°). Low affinity rabbit sites show similar effects. However, D_2O exchanged relatively slowly with the high affinity rabbit site at 20° ($\sim$ 2 min), the rate being substantially slower at 5° ($\sim$ 20 min). We believe that the effect of D_2O on the fluorescence of bound fluorescein ligand (i.e. enhancement) is a distinctive measure of low and high affinity sites. High affinity sites characteristically show minimal fluorescence enhancement and slow equilibration with D_2O. Low affinity sites show relatively high levels of fluorescence enhancement and rapid equilibration in D_2O. Chicken antibodies (even their highest affinity subpopulations) more closely resemble low affinity rabbit IgG active sites than they do the highest affinity rabbit antibody molecules. The exact mechanism whereby deuterium oxide causes an enhancement of fluorescence by antibody bound fluorescyl ligand is not known. However, studies are in progress to determine the mechanism.

REFERENCES

1.   Kubo, R. T., Zimmerman, B. and Grey, H. M. in Phylogeny of Immunoglobulins (M. Sela, Ed.) (Academic Press, New York, 1973).

2. Nisonoff, A., Hopper, J. E. and Springer, S. B. in The Antibody Molecule (Academic Press, New York, 1975).

3. Lopatin, D. E. and Voss, E. W., Jr. Biochemistry $\underline{10}$:208 (1971).

4. Watt, R. M. and Voss, E. W., Jr. Immunochemistry, (In Press).

5. Eisen, H. N. in Methods in Immunology and Immunochemistry (C. A. Williams and M. W. Chase, Eds.) (Academic Press, New York, (1967).

6. Hoffmeister, M. J. and Voss, E. W., Jr. Immunochemistry $\underline{11}$:641 (1974).

7. Voss, E. W., Jr. and Eisen, H. N. Fed. Proc. $\underline{27}$:684 (1968).

8. Voss, E. W., Jr. and M. M. Sige. J. Immunol. $\underline{109}$:5 (1972).

9. Mitchell, J. E., Conrad, H. E. and Voss, E. W., Jr. Immunochemistry $\underline{13}$:659 (1976).

10. Velick, S. F., Parker, C. W. and Eisen, N. H. Proc. Nat. Acad. Sci. (U.S.) $\underline{46}$:1470 (1960).

11. Vesterberg, O. and Svensson, H. Acta Chem. Scand. $\underline{20}$:820 (1966).

12. Sonoda, S. and Schlamowitz, M. Immunochemistry $\underline{7}$:885 (1970).

13. Spencer, R. D. and Weber, G. Ann. N. Y. Acad. Sci. $\underline{158}$:361 (1969).

14. Lopatin, D. E. and Voss, E. W., Jr. Immunochemistry $\underline{11}$:461 (1974).

15. Eisen, H. N. and Siskind, G. W. Biochemistry $\underline{3}$:996 (1964).

16. Sips, R. J. Chem. Phys. $\underline{16}$:490 (1948).

17. Lakowicz, J. R. and Weber, G. Biochemistry $\underline{12}$:4161 (1973).

18. Stryer, L. J. Am. Chem. Soc. $\underline{88}$:5708 (1966).

19. Andersson, L., Rehnström, A., and Eaker, D. L. Eur. J. Biochem. $\underline{20}$:371 (1971).